OXFORD MEDICAL PUBLICATIONS

Duchenne Muscular Dystrophy

OXFORD MONOGRAPHS ON MEDICAL GENETICS

General Editors:

Former Editors:

ARNO G. MOTULSKY

J. A. FRASER ROBERTS

PETER S. HARPER

C. O. CARTER

MARTIN BOBROW

CHARLES SCRIVER

1. R. B. McConnell: *The genetics of gastro-intestinal disorders*
2. A. C. Kopeć: *The distribution of the blood groups in the United Kingdom*
3. E. Slater and V. A. Cowie: *The genetics of mental disorders*
4. C. O. Carter and T. J. Fairbank: *The genetics of locomotor disorders*
5. A. E. Mourant, A. C. Kopeć, and K. Domaniewska-Sobczak: *The distribution of the human blood groups and other polymorphisms*
6. A. E. Mourant, A. C. Kopeć, and K. Domaniewska-Sobczak: *Blood groups and diseases*
7. A. G. Steinberg and C. E. Cook: *The distribution of the human immunoglobulin allotypes*
8. D. Tills, A. C. Kopeć, and R. E. Tills: *The distribution of the human blood groups and other polymorphisms: Supplement 1*
10. D. Z. Loesch: *Quantitative dermatoglyphics: classification, genetics, and pathology*
11. D. J. Bond and A. C. Chandley: *Aneuploidy*
12. P. F. Benson and A. H. Fensom: *Genetic biochemical disorders*
13. G. R. Sutherland and F. Hecht: *Fragile sites on human chromosomes*
14. M. d'A. Crawfurd: *The genetics of renal tract disorders*
16. C. R. Scriver and B. Childs: *Garrod's inborn factors in disease*
17. R. J. M. Gardner and G. R. Sutherland: *Chromosome abnormalities and genetic counseling*
18. M. Baraitser: *The genetics of neurological disorders,* second edition
19. R. J. Gorlin, M. M. Cohen, and L. S. Levin: *Syndromes of the head and neck,* third edition
20. R. A. King, J. I. Rotter, and A. G. Motulsky: *The genetic basis of common diseases*
21. D. Warburton, J. Byrne, and N. Canki: *Chromosome anomalies and prenatal development: an atlas*
22. J. J. Nora, K. Berg, and A. H. Nora: *Cardiovascular diseases: genetics, epidemiology, and prevention*
23. P. Maroteaux: *Bone disorders of children*
24. A. E. H. Emery: *Duchenne muscular dystrophy,* second edition
25. E. G. D. Tuddenham and D. N. Cooper: *The molecular genetics of haemostasis and its inherited disorders*
26. A. Boué: *Fetal medicine*

OXFORD MONOGRAPHS ON MEDICAL GENETICS No 24

Duchenne Muscular Dystrophy

Second Edition

ALAN E. H. EMERY

MD, DSc, PhD, FRCP, FLS, FRS(E)

Emeritus Professor of Human Genetics,
Honorary Fellow, University of Edinburgh, UK;
Visiting Fellow, Green College, Oxford, UK;
Research Director, European Neuromuscular Centre,
Baarn, The Netherlands

OXFORD   NEW YORK   TOKYO
OXFORD UNIVERSITY PRESS
1993

Oxford University Press, Walton Street, Oxford OX2 6DP

Oxford   New York   Toronto
Delhi   Bombay   Calcutta   Madras   Karachi
Kuala Lumpur   Singapore   Hong Kong   Tokyo
Nairobi   Dar es Salaam   Cape Town
Melbourne   Auckland   Madrid
and associated companies in
Berlin Ibadan

Oxford is a trade mark of Oxford University Press

Published in the United States
by Oxford University Press Inc., New York

First edition published 1987
Revised edition published 1988
Second edition published 1993

A catalogue record for this book is available from the British Library

Library of Congress Cataloging in Publication Data
Emery, Alan E.H.
Duchenne muscular dystrophy/Alan E.H. Emery. — 2nd ed.
p.   cm. — (Oxford monographs on medical genetics; no. 24)
(Oxford medical publications)
Includes bibliographical references and index.
1. Duchenne muscular dystrophy. I. Title. II. Series.
III. Series: Oxford medical publications.
[DNLM: 1. Muscular Dystrophy.   WE 559 E53d]
RJ482. D78E44   1993   616.7'48 — dc20   92-49084
ISBN 0-19-262370-2

Typeset by Colset Pte Ltd, Singapore
Printed in Great Britain by
Biddles Ltd, Guildford & King's Lynn

Po 4279

To

Kyle Grace

memories of whose ever-cheerful

disposition were a continual

source of encouragement

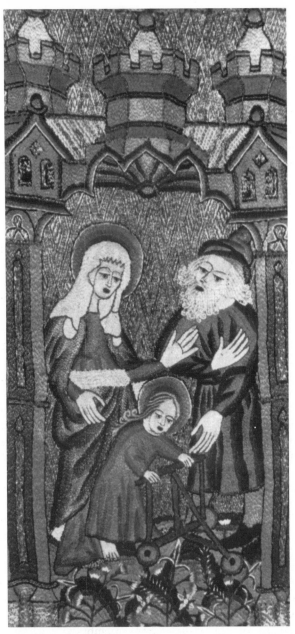

Detail of an orphrey on a fourteenth century dalmatic in The Burrell Collection, Glasgow. (Reproduced with permission.)

Foreword

JOHN WALTON (LORD WALTON OF DETCHANT)

President, World Federation of Neurology;
former Warden, Green College, Oxford;
former Professor of Neurology, University of Newcastle upon Tyne;
Chairman, Muscular Dystrophy Group of Great Britain and
Northern Ireland

As I said in my foreword to the first edition of this book, published in 1987, Professor Emery has made outstanding contributions to our knowledge of neuromuscular disease over the last four decades, especially in the field of genetics. I remarked that it was entirely appropriate that he should have chosen to devote his very considerable talents to undertaking a detailed and scholarly survey of the literature on Duchenne muscular dystrophy, enlivened by the fruits of his personal experience, in order to present a current review of present knowledge of this disease.

That first edition was warmly welcomed by the neurological, paediatric, and genetic communities, and I have no doubt that the same will prove to be true of this much revised and updated second edition, which I have greatly enjoyed reading. As before, the book begins with a fascinating and scholarly historical introduction, before going on to discuss the clinical features, diagnostic methods, differential diagnosis, and non-muscular manifestations of the disease, and subsequently its biochemistry, pathogenesis, genetics, and molecular pathology. Very properly, the last few chapters deal with prevention, genetic counselling, and management, and there are a number of exceptionally useful appendices, one of which lists the various Muscular Dystrophy Associations which have been established to aid research and patient care and welfare in countries throughout the world.

Since the first edition was published, new knowledge of this disease and of its aetiology and pathogenesis has accumulated at a remarkable rate. Localization, identification, and characterization of the gene responsible for the disease and of the missing protein product, dystrophin, which leads to incompetence of the muscle fibre membrane and in turn to the pathological cascade of change in the muscle fibres which causes them to become weak and to waste progressively, came about in the very year the first edition appeared. Since that time the use of monoclonal antibodies against dystrophin in immunochemical staining of muscle biopsy specimens has contributed immeasurably to accurate diagnosis. Carrier detection and, in consequence, genetic counselling, antenatal diagnosis, and hence prevention of the disease have become much more precise and feasible, and all of us interested in the field are now confident that effective gene transfer is within sight, if not immediately, probably within the next decade. All of these features and many more are handled lucidly yet comprehensively in Professor Emery's inimitable style. This second edition, like the first, presents an invaluable state-of-the-art review at a time when the prospects not only of more effective prevention but also of effective treatment for this tragic disease have begun to raise justifiable hopes in the minds of those with the condition and of their parents, families, and those who care for them. Neurologists, paediatricians, geneticists, biochemists, pathologists, nurses, physiotherapists, occupational therapists, social workers, teachers, and many other members of the caring community will find much in this book to inform, inspire, and encourage them. I am confident that it will be deservedly successful.

Preface

While preparing the first edition of this book the gene for Duchenne muscular dystrophy was located, and subsequently Becker muscular dystrophy was shown to be allelic. Gene-specific probes became available and around the time the book was published the protein product of the Duchenne gene had been identified and called dystrophin. Since then the subject has attracted considerable interest among medical scientists. It has been estimated, for example, that over 250 papers have been published on dystrophin in the three years following its identification (Rojas and Hoffman 1991). It would be quite impossible to review all this material in detail. Instead I have concentrated on those areas likely to be most helpful in our understanding of the detailed pathogenesis of the disease, in providing methods for carrier detection and prenatal diagnosis, and in particular give pointers for possible new ways of approaching treatment. This is clearly a very exciting period in the history of the disease. For the very first time we can now begin to have a clearer picture of pathogenesis and more rational ideas regarding treatment.

In preparing this new edition I am particularly grateful to Professor Valerie Askanas, Dr Kate Bushby, Dr Kay Davies, Professor Victor Dubowitz, Dr Eric Hoffman, Professor George Karpati, Dr Don Love, and Dr Louise Nicholson for much useful advice, to Mrs Isobel Black for her excellent secretarial assistance, and to my wife Marcia for her tireless help with the ever-increasing bibliography. Finally I should very much like to thank the staff of Oxford University Press for their continued support and encouragement.

Edinburgh and Oxford   A. E. H. E.
July 1992

Contents

1. Introduction   1

2. History of the disease   6
   Early beginnings   6
   Edward Meryon   11
   Duchenne de Boulogne   12
   William R. Gowers   15
   Wilhelm Heinrich Erb   19
   Recognition of heterogeneity   20
   Recent developments   23

3. Clinical features   26
   Onset   26
   Muscle pseudohypertrophy   30
   Distribution of muscle weakness   31
   Early signs   32
   Progression   34
   Assessment of motor ability   35
   Later stages   37
   Disorders in affected boys other than muscular dystrophy   41
   Summary and conclusions   41

4. Confirmation of the diagnosis   45
   Serum creatine kinase   45
   Creatine kinase isoenzymes   48
   Other serum enzymes   48
   Electromyography (EMG)   50
   The normal EMG   51
   The EMG in muscular dystrophy   52
   The EMG in other disorders   53
      Other forms of muscular dystrophy   53
      Spinal muscular atrophy   53
      Polymyositis   55
   Muscle pathology   55
      Biopsy technique   56
      Preclinical stage   56
      Later stages   61
   Muscle histochemistry   64
   Muscle innervation   68

Electronmicroscopy   68
DNA and dystrophin studies   69
DNA studies on peripheral blood   69
Dystrophin studies on muscle biopsy material   74
Other investigations   77
Summary and conclusions   77

5. Differential diagnosis   80

The congenital muscular dystrophies   80
Congenital myopathies   81
Other X-linked muscular dystrophies   82
  Becker type muscular dystrophy   82
  Apparent Duchenne and Becker muscular dystrophies in the
    same family   87
  Dystrophin in Becker muscular dystrophy   87
  Mabry type muscular dystrophy   88
  X-linked muscular dystrophy with early contractures and
    cardiomyopathy (Emery–Dreifuss type)   88
  X-linked myopathy with autophagy   90
  Quadriceps myopathy   90
  X-linked scapulo-peroneal muscular dystrophy   91
Autosomal recessive limb girdle muscular dystrophy of
  childhood   91
The manifesting carrier of Duchenne muscular dystrophy   97
Heterozygous identical twins   101
The spinal muscular atrophies   102
Summary and conclusions   106

6. Involvement of tissues other than skeletal muscle   108

Smooth muscle   109
Cardiac muscle   109
Vascular system   114
Central nervous system   115
  IQ of affected boys   115
  Partition of IQ   117
  Behaviour and emotional disturbances   118
  Neurological investigations   118
Skeletal system   120
Gastrointestinal system   121
Other manifestations   122
Dystrophin synthesis and phenotype   123
Retinal neuro transmission   123
Summary and conclusions   124

7. Biochemistry of Duchenne muscular dystrophy   125

Selection of material, patients, and controls   125
Molecular basis   126

— Muscle tissue 126
    Muscle wasting 127
    Enzyme changes in dystrophic muscle 131
    Membrane enzymes 133
    'Dedifferentiation' 134
Cultured myoblasts 137
Cultured fibroblasts 140
Peripheral blood leucocytes 140
Serum 141
    'Toxic plasma factor' 141
Urine 142
Animal models 143
    Muscular dystrophy in the mouse 144
    Muscular dystrophy in the cat 146
    Muscular dystrophy in the dog 146
Summary and conclusions 146

8. Genetics 148
Mode of inheritance 148
    Paternal inheritance 149
    Penetrance 149
    Heterozygous advantage and fetal loss 150
Incidence 150
    Changes in incidence in recent years 156
Mutation rate 159
    Indirect estimation of mutation rate 159
    Direct estimation of mutation rate 159
    Parental age and mutation rate 160
    Sex difference in mutation rate 161
Clinical heterogeneity 165
Summary and conclusions 167

9. Molecular pathology 168
Localization of the Duchenne gene 169
Linked DNA markers 175
Isolation of the Duchenne gene 179
    Deletions 180
    Origin of deletions 181
Molecular pathology and phenotype 182
    Frame-shift hypothesis 182
    Mutation site 182
The dystrophin gene 186
Dystrophin 187
Summary and conclusions 188

10. Pathogenesis   190

Vascular abnormalities   190
Neurogenic abnormalities   191
Membrane abnormalities   191
Calcium abnormalities   199
Immune factors   205
Conclusions   208

11. Prevention   209

Ascertainment of families at risk   209
  Population screening   209
  Genetic registers   212
Carrier detection   215
  Definition of carrier status   215
  Biological considerations   216
  Methodological considerations   216
  Carrier detection tests   217
  Clinically manifesting carriers   218
  Muscle pathology   221
Serum creatine kinase   222
Linked DNA markers   228
Calculation of risks   229
Direct carrier detection   238
  Dosage   238
  Junction fragments   238
  In situ hybridization   239
  Lymphocyte RNA   240
  Automated DNA analysis   240
  The future   240
Muscle dystrophin   241
Prenatal diagnosis   243
  Fetal muscle biopsy   245
  Fetal muscle dystrophin   245
Germ-line mosaicism   246
Ova transfer and blastocyst biopsy   249
Summary and conclusions   249

12. Genetic counselling   251

Nature of genetic counselling   251
Non-directive counselling   253
Timing of counselling – the coping process   254
Who should be offered genetic counselling?   255
Effects of genetic counselling   256
Summary and conclusions   258

13. Management   260

General management   260
   Active exercise   261
   Passive exercise and physiotherapy   262
   Chronic low frequency electrical stimulation   264
Scoliosis   265
   Prolongation of ambulation   267
   Standing frames   269
   Swivel walkers   270
Aids for the disabled   270
Surgery   270
Surgical–anaesthetic risks   273
Fractures   275
Respiratory problems   275
Assisted ventilation   276
Cardiac problems   277
Psychological problems   278
Educational and social needs   280
Drug therapy   282
   Early drug trials   282
   Evaluation of drug trials   283
   Design of drug trials   284
   Statistical considerations   285
Recent drug trials   290
Myoblast transfer   290
Gene therapy   293
Comprehensive management   294
Summary and conclusions   295

Appendices   297
Appendix A.   Duchenne's obituary   297
Appendix B.   MRC grading of muscle strength   299
Appendix C.   Swinyard grade   300
Appendix D.   Vignos grade   301
Appendix E.   Hammersmith motor ability score   302
Appendix F.   CIDD group grade   303
Appendix G.   Intragenic RFLPs   304
Appendix H.   Muscular dystrophy associations and groups in
                 various countries   306

References   310

Index   380

1 Introduction

Duchenne muscular dystrophy is the second most common genetic disorder in humans and has been recognized as a distinct entity for over a hundred years. In the last thirty years or so it has generated a great deal of interest among research workers and in their bibliography of what they considered to be the more important publications on the subject up to 1985, Herrmann and Spiegler (1985) listed no less than 789 references. Yet despite all the interest, the cause remained elusive until 1987. This was in part due to the fact that the tissue which is predominantly affected, namely skeletal muscle, is complex as must also be the genetic repertoire responsible for its normal development and functioning.

There are 434 different muscles in the human body which in the adult contribute to over 40 per cent of the total body weight. Much has been written on the development and morphology of muscle, and an excellent review is given by Landon (1982), but here only some general principles need be emphasized. The essential element of muscle is the *muscle fibre* (myofibre) which has been defined as '. . . a multinucleated cell that contains a large number of myofibrils embedded in a matrix of undifferentiated protoplasm, all enclosed within a fine sheath, the sarcolemma' (Adams 1975, p. 15). Muscle fibres are grouped together into fascicles and a network of collagen fibres surrounds each fascicle (perimysium), and extends between individual muscle fibres (endomysium). Each muscle fibre, which vary in length from one muscle to another, is bounded by the plasma membrane (*plasmalemma*) and an outer basement membrane (*basal lamina*). The latter along with the endomysium constitute the *sarcolemma* though this term is sometimes also used when referring to the plasma and basement membranes together (Fig. 1.1). Each multinucleated muscle fibre is formed during development by the fusion of several dividing mononucleated myoblasts derived from the myotomes. After fusion the nuclei of the fibre do not divide again and lie in the cytoplasm (*sarcoplasm*) along with the contractile elements. Small mononucleated *satellite cells* are situated between the plasma and basement membranes of the muscle fibre. These cells contain many ribosomes and are particularly frequent in diseased muscle, though how this occurs is unknown. They are believed to be a persistent population of myoblastic stem cells which retain the ability to divide and are a source of additional muscle fibre nuclei during growth and regenerative repair (Fig. 1.2). A muscle fibre contains many *myofibrils* which are the contractile elements of muscle and display alternating dark (A) and light (I) bands, and through the centre of

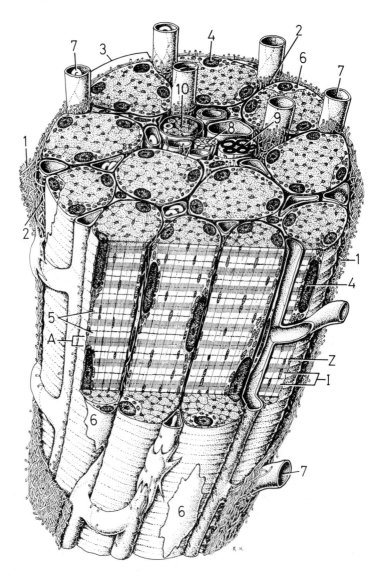

Fig. 1.1 Diagrammatic representation of a small fascicle of muscle fibres. (1, perimysium; 2, endomysium; 3, muscle fibre (myofibre); 4, nucleus; 5, contractile myofibrils; 6, satellite cells; 7, capillaries.) (From Krstić (1978) reproduced with kind permission of the author and publishers.)

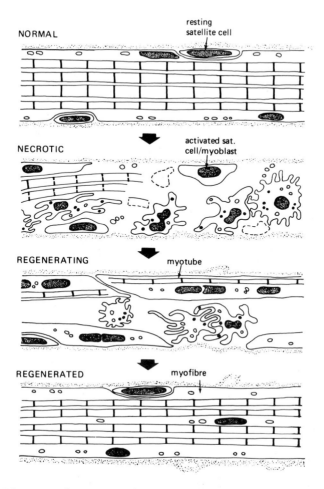

Fig. 1.2 Diagrammatic representation of a satellite cell and its role in muscle fibre regeneration. (Reproduced by kind permission of Professor M. J. Cullen.)

the latter is the dense Z-line (band or disc) (*see* Fig. 1.1). The myofibrils are themselves composed of thick and thin *myofilaments*. During contraction and relaxation of the muscle, thin filaments slide between the thick filaments. In addition to nuclei and myofibrils, the sarcoplasm of a muscle fibre contains mitochondria, glycogen granules, lipid bodies, ribosomes, the transverse system of tubules (*T-system*), and the *sarcoplasmic reticulum*. The latter is equivalent to the endoplasmic reticulum of cells in other tissues and forms a network of tubules which run between the myofibrils. The T-system consists of transversely arranged, fine, interconnecting, tubular extensions of the plasma membrane. A single T-tubule and two dilated ends of the sarcoplasmic reticulum form so-called '*triads*' which are concerned with the excitation and contraction of muscle fibres. A nerve impulse, via the neuromuscular junction, produces depolarization of the muscle cell surface membrane which then spreads inwards along the T-system to the triads. This results, in the rapid release of calcium from the sarcoplasmic reticulum into the sarcoplasm, which in turn then results in the interaction between thick and thin filaments producing muscle contraction (Fig. 1.3).

Any attempt to mention all the reported findings in this disease would be in danger of turning into a mere catalogue because so many appear to be unrelated and often contradictory. Futhermore, on present knowledge it is difficult to find a satisfactory explanation for all the various observations which have been reported.

However, now the defective gene and its normal product (dystrophin) have been identified research in future will no doubt provide explanations for many observations which so far have been difficult to explain. For example, how so does the absence of dystrophin in Duchenne muscular dystrophy lead to high serum levels of sarcoplasmic enzymes, the enzyme profiles in affected muscles, and the progressive nature of the disease?

During the process of selecting and emphasizing certain findings for the sake of clarity, it is inevitable that the resultant picture may be over-simplified, somewhat idiosyncratic, and probably inconsistent. The only defence is that voiced by Miguel de Unamuno in Erwin Schrödinger's book *What is life?* (1944) which Watson and Crick and many others found so illuminating:

If a man never contradicts himself, the reason must be that he virtually never says anything at all.

The references have been selected because they are of historical interest, or present helpful and detailed reviews, or are considered to be particularly seminal in regard to pathogenesis. Apart from Herrmann and Spiegler's bibliography (1985), the Muscular Dystrophy Association of America up to 1990 published monthly abstracts from the world literature on clinical and basic science research into muscular dystrophy and related disorders. Unfortunately there is currently no longer any such abstracting service.

Finally, there have been several monographs in recent years which present detailed reviews of the muscular dystrophies and related disorders in general, such as Swash and Schwartz (1988), Dubowitz (1988, 1989), Walton (1988), and Jerusalem and Zierz (1991) as well as several which deal with specific aspects of the disease, especially muscle pathology (Mastaglia and Walton 1982; Schröder 1982; Carpenter and Karpati 1984; Kakulas and Adams 1985; Dubowitz 1985). The comprehensive text of Engel and Banker (1986) covers the anatomy, biochemistry, and physiology of normal muscle as well as detailed reviews of various neuromuscular disorders.

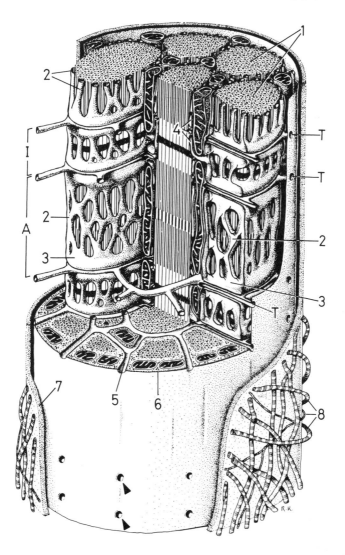

Fig. 1.3 Diagrammatic representation of a single muscle fibre. (1, myofibril; 2 and 3, sarcoplasmic reticulum; T and 5, transverse tubular system; 4, triads; 6, plasma membrane; 7, basement membrane; 8, endomysium.) (From Krstić (1978) reproduced with kind permission of the author and publishers.)

This book, which is partly based on cases and families studied by the author, is not intended for the expert in any particular field, but rather for those with more catholic interests who are involved in this distressing and perplexing disease, which Gowers himself (1879*b*) referred to as being '. . . one of the most interesting and at the same time most sad'.

2 History of the disease

Early beginnings

Muscular dystrophy has no doubt afflicted humans from earliest times. Since the ancient Egyptians in their wall paintings often depicted physical abnormalities with some care, so that they can often be identified as diseases we now recognize, such as paralytic poliomyelitis and congenital dwarfism, it is just possible that they might have portrayed muscular dystrophy. In fact it has been suggested (Pöch and Becker 1955) that this might be so in a relief painting on the wall of a tomb in ancient Egypt, dating from the eighteenth Dynasty of the New Kingdom, that is, about 1500 BC (Fig. 2.1). The subject depicted on the wall of the Temple of Hatshepsut is the Queen of Punt who

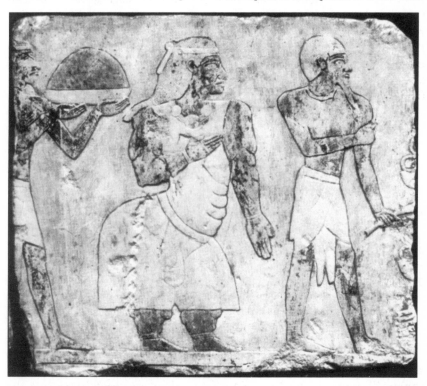

Fig. 2.1 Egyptian relief painting from the eighteenth Dynasty. (Reproduced by kind permission of Professor P. E. Becker.)

shows lumbar lordosis and who, it has even been suggested, may also have some calf enlargement. However in comparison with the adjoining figure she seems generally fatter, and perhaps what is shown is no more than generalized obesity, which is also the opinion of an expert Egyptologist (Riad 1955). However on the wall of a tomb (No. 17 in Newberry 1893) at Beni Hasan, dating from the Middle Kingdom (*circa* 2800–2500 BC), the author noticed that there are depicted two figures of interest (Fig. 2.2). The first has bilateral club foot. In the middle, however, is a boy with what could just possibly be muscular dystrophy. He has lost the normal arch of his feet, which is usually clear in Egyptian wall paintings as seen in the figure to the right. Also, his calves seem somewhat enlarged, and he may have some degree of (pseudo) hypertrophy of certain upper limb muscles. On the other hand as the hieroglyph above his head implies he may have been a dwarf.

The *Transfiguration* was Raphael's last great work, and was unfinished when he died on Good Friday, 1520, at the untimely age of 37. Vasari, in his *Lives of the Artists*, considers the boy in the painting to be 'possessed by a devil', an idea which may have prompted subsequent observers to suggest that it could illustrate a case of epilepsy. However, Duchenne himself, after whom the commonest form of muscular dystrophy is named, when visiting the National Hospital for Nervous Diseases in London where a reproduction of the painting hung, commented at the time that the boy depicted by the artist might be suffering from pseudohypertrophic muscular dystrophy (Fig. 2.3).

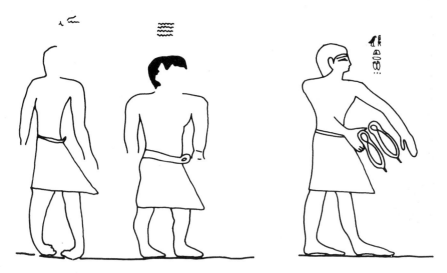

Fig. 2.2 Drawings from a tomb at Beni Hasan (*circa* 2800–2500 BC).

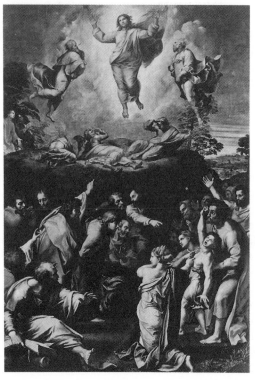

Fig. 2.3 Raphael's *Transfiguration*. (Reproduced by kind permission of the *Musei Vaticani*.)

It is also interesting to note, as Lord Walton has pointed out (Walton 1990), that William Harvey (1578–1657) should be remembered not only for his observations on the circulation of the blood but also for his studies in neurology and the structure and function of muscles. He showed, for example, that muscles can be distinguished by their structure, according to whether they are primarily fleshy, tendinous, sinewy, or membranous, as well as their action in causing movement.

However, the first clinical descriptions of dystrophy itself, at least in the English language, can be attributed to Charles Bell. He was born in Fountainbridge in Edinburgh in 1774, where he studied medicine and subsequently worked as a surgeon–anatomist, often illustrating his works with his own carefully executed drawings. At the age of thirty he moved to London where he spent most of his working life, and was a Founder of the Middlesex Medical School. He returned to Edinburgh to the Chair of Surgery in 1835, and died in 1842 from angina. He is best remembered for being the first to describe paralysis of the facial nerve (Bell's palsy) and, with the French experimental physiologist, François Magendie, for discovering

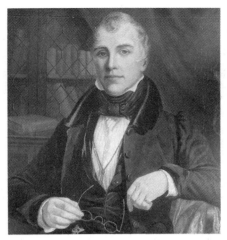

Fig. 2.4 Sir Charles Bell. (Reproduced by kind permission of the National Galleries of Scotland, Edinburgh.)

the distinct functions of the posterior (sensory) and anterior (motor) nerve roots of the spinal cord (Fig. 2.4).

Among his numerous publications is his *The nervous system of the human body* first published in 1830 and which subsequently ran to several editions. In it he describes (Case 89) a young man of eighteen with wasting and weakness of the quadriceps muscles which began some 8 years previously and which

. . . disabled him from rising; and it is now curious to observe how he will twist and jerk his body to throw himself upright from his seat. I use this expression, for it is a very different motion from that of rising from the chair.   (Bell 1830, p. CLXIII)

There was no sensory loss. Without muscle pathology the diagnosis cannot be certain, but the description would certainly be compatible with muscular dystrophy.

Gowers (1879*b*), whose seminal contributions to the subject will be dealt with in more detail later, refers to the possibility of the disease having been described in 1838 by Coste and Gioja in the *Annali Clinici dell'Ospedale degli 'Incurabili di Napoli* which was abstracted in Schmidt's *Jahrbücher* (Schmidt 1838). But this was a mistake. Recent research by Professor Giovanni Nigro of the University of Naples (Nigro 1986) has revealed that the cases in question were presented by Professor Gaetano Conte (*not* Coste) with the help of a Dr L. Gioja and reported in the journal in fact in 1836 (Conte and Gioja 1836). Two brothers apparently first manifested the disease at age 8, had enlarged calves and progressive muscle wasting and weakness, which particularly affected the lower limbs, and subsequently developed contractures of the knees and hips. The elder brother died of

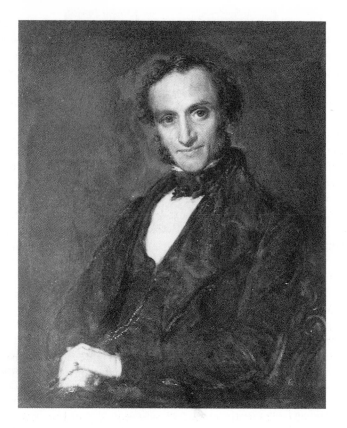

Fig. 2.5 Dr Edward Meryon (by John Linnell, private collection).

cardiac failure. Sensory functions were intact and mentation was normal. The clinical features are presented in detail and the original publication has now been reproduced in full in *Cardiomyology* (Vol. **V** (No. 1) 1986, pp. 1–30). It seems very likely that these two brothers probably had muscular dystrophy though there is no report of muscle pathology. But certainly Professor Gaetano Conte, who was born in Naples in 1798 and dedicated most of his life to the study of 'scrofole' (?dystrophy), must rank among the pioneers in the history of the subject.

However, in 1847 a Mr Partridge presented a case to the Pathological Society of London (reported in the *London Medical Gazette* Vol. 5, p. 944) of a boy who, from about the age of nine, had developed progressive muscle wasting and weakness, had enlarged calves and muscle contractures and who died after an attack of measles at age 14. Examination of muscle tissue at autopsy revealed widespread fatty degeneration. In the same year, 1847, Dr

W. J. Little, a physician at the London Hospital, studied two affected brothers aged 12 and 14 which he reported in detail in 1853 in a book entitled *On the nature and treatment of the deformities of the human frame*. Both brothers presented a similar picture. Onset was in early childhood with a tendency to walk on the toes and a peculiar gait with the '. . . head and body having been inclined backwards'. There was progressive muscle wasting and weakness affecting the neck, trunk, and upper and lower extremities associated with enlargement of the calf muscles and contractures 'behind the heels'. Sensation was normal. Both boys were unable to walk by the age of 11. The elder died at 14 and at autopsy, examination of the gastrocnemius and soleus muscles (and some other muscles as well) revealed that the muscle tissue had been largely replaced by fat ('adipose degeneration'). The brain and spinal cord appeared normal. These findings would certainly be consistent with the diagnosis of the severe form of muscular dystrophy which predominantly affects boys. However, the fullest and earliest description of this disorder must be credited to Dr Edward Meryon of St. Thomas's Hospital, London (Fig. 2.5).

Edward Meryon

Edward Meryon was born in 1809 and studied medicine in Paris and University College, London. He qualified as a Member of the Royal College of Surgeons in 1831, proceeding to an MD degree in 1844. His chief appointments were at St. Thomas's Hospital and the Hospital for Nervous Diseases where it is just possible he may have been acquainted with the young William Gowers. He was apparently a man of wide learning and published several books relating to the nervous system. He also embarked on a *History of medicine* but unfortunately did not get beyond a first volume. In Feiling's *History of the Maida Vale Hospital* the only reference to him reads: 'Edward Meryon although not really distinguished in medicine, was clearly a well-known figure in London society at the time' (Feiling 1958, p. 5). He died at his home in Mayfair in 1880, at the age of 71 (Emery and Emery 1993).

In a communication addressed to the Royal Medical and Chirurgical Society in December 1851 and which was published in the Transactions of the Society the following year, Meryon described eight affected boys in three families. Interestingly, one of the two affected brothers in the second family is the case on which Partridge had earlier reported his autopsy findings in 1847. Meryon was particularly impressed by the familial nature of the condition and its predilection for males, and in his book *Practical and pathological researches on the various forms of paralysis* published in 1864, he details a family in which there were four affected cousins with the disorder having been transmitted through three sisters. Secondly, he subjected muscle tissue to microscopic examination and reported that . . .

the striped elementary primitive fibres were found to be completely destroyed, the sarcous element being diffused, and in many places converted into oil globules and granular matter, whilst the sarcolemma and tunic of the elementary fibre was broken down and destroyed.   (Meryon 1852, p. 76)

He therefore used the term 'granular degeneration' for the microscopic changes he observed. Thirdly, he observed that

. . . the relative proportion of the grey matter to the white in the cord, and the ganglionic cells of the former, and the tubular structure of the latter, as well as of the nerves and the white substance within the neurolemma, wherever examined by the microscope, all bore evidence of the healthy condition of the nervous system.
                                                  (Meryon 1852, p. 78)

Thus, he concluded that this was a familial disease which primarily affected muscle tissue and was not a disease of the nervous system. Meryon's clear delineation of the disorder and his understanding of its nature were very significant contributions. It is therefore unfortunate that he has not always been given the credit he deserves and that his work is completely over-shadowed by that of Duchenne.

Duchenne de Boulogne

Guillaume Benjamin Amand Duchenne, Duchenne de Boulogne as he signed himself in order not to be confused with Duchesne of Paris, was born in the town of Boulogne-sur-Mer on 17 September 1806 (Fig. 2.6). He studied

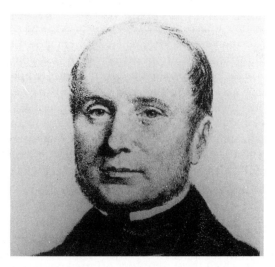

Fig. 2.6 Duchenne de Boulogne. (Reproduced from *The founders of neurology*, edited by Webb Haymaker, 1953. Courtesy of Charles C. Thomas, Publishers, Springfield, Illinois.)

medicine in Paris where his teachers included Cruveilhier, Dupuytren, and Laennec. He then returned to Boulogne with the intention of being a family doctor (Guilly 1936). However, this proved a very unhappy time, for his young wife died of puerperal sepsis 14 days after giving birth to their son Emile in 1833, and for several years afterwards he remained depressed and lost interest in his work. In 1839 he remarried, this time to a widow, but this does not seem to have been a happy marriage. Then in 1842, at the age of 36, he returned to Paris where he spent the rest of his life. Cuthbertson (1977) suggests there may have been three factors instrumental in his return to Paris and to neurology: his growing interest in the possible therapeutic effects of electricity, his own family history of a 'nervous' disease, and his disastrous second marriage. Whatever the reasons he quickly settled in Paris where he became a sort of itinerant physician mainly at the Salpêtrière. He never held an official hospital or academic appointment and was therefore completely free to pursue his obsessional interests in the electrical stimulation of muscle, muscle function, and neuromuscular diseases. He studied the mechanisms of facial expression, a subject which had also interested Charles Bell some years previously. His painstaking observations led to clear descriptions of several disorders, his name now being most closely associated with progressive muscular atrophy (with Aran) and progressive bulbar palsy (both part of the motor neurone disease complex), and of course pseudohypertrophic muscular dystrophy. He devised a strength gauge or dynamometer and a special needle-harpoon for muscle biopsy. His numerous publications have been translated, edited, and condensed for the New Sydenham Society by Poore (1883). The last five years of his life saw him famous but tragic: his wife died in 1870 and his son shortly afterwards from typhoid fever. He suffered a cerebral haemorrhage in August 1875, and Potain and Charcot never left him during the last weeks of his illness, taking it in turns to sleep by his bed. He died on 17 September 1875 on his 69th birthday. On 30 October the Paris correspondent of the *Lancet* (see Appendix A), commenting on Duchenne's life and work, wrote that despite many adverse circumstances

. . . his reputation has come out clear and bright as an honest, hard-working, acute, and ingenious observer, an original discoverer, a skilful professional man, and a kind-hearted, benevolent gentleman.

Despite his abounding interest in research, it seems he never lost a bedside manner.

Duchenne's interest in muscular dystrophy was first aroused in 1858 when his attention was drawn to a case, details of which he published in 1861 in the second edition of his book *De l'électrisation localisée* (Duchenne 1861). Later, in 1868, he reviewed in considerable detail his original case plus 12 further cases, two of whom were young girls, and referred to a further 15 cases in the German literature (Duchenne 1868). By 1870 he had seen some

40 cases of the disease, not counting those he saw when he visited the London hospitals around this time (Fig. 2.7).

Duchenne defined the disease as being characterized by: progressive weakness of movement, first affecting the lower limbs and then later the upper limbs; a gradual increase in the size of many affected muscles; an increase in interstitial connective tissue in affected muscles with the production of abundant fibrous and adipose tissue in the later stages. The onset was in childhood or early adolescence, was more prevalent in boys than girls, and could affect several children in the same family. Though Meryon had studied

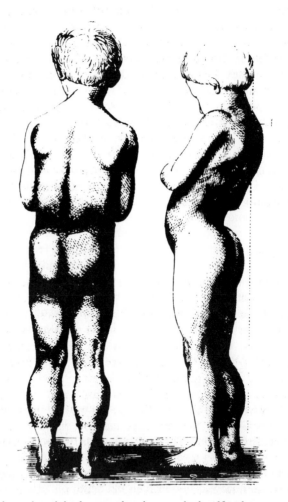

Fig. 2.7 Duchenne's original case, showing marked calf enlargement and lumbar lordosis. (From *Arch. Gén. Méd.* Vol. 11, p. 8 (1868).)

the histology of affected muscles, his observations had been limited to material obtained at autopsy. Duchenne on the other hand, used his needle-harpoon (*enporte-pièce histologique*) to obtain biopsy specimens in life. In fact, using this technique, he was able to study material from the same patient at different stages of the disease. His observations led him to conclude that the fundamental anatomical lesion was hyperplasia of the interstitial connective tissue which therefore prompted him to use the term *paralysie myosclérosique* as an alternative to *paralysie musculaire pseudo-hypertrophique*. Previously, a pathological diagnosis could only be made at autopsy so-called diagnosis of Morgagni. But Duchenne's technique meant such a diagnosis could be made in life. He believed, correctly, that unlike progressive (spinal) muscular atrophy of childhood the disease was not caused by a lesion in the spinal cord. In this matter it is rather disappointing that Duchenne felt he should dismiss Meryon's contributions when he says that the latter confused the disease with progressive muscular atrophy, and therefore thought it had a neurogenic basis, which as we have seen he did not, and Duchenne goes further by giving the date of Meryon's address to the Royal Medical and Chirurgical Society as 1866 when in fact it was some 15 years earlier in 1851. Duchenne carefully weighed the available evidence regarding the possible aetiology of the disorder, particularly with regard to possible neurological or vasomotor factors, but had to conclude, just as we would have done until relatively recently '. . . la pathogénie de la paralysie pseudo-hypertrophique est très obscure; elle doit être réservée . . .'.

William R. Gowers

Considerable interest now began to be shown in the disease and numerous case reports appeared in the French, English, German, American, Australian, and Danish literature (Dubowitz 1978). However, the next physician to enter the stage who made a significant contribution to the subject was William R. Gowers. Gowers was born in 1845 and spent all his life in London. He had a brilliant undergraduate career at University College Hospital where he was awarded medals in almost every subject of the medical curriculum and graduated with first class honours. He later became Professor of Medicine at University College, as well as being a physician at the National Hospital for Nervous Diseases. He was a man of immense intellect and wide interests. He was a knowledgeable botanist and an authority on mosses, an accomplished artist (he exhibited at the Royal Academy), and an obsessional shorthand writer. He introduced into medicine a number of new terms such as 'knee jerk', 'fibrositis', and 'abiotrophy'. He described several clinical signs including the nasal smile in myasthenia gravis, as well as the so-called Gowers' manoeuvre. He also invented a haemocytometer which was widely used for many years. It is understandable that in his day he was therefore widely admired and respected. He remained, however, a reserved and very private individual with few intimate friends. He died in 1915 at the age of 70 (Critchley 1949) (Fig. 2.8).

Gowers' interest in muscular dystrophy was kindled when working as a premedical student apprentice to a Dr Thomas Simpson in Coggeshall, Essex. Here he came across a family with four brothers afflicted with a '. . . strange disorder of locomotion with wasting of some muscles and enlargement of others'. Later he learned that the disease had been described in 1852 by Meryon and in 1879 he delivered a series of lectures on the disorder at the National Hospital which were published in *Lancet* (Gowers 1879*a*) and

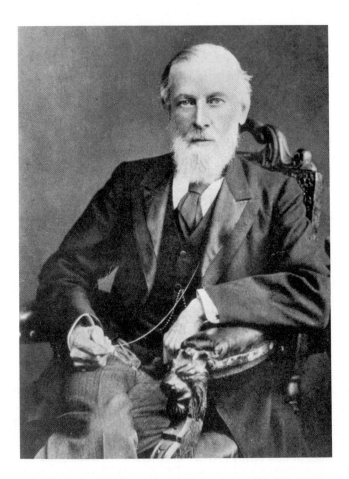

Fig. 2.8 Sir William Gowers. (Reproduced by kind permission of Dr Macdonald Critchley.)

subsequently made into a monograph (Gowers 1879*b*). The latter was based on information from 220 cases, which included 24 he had seen himself, 20 seen by colleagues, and the remainder from the literature. In deference to Duchenne he referred to the disease as 'pseudohypertrophic muscular paralysis', and in his monograph he attempted to give as complete a picture of the disease as possible with detailed discussions of the clinical features, pathology, prognosis, and possible treatment. As with all of Gowers' writings, clarity, thoughtfulness and good prose are evident. This is illustrated in the graphic opening paragraph:

The disease is one of the most interesting and at the same time most sad, of all those with which we have to deal: interesting on account of its peculiar features and mysterious nature; sad on account of our powerlessness to influence its course, except in a very slight degree, and on account of the conditions in which it occurs. It is a disease of early life and of early growth. Manifesting itself commonly at the transition from infancy to childhood, it develops with the child's development, grows with his growth – so that every increase in stature means an increase in weakness, and each year takes him a step further on the road to a helpless infirmity, and in most cases to an early and inevitable death.

The interest in the book lies mainly in the detailed presentation of the clinical features of the disease, and describes what is nowadays usually referred to as Gowers' manoeuvre or Gowers' sign (Fig. 2.9). Weakness of the hip and knee extensors causes difficulty in rising from the floor or a chair. As a result, when getting up, patients

. . . first put the hands on the ground (1), then stretch out the legs behind them far apart, and, the chief weight of the trunk resting on the hands, by keeping the toes on the ground and pushing the body backwards, they manage to get the knees extended so that the trunk is supported by the hands and feet, all placed as widely apart as possible (2). Next the hands are moved alternately along the ground backwards so as to bring a larger portion of the weight of the trunk over the legs. Then one hand is placed upon the knee (3), and a push with this and with the other hand on the ground is sufficient to enable the extensors of the hip to bring the trunk into the upright posture.

Gowers recognized that this had also been noted by Duchenne: 'If he bent forward he could only recover his position by catching hold of the furniture, or by supporting his hands on his thighs' (Poore 1883, p. 184). At first Gowers thought the action of putting the hands on the knees, then grasping the thighs higher and higher ('climbing up his thighs') so as to extend the hips and push up the trunk was pathognomonic for the disease. However, he later realized that it could also be seen in other diseases in which the same muscle groups were affected.

Gowers also emphasized that the disease was primarily a disease of muscle and that the spinal cord was unaffected. Further, he was impressed by the predilection for males and was clearly convinced of the hereditary nature of

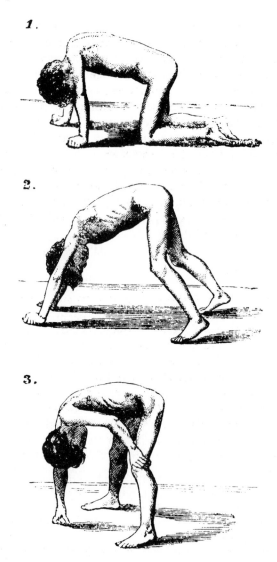

Fig. 2.9 Gowers' sign or manoeuvre. (From W. R. Gowers' *Pseudo-hypertrophic muscular paralysis*, 1879.)

the disorder. Of the total of 220 cases only 30 were females and these were usually less severely affected. Although isolated cases were common, he was impressed by the frequency with which other relatives could be affected (of the 220 cases, 102 were isolated and 118 were grouped in 39 families). Perhaps his most revealing observation was that '. . . the disease is almost never to be heard of on the side of the father; when antecedent cases have occurred they have almost invariably been on the side of the mother'. Gowers also observed that a woman could have affected sons by different husbands, but found no instance in which members of the father's family suffered from the disease. He concluded that limitation to males and inheritance only through the mother was the same as haemophilia. This pattern of inheritance was already recognized at the time, and sometimes referred to as Nasse's law (Nasse 1820), although in fact it had been appreciated since the days of the Talmud some 1500 years earlier. The Jews excused from circumcision the sons of all the sisters of a mother who had a son with the 'bleeding disease'. The sons of the father's sibs were not so excused. The genetic basis for this mode of inheritance was appreciated through the rediscovery of Mendelism in 1900 and its cytological basis (X-linkage) recognized a few years later (reviewed in McKusick 1964).

Wilhelm Heinrich Erb

By this stage in the story it was now quite clear that the disease primarily affected skeletal muscle and was hereditary. However, it was also clear that not all cases presented with exactly the same clinical features: females were occasionally affected and sometimes the disease in males would pursue a more benign course with survival into at least the third decade (for example, Gowers' cases 23, 35, and 36). This raised the possibility that perhaps after all there was more than one disease, an idea first pursued by Erb.

Wilhelm Heinrich Erb (Fig. 2.10) was born in 1840 in Bavaria and studied medicine at Heidelberg, Erlangen, and Munich. His subsequent professional life was spent almost entirely in Heidelberg. Erb was without doubt one of the greatest clinical neurologists of all time (Kuhn and Rüdel 1990). But he was also a great clinical teacher — the archetype of the time: severe, cultured, and always impeccably dressed. He died of a heart attack when he was 81; it is said whilst listening to Beethoven's *Eroica*.

Erb was greatly influenced by the studies of Duchenne, both with regard to the possible diagnostic and therapeutic uses of electricity in neurology, as well as his work on muscle disease. His pathological studies convinced him that the disease was due to a degeneration of muscle tissue and coined the term 'Dystrophia muscularis progressiva' or progressive muscular dystrophy, a term which has been used ever since (Erb 1884). Many of the cases he studied were clearly different from cases described by Duchenne and he was well aware of this. In fact he is credited with being the first to attempt to classify this group of diseases (Erb 1891). The details of his classification would now be questioned, but the idea that this was not one disease but a heterogeneous group of disorders was certainly true.

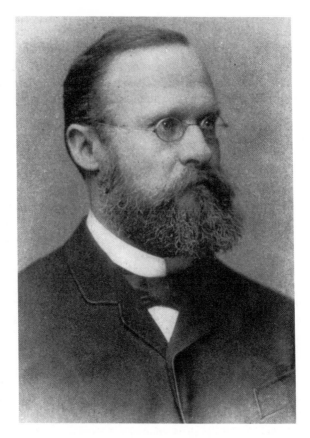

Fig. 2.10 Wilhelm Heinrich Erb. (Reproduced from *The founders of neurology*, edited by Webb Haymaker, 1953. Courtesy of Charles C. Thomas, publishers, Springfield, Illinois.)

Recognition of heterogeneity

Over the next few decades, as physicians began to study their patients in increasing detail, attempts began to be made to categorize different types and to classify them according to various clinical criteria, such as distribution of muscle weakness, age at onset and progression, and later was added the mode of inheritance. Although there were a few who continued for a while to believe that muscular dystrophy was essentially one disease (for example, Milhorat and Wolff 1943), this view was gradually abandoned.

However, there is a serious problem in considering heterogeneity within a group of disorders such as the muscular dystrophies. Differences between disease entities may be more apparent than real: variations within a spectrum and not necessarily a reflection of true genetic differences. This is constantly to be borne in mind when attempting to resolve apparent heterogeneity. The sentiments of Francis Bacon in 1620 are therefore apt:

The steady and acute mind can fix its contemplations and dwell and fasten on the subtlest distinctions: the lofty and discursive mind recognises and puts together the finest and most general resemblances. Both kinds however easily err in excess, by catching the one at gradations the other at shadows.

Those who contributed most significantly to our present ideas on classifying the muscular dystrophies include Bell (1943), Tyler and Wintrobe (1950), Levison (1951), Stevenson (1953), Becker (1953, 1964), Lamy and de Grouchy (1954), Walton and Nattrass (1954), and Morton and Chung (1959). How heterogeneity within this group of diseases was gradually resolved makes a fascinating byway in the history of medicine. However, there would be little value here in summarizing the detailed findings of these earlier studies, which in any event have been critically reviewed by Walton and Nattrass (1954). More recent classifications have been proposed by Emery and Walton (1967), Becker (1972), and by Walton and Gardner-Medwin (1988). One favoured by the author (Emery, 1990*a*) is reproduced in Table 2.1.

At this point perhaps it would be appropriate to consider which disorders are included under the heading 'muscular dystrophies'. For practical purposes a useful definition is *a group of inherited disorders which are characterized by a progressive muscle wasting and weakness, in which the muscle histology has certain distinctive features (muscle fibre necrosis, phagocytosis, etc.) and where there is no clinical or laboratory evidence of spinal cord or peripheral nervous system involvement or myotonia.* Excluded are, therefore, the myotonic syndromes and the various congenital myopathies. However, such a definition encompasses disorders which vary considerably in their onset, severity, and distribution of muscle involvement. At one extreme there is the rapidly progressive form of congenital muscular dystrophy which is present at birth with generalized muscle involvement and leads to death within a few months. At the other extreme there is ocular muscular dystrophy where onset is in adult life, the disease is often limited to the extra-ocular muscles and may be no more than a minor inconvenience.

Here we shall concentrate on that form of dystrophy which is associated with the name of Duchenne. Until fairly recently eponyms were retained for several other forms of dystrophy such as the scapulohumeral (Erb), pelvifemoral (Leyden–Möbius), and the facioscapulohumeral

Table 2.1 *Clinical and genetical classification of the muscular dystrophies*

---

1. *X-linked dystrophies*
a. Proximal
    (i) Duchenne
    (ii) Becker
    (iii) Mabry
b. With early contractures and cardiomyopathy (Emery–Dreifuss)
c. Myopathy with autophagy (Finnish)
d. Quadriceps myopathy?
2. *Autosomal recessive dystrophies*
a. Proximal
    (i) Congenital forms
        Rapidly progressive
        Slowly progressive (numerous variants)
    (ii) Childhood form(s)
    (iii) Adult forms
        Limb girdle
        Scapulohumeral
b. Quadriceps
    Quadriceps myopathy?
3. *Autosomal dominant dystrophies*
a. Facioscapulohumeral
b. With early contractures and cardiomyopathy (Emery–Dreifuss)
c. Scapuloperoneal
d. Proximal
    (i) Dominant limb girdle dystrophy
    (ii) Hereditary myopathy limited to females (Henson)
    (iii) Hereditary myopathy limited to males (De Coster)
e. Distal
    (i) Childhood form
    (ii) Adult form
f. Ocular
    (i) Ocular form
    (ii) Oculopharyngeal forms (AD, AR)

(Landouzy–Dejerine) forms. But this habit has now been largely abandoned in favour of a clinical–genetical nomenclature. However, there remains one important exception; the retention of Becker's name for the X-linked form of the disease which clinically resembles Duchenne muscular dystrophy but is more benign, affected individuals often surviving into middle age.

Becker was, until his retirement in 1975, Professor of Human Genetics at the University of Göttingen, a position he had held since 1957 (Fig. 2.11). Although by training a neurologist and psychiatrist, most of his work has

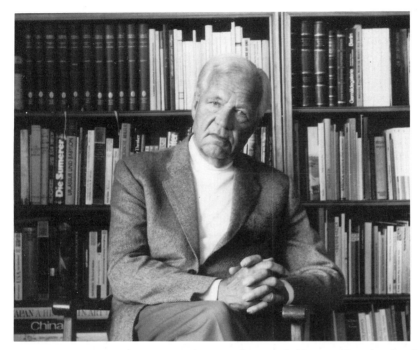

Fig. 2.11 Peter Emil Becker. Emeritus Professor of Human Genetics in the University of Göttingen.

centred on human genetics. The dystrophy which bears his name was first brought to his attention by Dr Franz Kiener, a psychologist in Regensburg, who sought Becker's advice on the disease which affected several of his own relatives. Together, they studied the family in detail (Becker and Kiener 1955) and a few years later Becker reported two further families with the same disease (Becker 1962). Patients with the disease had been observed previously by others, but it was Becker who showed that it was clearly a separate clinical and genetic entity. It is now known that Duchenne and Becker types of muscular dystrophy are due to mutations at the same locus on the X chromosome. That is, they are allelic.

Recent developments

Some important landmarks in the history of Duchenne muscular dystrophy are listed in Table 2.2. The most exciting developments occurred just over 10 years ago with the mapping of the defective gene to a specific locus on the short arm of the X chromosome (Xp21). And within two or three years

Table 2.2 *Landmarks in the history of Duchenne muscular dystrophy*

Nineteenth century	DMD recognized as a specific clinical disorder (Bell 1830; Conte and Gioja 1836; Meryon 1852; Duchenne 1861, 1868; Gowers 1879*a, b*)
1955	BMD recognized as a distinct X-linked muscular dystrophy (Becker and Kiener 1955)
1959–60	SCK raised in patients (Ebashi *et al.* 1959; Dreyfus *et al.* 1960) and in female carriers (Schapira *et al.* 1960)
1978–83	DMD mapped to Xp21 by X/A translocations (Verellen *et al.* 1978; Lindenbaum *et al.* 1979) and DNA markers (Murray *et al.* 1982; Davies *et al.* 1983)
1983–84	BMD and DMD shown to be allelic (Kingston *et al.* 1983, 1984)
1985	Gene-specific probes (PERT, Kunkel *et al.* 1985; XJ, Ray *et al.* 1985)
	Gene deletions detected (Monaco *et al.* 1985)
1987–88	cDNA cloned and sequenced (Koenig *et al.* 1987, 1988)
	Protein product (dystrophin) identified (Hoffman *et al.* 1987*a*)
	Dystrophin localization and functional studies begin (Sugita *et al.* 1988; Zubrzycka-Gaarn *et al.* 1988)
1989–90	Myoblast transfer experiments in mouse (Patridge *et al.* 1989) and humans (Karpati 1990; Law *et al.* 1990)
1990–91	Direct gene transfer (Wolff *et al.* 1990; Dickson *et al.* 1991)

gene-specific probes became available, culminating in the identification and characterization of the defective protein in Duchenne and Becker muscular dystrophies, namely dystrophin. Many individuals have played important roles in these studies, the most notable being Dr Kay Davies of Oxford, Dr Lou Kunkel of Boston, Dr Ron Worton of Toronto, and Dr Eric Hoffman of Pittsburgh (Fig. 2.12). These developments will be discussed in detail in the text.

Based on these various findings rational new approaches to therapy are beginning to be considered. The prospects are now more hopeful than ever that, in the not too distant future, an effective therapy will be found for this tragic disease.

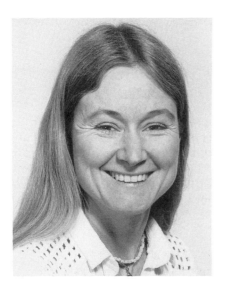
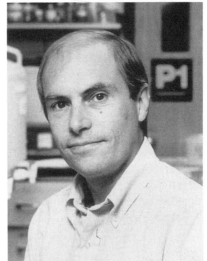
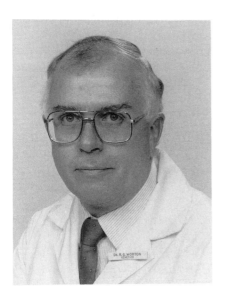
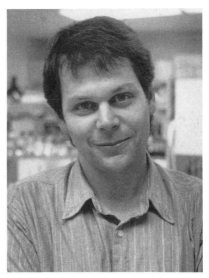

Fig. 2.12 Investigators who have played leading roles in recent research which has led to the localization and characterization of the Duchenne gene and its product. (*Above*: Dr Kay Davies and Dr Lou Kunkel; *below*: Dr Ron Worton and Dr Eric Hoffman.)

3 Clinical features

In the preclinical stage of Duchenne muscular dystrophy, before there are any signs of the disease, muscle histology is abnormal. Furthermore, significant histological and histochemical abnormalities have now been detected in muscle tissue from fetuses at risk for Duchenne muscular dystrophy as early as the second trimester of pregnancy (see Chapter 4). The disease is therefore already manifest in the fetus. Postnatally, however, the onset of clinical signs and symptoms is insidious and parents may be unaware that anything is wrong for some time.

Onset

Occasionally mothers volunteer that their affected son seemed 'floppy' at birth and in infancy. However, this is never as pronounced or as frequent as in the congenital forms of muscular dystrophy (Fig. 3.1) or infantile spinal muscular atrophy (Werdnig–Hoffmann disease).

The term amyotonia congenita (myatonia congenita, Oppenheim disease)

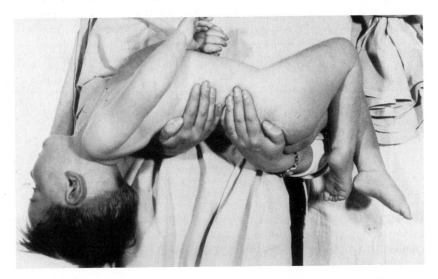

Fig. 3.1 A 3-year old boy with a relatively non-progressive form of congenital muscular drystrophy. He has generalized hypotonia with retarded motor development and can still not sit without support. (From Emery (1990a) with permission.)

has been applied to the syndrome of generalized muscular hypotonia, feebleness of voluntary movements, and depressed or absent tendon reflexes which is present at birth or is manifest shortly after birth. In one careful follow-up study (Walton 1956) of all infants affected in this way, over 60 per cent proved to have Werdnig–Hoffmann disease, 20 per cent a myopathy of one form or another, and the remainder had a variety of conditions including cerebral palsy and mental handicap. Three of the 109 cases in the study went on to develop Duchenne muscular dystrophy. However, in many cases of amyotonia, no cause is found, and these have been referred to as 'benign congenital hypotonia' because most of them resolve completely in childhood (Dubowitz 1978). However, this diagnosis should be accepted with some caution because refinements in muscle histochemistry and biochemistry in recent years have revealed several specific myopathies which can present in this way (Brooke *et al*. 1979).

'Failure to thrive' may, in some cases, be associated with the subsequent development of Duchenne muscular dystrophy (Call and Ziter 1985) as may also speech delay, and most boys show a delay in motor development in early childhood (Dubowitz 1963a; Gardner-Medwin *et al*. 1978). Any male infant who fails to thrive or where there is delay in motor, mental, or speech development for no apparent reason should have his serum creatine kinase level determined (p. 46) in order to exclude the possibility of Duchenne muscular dystrophy.

Often mothers notice that there is a delay in learning to walk. Of 114 cases in which this information was reliably documented, in 64 (56 per cent) walking was delayed until at least 18 months (Table 3.1) and roughly a quarter did

Table 3.1 *Distribution of age in learning to walk in 114 affected boys*

Age (months)	No.	Cumulative %
8–9	1	0.9
10–11	3	3.5
12–13	10	12.3
14–15	20	29.8
16–17	16	43.8
18–19	26	66.6
20–21	6	71.9
22–23	3	74.5
24–25	21	92.9
26–27	1	93.8
28–29	0	93.8
30–31	3	96.4
32–33	0	96.4
34–35	0	96.4
36	4	99.9

Table 3.2 *Percentile distribution of age at apparent onset in 144 affected boys*

Percentile	Age (years)
25	<2
50	2.4
60	2.8
70	3.4
75	3.7
80	4.1
90	5.1
95	6.1
99	7.8

not walk until they were at least 2 years old. In normal children, by comparison, the average age in learning to walk is about 13 months, and 97 per cent are walking by 18 months (Neligan and Prudham 1969).

Approximate percentiles for age at apparent onset in 144 cases are given in Table 3.2. In this and other age-related events based on cases studied by the author, percentiles were obtained by fitting the best curve to the data. It will be seen that in 90 per cent of cases onset is before school age (about 5 years). These data, however, should be accepted with a little caution because age at onset is notoriously difficult to assess with any accuracy, although parents can usually give a good idea as to when they first noticed that something seemed to be wrong with their son.

It is often stated that if the parents have already had an affected son, the onset of the disorder in a second affected son is noted to be earlier because they are conscious of the possibility. But this is by no means always true as shown in Table 3.3 where age at onset is given for affected brothers in cases

Table 3.3 *Age (years) at onset in affected brothers*

Case no.	1st born	2nd born	3rd born
11	2	7	—
90	5	3	—
100	$2\frac{1}{2}$	5	—
111	$2\frac{1}{2}$	4	—
121	$1\frac{3}{4}$	$1\frac{1}{2}$	—
528	$1\frac{1}{2}$	6	—
587	4	$2\frac{1}{2}$	—
593	$7\frac{1}{2}$	$7\frac{1}{2}$	—
1761	$4\frac{1}{2}$	$4\frac{1}{2}$	$4\frac{1}{2}$
2009	3	$1\frac{1}{2}$	—

where this information was personally recorded *at the time the diagnosis was confirmed* in each case.

On close questioning in almost all cases, the affected child *was never able to run properly*. Other complaints at the time of onset included waddling gait, walking unsteadily with a tendency to fall easily, walking on toes, and difficulty in climbing stairs. In a few instances weakness was first noticed after the child had sustained a fracture following a fall. Sometimes the parents noted a tendency to 'throw out his leg' when walking, for the 'feet

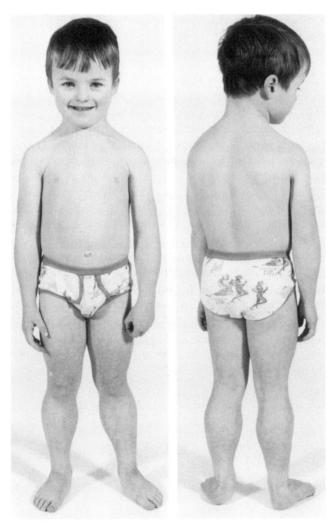

Fig. 3.2 A 4-year-old boy with Duchenne muscular dystrophy. Note the enlarged calves.

to turn in', or their attention was even drawn to enlargement of the calf muscles (Fig. 3.2).

However, although most cases in the present series presented in early childhood, there were five cases (which were all isolated cases) where onset was apparently delayed until the age of 8 or 9. This exceptionally late onset raises the possibility that these cases might not in fact be Duchenne muscular dystrophy but the more benign Becker type of muscular dystrophy in which age at onset is often somewhat later. However, the subsequent clinical course in all but case 144 would be compatible with the diagnosis of Duchenne muscular dystrophy (Table 3.4). In any event, apart from the clinical course, a distinction between these two disorders can now be made on the basis of DNA studies (p. 87).

Muscle pseudohypertrophy

The most obvious feature in the early stages of the disease is enlargement of the calf muscles which are often said to feel 'firm' or 'woody'. Of 89 cases where the size of the calves was noted at some time in the course of the disease, in at least 85 (96 per cent) they seemed much larger than normal. However, such enlargement may also involve the masseters, deltoids, serrati anterior, and quadriceps, and occasionally other muscles as well. Macroglossia is not uncommon. Muscle enlargement, at least in part, is due to an excess of adipose and connective tissue, and therefore the term 'pseudohypertrophy' is widely used. But true (work) hypertrophy may also play a role as a compensation for weakness in other muscles (Bertorini and Igarashi 1985). However, in Duchenne muscular dystrophy it is difficult to imagine this as being an important factor because in some cases such muscle enlargement can be extensive (Fig. 3.3). Interestingly, if in an affected boy a limb becomes affected by poliomyelitis then there is no pseudohypertrophy in that limb and therefore, presumably, it depends on an intact nerve supply (Tyler 1950). Pseudohypertrophy is not pathognomonic for Duchenne muscular dystrophy since it can also occur in some other forms of dystrophy and even occasionally in spinal muscular atrophy.

Table 3.4 *Cases with delayed onset*

| Case no. | Age (years) | | | Comments |
	Onset	Chairbound	Death	
144	8	—	—	Now age 10 and moderately affected
124	8	11	20	—
1741	8	12	—	Parents not good witnesses
2197	9	11	—	Severely mentally retarded (IQ < 50)
112	9	12	21	—

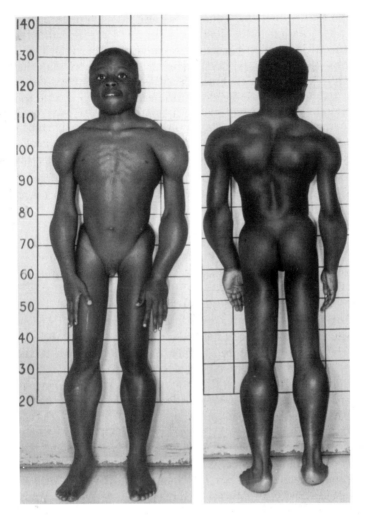

Fig. 3.3 Extensive muscle enlargement (pseudohypertrophy) in a case of Duchenne muscular dystrophy. (Reproduced by kind permission of Dr Sarah Bundey.)

Distribution of muscle weakness

Muscle involvement is always bilateral and symmetrical. In general, in the early stages of the disease, the lower limbs are affected more than the upper limbs, and the proximal muscles more than the distal muscles. At this stage certain muscles are predominantly affected. These include the latissimus dorsi, sterno-costal head of the pectoralis major, brachioradialis, biceps, triceps, iliopsoas, glutei, and quadriceps muscles. The involvement is highly selective. For example, the quadriceps are more affected than the hamstrings, triceps more than biceps, wrist extensors more than flexors, neck flexors more than extensors, dorsiflexors of the feet more than the plantar flexors. Even within a single muscle there is differential involvement. For example, the sterno-costal head of the pectoralis major muscle is more affected than the clavicular head, but in contrast the clavicular head of the sternomastoid muscle is more affected than the sternal head. This differential muscle involvement, which has been elaborated upon by Bonsett (1969), becomes less clear as the disease progresses so that ultimately such patterns are no longer obvious. Later slight facial weakness often develops and the intercostal muscles also become affected, but sphincter control, chewing, and swallowing are never affected.

Early signs

This pattern of muscle involvement results in several well-defined physical features associated with the disease. Weakness of the gluteus medius and minimus muscles (which abduct the hip and hold the pelvic bone down to the greater trochanter of the femur) results in the pelvis tilting down toward the unsupported side when an affected child raises his leg from the ground. To compensate for this he inclines toward the supporting leg. As he moves forward this action is continually repeated and results in the broad-based, waddling gait which is so characteristic of Duchenne muscular dystrophy. But, as Professor Dubowitz has pointed out, 'not everything that waddles is muscular dystrophy' for other conditions can also produce this type of gait (for example, spinal muscular atrophy). Weakness of the gluteus maximus muscle (which powerfully extends the hip) results in a tendency for the pelvis to tilt forward and in order to compensate for this a lumbar lordosis develops. In order to maintain his balance, and possibly because of an imbalance between the dorsiflexors and plantar flexors, he also tends to walk on his toes. However, the mechanical effects of muscle weakness on the gait in this disorder are complex and have been analysed in considerable detail by Sutherland and colleagues (1981).

Weakness of the knee and hip extensors results in the classical Gowers' manoeuvre: the child climbs up his thighs in order to extend the hips and push up the trunk (Fig. 2.8 and 3.4). However, it may be impossible to elicit this sign before the age of 4 or 5. Even before this age I have found that an affected child is unable to rise from a sitting position on the floor if he is asked to *keep his arms folded* (which prevents him from pushing on his thighs or on the floor) whereas a normal child can accomplish this quite easily.

In the early stages of the disease it may also be difficult to elicit weakness of the pectoral girdle musculature by formal testing. However, if the child is grasped around the chest from behind and an attempt made to lift him there is a tendency to 'slide-through' the examiner's arms. Also, by placing the examiner's hands inside the upper arms a normal child can be held up with comparative ease, but not an affected child. Both these signs are positive by the age of 4 and sometimes earlier. As the disease progresses, winging of the scapulae becomes apparent.

The affected muscles are not tender (which could suggest myositis) and there is no voluntary or percussion myotonia. As the muscles become weaker and wasted, the corresponding tendon reflexes become depressed, though good ankle jerks are retained for a long time and are the last of the tendon reflexes to disappear. The plantar responses are always flexor and there is no sensory loss.

In the early stages of the disease, apart from the obvious difficulties of trying to keep up with his peers, affected boys usually make few complaints apart from occasionally cramp and perhaps stiffness, particularly in the calf muscles. However, when such symptoms are severe this raises the possibility

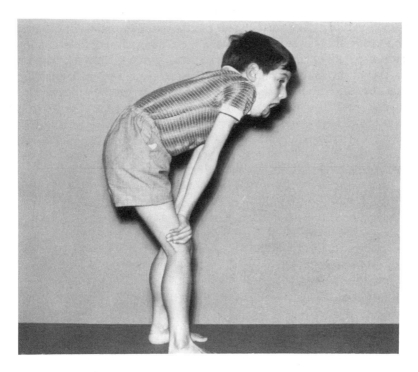

Fig. 3.4 Gowers' sign or manoeuvre.

of some other myopathy (such as McArdle's syndrome or carnitine palmityl-transferase deficiency) or perhaps myositis. More than a third of affected boys show some degree of intellectual impairment and some are severely mentally retarded. This aspect of the disease will be dealt with later (p. 115).

Progression

The weakness is progressive but nevertheless often shows periods of apparent arrest. It is because of this fluctuation that the assessment of the efficacy of any suggested therapy has to be evaluated with considerable care.

As the disease progresses the lumbar lordosis becomes more exaggerated and the waddling gait increases. Shortening of the heel cords (Achilles tendon) becomes more marked and an equinovarus deformity develops, though this is more obvious when the boy becomes confined to a wheelchair.

Although, initially, an affected boy may find he only needs a wheelchair at certain times (for example when going outside) inevitably he will become permanently confined to a wheelchair. The age at which this occurs is more precise and much better documented than the age at onset (Table 3.5). In the present series, with very few exceptions which have been excluded, no attempts had been made to prolong ambulation by various orthopaedic measures and therefore the data relate to the natural progress of the disease.

Of the 120 affected boys in which the age at becoming confined to a wheelchair was reliably known, in 95 per cent of cases this occurred by the age of 12. Age at becoming confined to a wheelchair was not significantly correlated with age at onset but was significantly correlated with age at death ($N = 55, r = 0.33, P < 0.02$). The difference in mean age at death in boys who became chairbound by 8 years of age ($N = 27$, mean 16.23, s.d. 2.66)

Table 3.5 *Percentile distribution of age at becoming confined to a wheelchair in 120 affected boys*

Percentile	Age (years)
10	6.7
20	7.4
30	7.8
40	8.2
50	8.5
60	8.9
70	9.3
75	9.6
80	10.0
90	11.0
95	11.9
99	13.2

compared with those who became chairbound after 8 years of age ($N = 28$, mean 17.77, s.d. 2.79) is statistically significant ($P < 0.05$). It would seem that *age at death after 15 increases roughly by one year for each year that a boy remains ambulant after the age of 7* up to the age of 10 or more (Table 3.6). In general terms, the earlier a boy becomes confined to a wheelchair, the poorer the prognosis.

Assessment of motor ability

It is often valuable to be able to chart the course of the disease in patients. A number of systems have been devised for doing this which depend on assessing either muscle strength or functional ability:
1. *Muscle strength*
   MRC grading (0–5)
   Ergometry
2. *Functional ability*
   Swinyard grade (1–8)
   Vignos grade (1–10)
   Hammersmith motor ability score (0–40)
   'CIDD' grade for upper limbs (1–6)

Details of the various grading systems are given in the Appendices B–F and will be discussed in more detail later. A very detailed functional scoring system has also been developed by Cornelio *et al.* (1982) which is expressed as the sum of single scores for gait, climbing stairs, getting up from a chair, and getting up from a seated position on the floor.

Since there is inevitably a subjective element in such methods, in order to make comparisons either between different patients or with the same patient over a period of time, they are best carried out by the same person. For many years I have assessed the Swinyard and Vignos grades of most patients examined (186 observations on 110 patients), and the results are given in Figs 3.5 and 3.6.

Table 3.6 *Age at death related to age at becoming confined to a wheelchair*

| | Age (years) confined to a wheelchair | | | |
	≤ 7	8	9	10 or more
No.	9	18	15	13
Mean	15.65	16.52	17.44	18.15
s.d.	3.36	2.29	2.65	3.00
No.	27		28	
Mean	16.23		17.77	
s.d.	2.66		2.79	

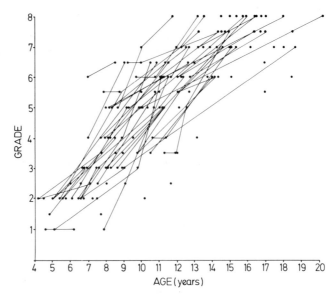

Fig. 3.5 Swinyard grade and age in boys with Duchenne muscular dystrophy. Points are joined for assessments on the same individual.

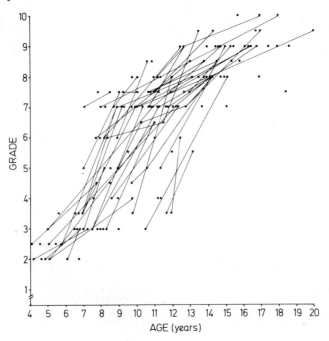

Fig. 3.6 Vignos grade and age in boys with Duchenne muscular dystrophy. Points are joined for assessments on the same individual.

Both grades correlate well with the progress of the disease. However, there is clearly considerable variation between different boys of the same age, and this has been well documented by others (Allsop and Ziter 1981; Cohen *et al.* 1982; Brooke *et al.* 1983). But apart from variations in motor ability between boys of the same age, affected boys also differ in their general appearance. Some retain their subcutaneous fat and muscle bulk whereas others become thin and atrophic. This is graphically demonstrated in the two boys of similar age shown in Fig. 3.7. The reason for this is not clear but there is a tendency for affected brothers to follow a similar pattern. In most cases sexual development is normal though puberty is delayed in a proportion of cases.

Later stages

As the disease progresses and muscle weakness becomes more profound, contractures increasingly develop, particularly flexion contractures of the

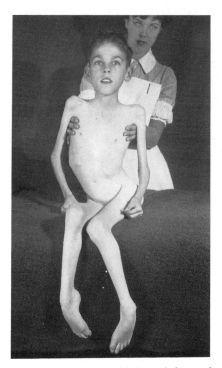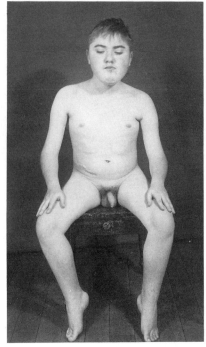

Fig. 3.7 A 13-year-old boy (*left*), and a 12-year-old boy (*right*) with Duchenne muscular dystrophy. (Reproduced by kind permission of Professor V. Dubowitz and W. B. Saunders Company, Publishers.)

elbows, knees, and hips. Later, movements of the shoulders and wrists also become limited. Talipes equinovarus deformity becomes marked with the talus bone protruding prominently under the skin on the dorsum of the foot. Unless adequate support is provided in the wheelchair a severe kyphoscoliosis develops. These various deformities have been well illustrated by Rideau (1979). Thoracic deformity poses the most serious problem as it restricts adequate pulmonary airflow on the compressed side (Fig. 3.8).

The respiratory problems are also aggravated by weakness of the intercostal muscles. About halfway through the course of the disease a gradual deterioration begins in pulmonary function with reduced maximal inspiratory and expiratory pressures. By the later stages there is a significant reduction in total lung capacity and an increase in residual volume. Oxygen tension (P_{O_2}) and carbon dioxide tension (P_{CO_2}) are usually normal and an increase in P_{CO_2} in a patient without respiratory infection indicates a bad prognosis (Inkley *et al.* 1974). However, differences in pulmonary function in the upright and supine positions are small, indicating that diaphragmatic

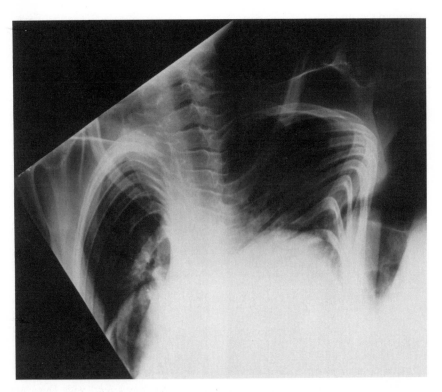

Fig. 3.8 Chest X-ray of an 18-year-old boy severely affected with Duchenne muscular dystrophy showing gross thoracic deformity.

function is relatively preserved. This may account for why respiratory failure develops late in the course of the disease and chronic alveolar hypoventilation appears to be rare. The effects on respiratory function are somewhat different in other forms of dystrophy (Newsom-Davis 1980).

Cardiac muscle is also affected, as will be discussed later, but it is rare for a boy to succumb to heart failure though occasional cases of sudden death may be attributable to cardiac involvement. In the present series of patients, 14 cases came to autopsy and the primary cause of death was given as pneumonia (11), 'respiratory failure' (1), diphtheria at age 8 (1), and acute cardiac arrhythmia (1).

That age at death might be in some way related to socio-economic factors is not borne out in the present study; when information on social class was

Table 3.7 *Age at death in Duchenne muscular dystrophy and social class of parents*

Age (years) at death	Social class					Total
	5	4	3	2	1	
< 10	–	–	1	–	–	*1*
10–14	1	1	4	2	–	*8*
15–19	4	15	11	5	1	*36*
20–24	2	–	1	–	–	*3*
Total	*7*	*16*	*17*	*7*	*1*	*48*

$(\chi^2 = 10.92; P > 0.05)$

Table 3.8 *Percentile distribution of age at death in 129 affected boys*

Percentile	Age (years)
10	12.0
20	13.4
30	14.3
40	15.0
50	15.5
60	16.2
70	17.0
75	17.6
80	18.1
90	19.5
95	20.5
99	23.5

available there was no apparent relationship with age at death (Table 3.7). Furthermore if we consider recent studies, there does not appear to be any significant difference in age at death in affluent compared with more deprived countries (Table 3.10, p. 42).

Age at death was not significantly correlated with age at onset but, as we have seen, it was correlated with age at becoming confined to a wheelchair. The percentile distribution of age at death is given in Table 3.8. In 90 per cent of cases this occurred before the age of 20.

These figures, however, could be biased towards earlier deaths since they exclude affected individuals who are still alive. However this seems unlikely to be important because in cases where year and age at death were well documented there was no significant difference between mean age at death in those who died between 1934 and 1963 compared with those who died between 1964 and 1973 (Table 3.9).

Gardner-Medwin in a detailed study of the natural history of the disease in the north-east of England (Gardner-Medwin 1982a) has suggested that recently boys with Duchenne muscular dystrophy might be surviving longer, perhaps because of some improvement in treatment. The present data do indicate a slight increase in mean age at death over the years. However, the mean age at death in the last 10 years ($N = 28$, mean 16.83, s.d. 2.53) does not differ significantly from the mean in the preceding 40 years ($N = 45$, mean 16.49, s.d. 3.03), although it is just significantly different ($0.02 < P < 0.05$) from the mean calculated from data given by Gowers in 1879 ($N = 25$, mean 15.36, s.d. 2.46) for cases that would now be categorized as Duchenne muscular dystrophy but excluding two of his cases who died accidentally in early childhood. But then some of Gowers' cases died of intercurrent infections, such as acute gastroenteritis and scarlet fever, which are uncommon causes of mortality in childhood in Britain nowadays. It would seem that if there has been any improvement in survival over the last 100 years this has been slight. However a large survey of 176 autopsy cases in Japan suggests that, compared with the past, *hospitalized* patients may survive longer, that pulmonary infection has become a less frequent cause of death, and that

Table 3.9 *Age at death and year at death recorded in 73 affected boys over the 50-year period 1934 to 1983 inclusive, compared with data from Gowers (1879b)*

	1934–1963	1964–1973	1974–1983	Gowers (1879b)
No.	13	32	28	25
Mean	16.27	16.63	16.83	15.36
s.d.	4.09	2.60	2.53	2.46

dystrophic changes in cardiac and respiratory muscles (resulting in cardiac failure and respiratory insufficiency) are now more closely related with a fatal outcome. The authors attribute these changes to the benefits of hospital care (Mukoyama *et al.* 1987). Furthermore, there is no doubt that survival can be significantly prolonged by various forms of assisted ventilation in the later stages of the disease and this will be discussed later (Chapter 13).

There is considerable variation in age at death, some boys succumbing as early as 8, while others survive into their mid-twenties. In the literature one case has been recorded as having fathered in his twenties a son and a carrier daughter (Thompson 1978), and another confirmed case survived, despite considerable physical handicap, to the age of 34 when he died an accidental death (Johnson *et al.* 1985). But such cases have been very much the exception.

Patterson and colleagues (1991) have analysed the actual *mode* of death and found that most boys died peacefully and often unpredictably. The authors emphasize that parents need to be apprised of this. The ages at which the three main events marking the disease occurred (onset, confined to a wheelchair, and death) in the present series are compared with those in other studies (Table 3.10). There is reasonable agreement between the various studies which are drawn from different populations, but all show considerable variation in these three main events.

The considerable variation in the disease is also illustrated in Table 3.11 from which it can be seen that some boys may become chairbound, or even die from the disease, before the apparent onset in other boys.

Disorders in affected boys other than muscular dystrophy

Several studies (Eiholzer *et al.* 1988; Zatz *et al.* 1988; and Rapaport *et al.* 1991*a*) have shown that affected boys are of normal length and weight at birth but subsequently growth is slower than normal and later they are often of short stature. Otherwise apart from mental handicap and problems directly relating to muscle weakness, most boys have very few health problems. The only other disorders recorded in the present series were recurrent urinary infections (2), left hydronephrosis with associated impaired renal function (1), unspecified congenital heart disease (1), undescended testes (1), and insulin-dependent diabetes mellitus (1); in the last case the same disease also affected the boy's father.

Summary and conclusions

Onset of the disease is insidious but an important hallmark in the very early stages is an inability to run properly. In over half the cases walking is delayed until at least 18 months of age. Manifestations of the disease are apparent

Table 3.10 *Ages at which the three main events marking Duchenne muscular dystrophy occur*

Region	Onset			Chairbound			Death				Reference
	No.	Mean	s.d.	No.	Mean	s.d.	No.	Mean	s.d.	Range	
Brazil	58	3.32	1.79	55	9.55	1.79	24	17.05	3.56	12–27	Zatz (1986)*
Canada	–	–	–	49	9.94	1.57	59	16.56	2.25	12–21	Murphy (1985)*
France	100	3.15	1.68	?	10.16	1.76	?	17.72	3.76	10–25	Rideau (1979)
Germany	41	3.07	2.24	42	9.36	2.62	40	14.71	3.76	8–23	Becker (1962)
Japan	105	3.7	1.9	128	10.8	1.9	65	18.0	2.9	–	Sugita (1985)*
Poland	483	2.3	1.46	234	10.1	1.90	58	18.1	3.31	–	Hausmanowa-Petrusewicz et al. (1986)*
Switzerland	88	2.89	1.29	83	9.81	1.50	47	17.79	3.22	11–29	Moser (1986)*
UK											
England (N)	144	2.6	–	86	9.5	–	–	18.7	–	13–28	Gardner-Medwin (1982a)
England (S)	64	3.07	1.75	56	9.05	2.02	7	15.57	2.82	11–18	Dubowitz (1978); (cases studied in 1960)
Scotland	144	3.26	1.74	120	9.39	1.69	129	16.27	3.12	8–25	Present series
USA											
Utah	46	3.76	2.15	–	–	–	25	17.68	3.34	13–25	Stephens and Tyler (1951)
Durham (NC)	70	2.87	1.52	47	9.32	1.89	11	17.12	3.38	11–24	Emery and Roses (unpublished 1988)

*Personal communication to the author.

Table 3.11 *Numbers of boys with Duchenne muscular dystrophy with different ages at onset, becoming confined to a wheelchair, and death (author's series)*

Age	Onset	Chairbound	Death
< 2	24	–	–
2	46	–	–
3	27	–	–
4	23	–	–
5	14	–	–
6	2	2	–
7	3	15	–
8	3	27	2
9	2	31	2
10	–	19	1
11	–	14	2
12	–	6	6
13	–	4	7
14	–	2	19
15	–	–	10
16	–	–	25
17	–	–	15
18	–	–	11
19	–	–	12
20	–	–	7
21	–	–	6
22	–	–	–
23	–	–	2
24	–	–	1
25	–	–	1
Total	*144*	*120*	*129*

in most cases before 5, but some remain apparently healthy until 8 or even 9 years of age. Pseudohypertrophy of the calf muscles is present in almost all cases and in some instances many other muscles are also affected. Wasting and weakness predominantly affects the proximal limb girdle musculature but early on muscle involvement is highly selective. A waddling gait, Gowers' sign, and 'sliding-through' the examiner's arms are useful diagnostic signs. However, even before Gowers' sign can be elicited, affected boys are unable to rise from a sitting position on the floor if asked to keep their arms folded. The age at becoming confined to a wheelchair (which is usually by the age of 12) is a prognostic sign in that age at death after 15 increases roughly by one year for each year that a boy remains ambulant after the age of 7 up to the age of 10 or more. Ninety per cent of boys die before the age of 20, usually from respiratory problems. However, as with the other main events in the natural history of the disorder, there is considerable variation from one individual to another. Apart from problems relating directly or indirectly to dystrophy, most affected boys have very few other health problems.

4 Confirmation of the diagnosis

It is unlikely that an experienced physician would have any difficulty in suspecting Duchenne muscular dystrophy in an otherwise healthy schoolboy who presents with a waddling gait, pseudohypertrophic calves, and a positive Gowers' sign. However, the diagnosis may not be so obvious in the very young or in those cases where onset is delayed until late childhood. Also, because of the uniformly poor prognosis and the parents' need for reliable genetic counselling, it is essential that the diagnosis be firmly established as soon as possible. This depends on the serum level of creatine kinase, electromyography, muscle pathology, and now DNA studies on peripheral blood leucocytes.

Serum creatine kinase

The enzyme creatine kinase (EC2.7.3.2) catalyses the reversible transfer of a phosphate group from creatine phosphate to adenosine diphosphate (ADP) forming creatine and adenosine triphosphate (ATP):

$$\text{Creatine phosphate} + \text{ADP} \rightleftharpoons \text{Creatine} + \text{ATP}$$

The International Union of Biochemistry suggested the systematic name ATP: creatine phosphotransferase with creatine kinase as the acceptable trivial name.

Over the years a number of methods have been developed for measuring the activity of the enzyme, each depending on one of three approaches. First, creatine is incubated with ATP in the reaction mixture and the formation of creatine phosphate (as inorganic phosphate) is determined (Kuby *et al.* 1954). Secondly, the amount of ADP produced in the reaction is determined by a series of coupled reactions, in the original method pyruvate kinase and lactate dehydrogenase systems being used (Tanzer and Gilvarg 1959). Thirdly, the preferred faster reaction may be utilized whereby creatine phosphate is incubated with ADP and the formation of creatine (or ATP) is determined (Ennor and Rosenberg 1954). We have favoured a modification of this last method (Rosalki 1967) where the amount of ATP generated is estimated by coupling the reaction with hexokinase and glucose-6-phosphate dehydrogenase (G6PD), the formation of reduced nicotinamide–adenine dinucleotide phosphate (NADPH) being finally determined:

$$\text{Creatine phosphate} + \text{ADP} \quad \rightleftharpoons \quad \text{Creatine} + \text{ATP}$$

$$\text{ATP} + \text{glucose} \quad \overset{\text{Hexokinase}}{\rightleftharpoons} \quad \text{Glucose-6-phosphate} + \text{ADP}$$

$$\text{Glucose-6-phosphate} + \text{NADP} \overset{\text{G-6-PD}}{\rightleftharpoons} \text{6-Phosphogluconate} + \text{NADPH}$$

A thiol compound (e.g. cysteine) is incorporated in the reaction mixture to enhance enzyme activity. The amount of activity in serum is expressed in International Units (iu) as the amount of enzyme which catalyses the transformation of 1 micromole of creatine phosphate/min/1000 ml of serum at 30 °C. Since there is very little enzyme in erythrocytes, assays on serum are not affected by haemolysis which is an important practical consideration.

In healthy infants in the immediate newborn period, the level of activity of serum creatine kinase (SCK) is often somewhat raised to around 200–300 iu. This may be due to muscular anoxia (Blum and Brauman 1975). But within a few days of birth, levels are reached which are not very different from older children (Zellweger *et al.* 1970). In young boys there is no significant correlation with age (Passos *et al.* 1985). However, in adolescence higher levels are not infrequent and may possibly be a reflection of increased muscle mass and physical activity at this period, otherwise values are the same as in adults. The distribution of SCK levels in normal young healthy adult men is positively skewed with a few individuals having high levels (Emery and Spikesman 1970*a*, *b*). But most values in young healthy adult men are less than 200 iu which is a little higher than in women (p. 225) presumably because the latter have less muscle mass.

Sibley and Lehninger in 1949 were the first to note that a serum enzyme (in this case aldolase) could be raised in patients with muscular dystrophy. Some 10 years later Ebashi and his colleagues in Tokyo (Ebashi *et al.* 1959) also showed that creatine kinase activity is raised in the serum of patients with muscular dystrophy, and this was confirmed the following year by Dreyfus in Paris (Dreyfus *et al.* 1960). Even at birth and before the disease becomes clinically evident, SCK levels are considerably higher in Duchenne muscular dystrophy than in normal boys – up to a hundred times higher. They *may* even be raised in the affected fetus by the second trimester of pregnancy (Edwards *et al.* 1984). However, as the disease progresses, levels fall but only approach normal values in the very late stages of the disease (Fig. 4.1).

The most likely explanation for the very high SCK levels in Duchenne muscular dystrophy is that the enzyme originates in muscle and escapes into the serum. The much lower levels in the later stages of the disease are no doubt due to the decrease in functioning muscle tissue and reduction in physical activity. Levels certainly decrease most around the time (age 8–10) when affected boys become confined to a wheelchair.

Grossly elevated SCK levels (50–100 times normal) occur not only in

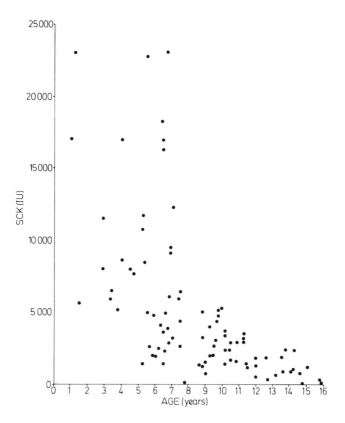

Fig. 4.1 SCK levels in boys with Duchenne muscular dystrophy.

Duchenne muscular dystrophy but also in the early stages of Becker muscular dystrophy (Emery and Skinner 1976), acute ischaemic muscle necrosis, and occasionally in the acute phase of polymyositis (Thompson 1971). Moderately elevated levels (up to 10 times normal) can occur in some other forms of muscular dystrophy (notably limb girdle and facioscapulo-humeral), spinal muscular atrophy (juvenile and adult forms), some individuals predisposed to malignant hyperpyrexia, and in certain non-hereditary disorders such as motor neurone disease, severe hypocalcaemia, hypothyroidism, and after myocardial infarction. Thus, a boy with evidence of proximal muscle weakness, with a waddling gait and a positive Gowers' sign, who is otherwise well and does not have polymyositis, but has a *grossly elevated* SCK level, is almost certainly suffering from Duchenne or Becker muscular dystrophy.

Creatine kinase isoenzymes

Creatine kinase exists in three molecular forms or isoenzymes. Each isoenzyme results from the dimeric association of two sub-units referred to as M and B, and the three isoenzymes are designated as MM, MB, and BB. The BB isoenzyme predominates in brain tissue, whereas the MM isoenzyme predominates in cardiac and skeletal muscle. The hybrid MB isoenzyme is a minor component in both cardiac and skeletal muscle. In normal serum the isoenzyme is very largely MM with only about 4 per cent being MB. This small MB fraction, however, is significantly increased in patients with Duchenne or Becker muscular dystrophy but does not distinguish between these two dystrophies (Vainzof *et al.* 1985). Though the MB form is found in cardiac muscle, its presence in serum in Duchenne muscular dystrophy is unrelated to cardiac involvement in the disease (Silverman *et al.* 1976) and presumably originates in dystrophic muscle in which there is more MB activity than in normal muscle.

Other muscle enzymes which exist as isoenzymes, and have been studied in detail in Duchenne muscular dystrophy, are lactate dehydrogenase, aldolase, and pyruvate kinase. Lactate dehydrogenase (LDH) exists as five isoenzymes (LDH 1–5). In the serum of patients with Duchenne muscular dystrophy there is a relative increase in the proportions of LDH 1–3 which reflects changes in the isoenzyme pattern in affected muscle tissue (Somer *et al.* 1973). There are muscle, brain, and liver forms of aldolase and the serum activity in Duchenne muscular dystrophy is predominantly that of the muscle type (Tzvetanova 1971). Pyruvate kinase (PK) exists as three isoenzymes (M_2, M_1, and L). In patients with Duchenne muscular dystrophy serum activity is mainly of the M_1 type which is the only PK isoenzyme found in skeletal muscle and brain and the major component in cardiac muscle (Zatz *et al.* 1978). Finally, carbonic anhydrase III and β-enolase are skeletal *muscle-specific* enzymes, and these too are elevated in the serum of affected boys (Carter *et al.* 1979, 1980; Mokuno *et al.* 1984). Thus, in all these instances the enzyme pattern in the serum of patients is similar to that in muscle tissue.

Other serum enzymes

Following the early studies in Paris (Schapira and Dreyfus 1963), several other enzymes have been found to be raised in Duchenne muscular dystrophy, though none to the same extent as creatine kinase. The highest levels (10–20 times normal) occur with aldolase, pyruvate kinase, carbonic anhydrase III, and β-enolase. Less dramatic increases have been found in a number of other enzymes including:

Lactate dehydrogenase
Phosphoglycerate mutase
Alanine aminotransferase (glutamic-pyruvic transaminase, GPT)
Aspartate aminotransferase (glutamic-oxaloacetic transaminase, GOT)
Phosphohexose isomerase
Phosphoglucomutase
α-Hydroxybutyrate dehydrogenase
Malate dehydrogenase

Most of these are major 'soluble' (sarcoplasmic) muscle enzymes. Their increase in serum in Duchenne muscular dystrophy probably reflects increased efflux through the muscle membrane, possibly augmented later in the disease process by release from fibres undergoing necrosis. Evidence supporting this idea has been critically assembled by Rowland (1980), who also provides an extensive bibliography. The evidence may be summarized as follows. (1) As already seen, the isoenzyme pattern of certain enzymes in serum closely resembles that of muscle tissue. (2) Under certain experimental conditions, it has been shown that enzymes are released from viable muscle tissue *in vitro*. (3) In patients aldolase levels have been shown to be slightly higher in the venous return than in the corresponding arterial supply of the lower limb. (4) Almost all of the enzymes that are increased in the serum of patients are cytoplasmic, whereas enzymes which are bound in some way to intracellular structures are not ordinarily found in the serum. (5) When the activity of an enzyme is increased in the serum of patients with Duchenne muscular dystrophy, it is almost always decreased in affected muscle, thus indicating that the enzyme originated from muscle. (6) The decline in serum enzyme levels as the disease progresses correlates well with the diminishing muscle mass. Finally, the idea is further supported by the fact that at least in some cases release is related to molecular size. The molecular weights of creatine kinase (81 000 daltons or 81 kDa) and aldolase (150 kDa) are considerably less than in AMP deaminase (320 kDa) and phosphofructokinase (400 kDa), which are also major muscle enzymes but which are virtually absent in serum of patients with Duchenne muscular dystrophy. However, some proteins with small molecular weights either do not appear at all in the serum of patients (adenylate kinase, 21 kDa), or only in relatively small amounts (myoglobin, 17 kDa).

The situation is therefore not simple and cannot be explained purely in terms of leakage from affected muscle. The serum level of an enzyme will be affected by its clearance rate, and its efflux from muscle will depend on its relative concentration in this tissue, its binding to intracellular structures and possibly some form of selective force at the level of the muscle membrane but about which little is yet known (Pennington 1977*a*).

From a practical point of view attempts to distinguish Duchenne and

Becker types of muscular dystrophy on the basis of serum levels of various enzymes have been uniformly unsuccessful.

Electromyography (EMG)

When muscle fibres contract they generate electrical activity. The electrical activity created by a group of muscle fibres activated by a single neurone, the so-called motor unit (Fig. 4.2), produces a motor unit action potential or simply action potential. Electromyography (EMG), among other things, is a technique for studying the electrical activity of contracting muscle fibres and provides useful information about the structure and functioning of motor units. It can therefore be a valuable diagnostic aid in neuromuscular disorders. It has the advantage over a biopsy that many different muscles and different parts of the same muscle can be studied. However, although changes in motor unit activity can give an idea of the severity and distribution of muscle involvement, it has been recognized for many years that these changes are not specific for any particular disease entity (Denny-Brown 1949). Furthermore, although some information can be gained from surface electrodes, usually the electrode is inserted into the muscle and cooperation by the patient is important. It can, therefore, be a difficult procedure to carry out on young children.

The technique of EMG involves inserting a fine concentric needle electrode through the skin into the muscle. The electrode is essentially a hollow needle surrounding an insulated core which is bared at the tip. The electrical activity generated when the electrode is inserted (insertion activity), when the muscle is at rest (spontaneous activity), and during voluntary muscle con-

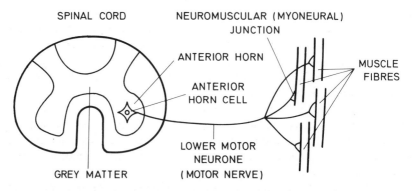

Fig. 4.2 The motor unit consists of an individual motor neurone (anterior horn cell) and the muscle fibres which it activates.

traction is suitably amplified and displayed on a cathode ray oscilloscope and often reproduced through a loudspeaker. A permanent record can be made on tape, and the information can also be fed into a computer for automated analysis.

The interpretation of electromyographic records requires much experience and in all but the most straightforward cases is best left to the expert. Here only a brief review can be given of the essential EMG changes helpful in diagnosing a suspected case of Duchenne muscular dystrophy. Further details, along with more sophisticated approaches, can be found for example in Buchthal and Rosenfalck (1963), Lenman and Ritchie (1970), and Yu and Murray (1984).

The normal EMG

When a needle electrode is inserted into a muscle, this evokes a discharge of action potentials, but this only lasts a brief period and is probably due to mechanical excitation of adjacent muscle fibres. At rest there is virtually no activity and the record is flat. However, on weak voluntary contraction of the muscle, action potentials are generated. They represent the potentials derived from groups of muscle fibres which are contracting nearly synchronously and are situated fairly close together and frequently activated by a single neurone. With minimal contraction and with the electrode position carefully adjusted, it is possible to record single action potentials. The wave form of the potential is determined by the number of phases or deflections across the base line. A potential with more than four phases is referred to as being polyphasic (Fig. 4.3).

The duration of the action potential, measured from the first deflection from the base line to its subsequent return to the base line, is averaged over a number of recordings, and in health ranges from about 4 to 15 ms. (Buchthal 1957). The amplitude (peak-to-peak) ranges from 100 μV to 1 mV, and normally less than about 5 per cent of the action potentials are polyphasic. However, these parameters are influenced by a number of factors including the type of electrode used, the depth of its insertion, the age and sex of the individual, the state of fatigue of the muscle, the ambient temperature, and the particular muscle being studied. Ideally, control values should be established using the same equipment, under the same conditions, and on individuals matched as closely as possible with the patients being investigated. Some representative normal values for the quadriceps and deltoid muscles in healthy young adults are given in Table 4.1. Values obtained in healthy children are less (Buchthal and Pinelli 1951; Buchthal 1957).

As the strength of voluntary contraction is increased, so more motor units are recruited and activated, giving rise to what is referred to as an *interference pattern* on the oscilloscope screen. The interference pattern is

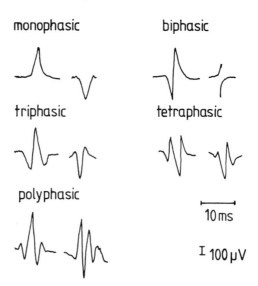

monophasic   biphasic

triphasic   tetraphasic

polyphasic

10 ms

100 μV

Fig. 4.3 Variations in the wave forms of action potentials recorded on minimal contraction of the gastrocnemius muscle in normal healthy adults.

reduced whenever the *number* of (activated) motor units is reduced as occurs in spinal muscular atrophy and in the late stages of muscular dystrophy.

The EMG in muscular dystrophy

Stemming from the early work of Buchthal and Kugelberg in the 1940s (Buchthal and Clemmesen 1941; Kugelberg 1947) the electromyographic features of muscular dystrophy came to be recognized: action potentials are smaller (reduced duration and amplitude) and polyphasic potentials more frequent than in normal. Many subsequent studies confirmed these earlier findings and have been reviewed by Buchthal and Rosenfalck (1963). Although muscular dystrophy may be suspected from inspection of the record as displayed on the oscilloscope, measurements of individual action potentials are less subjective and far more valuable. The changes observed are due to a general loss of active muscle fibres so that the *size* of each motor unit is reduced and as a result the action potentials are smaller. Later, as the disease progresses and muscle tissue is replaced by fat and connective tissue, so the *number* of motor units decreases and eventually there may be areas where very little if any activity can be recorded.

More recently several other electromyographic techniques have been introduced which can be of diagnostic value. The *single fibre EMG* electrode records activity from only a few fibres of a motor unit. It gives an idea

Table 4.1 *Some values (mean ± s.d.) for the amplitude and duration of motor unit action potentials in healthy young adults (Emery et al. 1973a)*

	Quadriceps			Deltoid		
	No.	Amplitude (μV)	Duration (ms)	No.	Amplitude (μV)	Duration (ms)
Males	15	384 ± 99	8.3 ± 1.2	12	318 ± 58	8.4 ± 0.8
Females	17	332 ± 61	7.2 ± 1.1	11	274 ± 37	8.6 ± 0.9

of the spatial distribution of muscle fibres and in Duchenne muscular dystrophy indicates an increase in fibre density early in the disease. However this and other sophisticated techniques such as *macro-EMG* and *scanning-EMG* are outside the scope of this discussion.

The EMG in other disorders

The EMG in other disorders which may have to be differentiated from a suspected case of Duchenne muscular dystrophy may be summarized as follows.

Other forms of muscular dystrophy

Other forms of dystrophy presenting in childhood and the various congenital myopathies all show a myopathic EMG which cannot usually be distinguished from Duchenne muscular dystrophy.

Spinal muscular atrophy

The electromyographic findings in this group of disorders are usually quite different from those found in myopathies. Characteristically there is prolonged insertion activity and fibrillation potentials are recorded at rest. These are small potentials with a duration of 0.5–2 ms and an amplitude of 30–150 μV, and occur at a rate of about 2–10 per second. They are probably, at least in part, due to the response of 'sensitized' denervated fibres to circulating acetylcholine. Occasionally these fibrillation potentials are reflected in a fine tremor of the base line of an ECG recording. In one case this drew my attention to the possible diagnosis (Fig. 4.4). This is rarely found in records from healthy individuals or patients with other neuromuscular disorders.

Other characteristics of the record in neurogenic atrophy include a reduced interference pattern, occasional 'giant' action potentials (high amplitude and long duration), and the mean action potential amplitude and

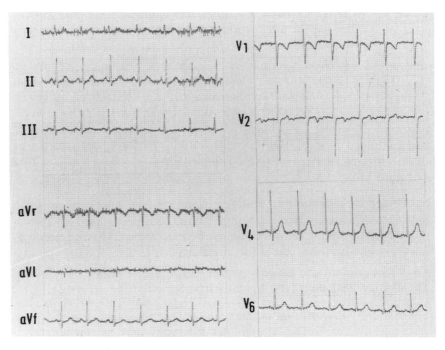

Fig. 4.4 ECG record of a boy aged 9 with Wohlfart–Kugelberg–Welander (type III) spinal muscular atrophy. Note the fine tremor particularly in the limb leads.

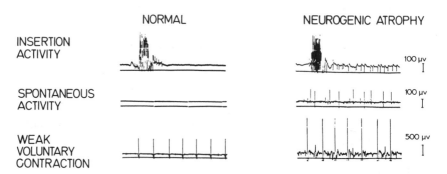

Fig. 4.5 Electromyographic features in neurogenic atrophy compared with normal: prolonged insertion activity, fibrillation potentials at rest, and occasional 'giant' potentials on voluntary contraction.

duration is generally increased (Gardner-Medwin *et al.* 1967; Hausmanowa-Petrusewicz *et al.* 1968*a*). These various changes find an explanation, at least in part, in the changes which result when denervation is followed by rein-nervation from surviving neurones. In some regions denervated muscle fibres become subsequently reinnervated by adjacent nerve fibres (collateral reinnervation) so increasing the size of the surviving motor unit.

The various features of the electromyographic record in neurogenic atrophy are compared with normal in Fig. 4.5. However, in such diseases the electromyographic record may sometimes appear almost normal or may even exhibit some myopathic features when the differentiation from dystrophy can be difficult.

Polymyositis

The other major disorder to be considered in the differential diagnosis is polymyositis. In the early stages of this disease there is prolonged insertion activity, and fibrillation potentials are present. The mean action potential duration and amplitude are reduced and polyphasic potentials are frequent.

Electromyographic features characterizing muscular dystrophy (and myopathies in general), spinal muscular atrophy, and polymyositis are sum-marized in Table 4.2. It would seem that the differentiation of muscular dystrophy from spinal muscular atrophy is fairly clear-cut, and in most cases this is true. It would also seem that polymyositis can be differentiated from muscular dystrophy on the basis of spontaneous activity. In general this is also true but it is not an entirely reliable difference because it may occur in dystrophy or be absent in polymyositis (Buchthal and Rosenfalck 1963).

Muscle pathology

A great deal has been written about the pathology of muscle in various neuromuscular disorders. Some texts give a concise account of the essential

Table 4.2 *The usual electromyographic features differentiating muscular dystrophy, spinal atrophy, and polymyositis*

	Muscular dystrophy	Spinal muscular atrophy	Polymyositis
Insertion activity	Very brief	Prolonged	Prolonged
Fibrillation potentials	–	+	+
Action potentials			
Duration	↓	↑	↓
Amplitude	↓	↑	↓
Polyphasic potentials	+	–	+
Giant potentials	–	+	–

changes observed in such disorders (Bethlem 1970; Hughes 1974) whereas others are extensive monographs which deal in detail with the various changes observed in the course of these diseases (Adams 1975, Mastaglia and Walton 1982; Schröder 1982; Carpenter and Karpati 1984; Dubowitz 1985; Kakulas and Adams 1985). Here only a brief description will be given of those changes in muscular dystrophy which are helpful in establishing the diagnosis.

Biopsy technique

A muscle biopsy is best carried out on a muscle which is moderately affected clinically. If a minimally affected muscle is chosen then the changes may be too slight to establish the correct diagnosis. On the other hand, if a severely affected muscle is selected it may also be impossible to establish a diagnosis because little may remain apart from fat and connective tissue. In the past the method of open excision under general anaesthesia was the method of choice. This was despite the recognized anaesthetic risks in patients who often have compromised respiratory and cardiac function. Although Duchenne himself had advocated the use of a biopsy needle 100 years ago, for a long time this did not meet with favour, largely because of the fear that being a 'blind' procedure, there might be the danger of damaging nerves or blood vessels. In fact, however, this has not proved the case and most now favour the use of a biopsy needle (Fig. 4.6) introduced with local anaesthesia under sterile conditions (Edwards *et al.* 1980; Heckmatt *et al.* 1984). Paraffin embedding of fixed material is still largely employed, but better results are obtained with liquid nitrogen and isopentane and studies made on cryostat sections. The latter procedure is associated with fewer artefacts and has the advantage that histochemical studies can also be carried out on the material. This is the method used here. Transverse sections are in general more informative than longitudinal sections, and useful stains are haematoxylin and eosin, or Gomori trichrome.

In a well established case of Duchenne muscular dystrophy, the changes observed in, say, the quadriceps or gastrocnemius muscles, include increased variation in fibre size, fibre necrosis with phagocytosis, and eventually replacement by fat and connective tissue (Fig. 4.7).

It is worthwhile considering some of these changes in a little more detail and tracing their development during the course of the disease.

Preclinical stage

Before there are any obvious clinical manifestations of the disease, there are already significant abnormalities in muscle pathology (Pearson 1962; Hudgson *et al.* 1967a; Bradley *et al.* 1972). Very early on the only significant abnormalities may be an increased variation in fibre size, and an increase in the number of prominent rounded fibres staining more densely with eosin — here referred to as *eosinophilic fibres*. In normal muscle these fibres are

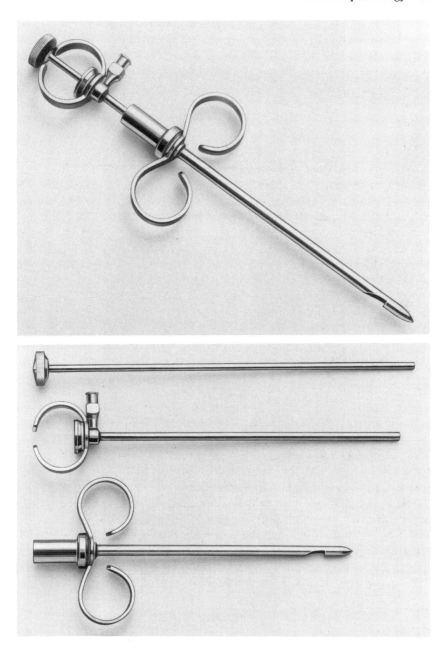

Fig. 4.6 The UCH skeletal muscle biopsy needle. (*Above*) the assembled instrument. (*Below*) the constituent parts which include the cutting cannula, with a side arm for applying suction, and the outer needle. (Instrument supplied by NI Medical, Redditch, Worcs., England.)

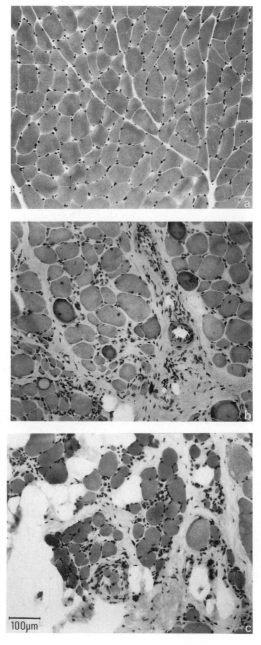

Fig. 4.7 Transverse cryostat sections of gastrocnemius muscle from (*a*) a healthy boy; (*b*) an early case of Duchenne muscular dystrophy; and (*c*) an advanced case of Duchenne muscular dystrophy (haematoxylin and eosin).

absent or very infrequent, and when present occur at the periphery of sections, indicating that they are artefactual. On the other hand, in Duchenne
muscular dystrophy, they are seen throughout sections and in some cases can
be particularly frequent (Fig. 4.8). These same fibres contain increased intracellular calcium as revealed by histochemical staining with alizarin red S, or
a fluorescent method with pentahydroxyflavone (Morin) (Fig. 4.9).

Increased intracellular calcium in skeletal muscle in Duchenne muscular
dystrophy has been demonstrated not only histochemically (Bodensteiner
and Engel 1978, Emery and Burt 1980) but also by X-ray microanalysis
(Maunder-Sewry *et al.* 1980), and by chemical methods (Bertorini *et al.*
1982). The proportion of calcium-positive fibres in Duchenne muscular
dystrophy is very variable and the highest proportion was found in a
preclinical case (Table 4.3). A significant increase in calcium-positive fibres
also occurs in Becker muscular dystrophy but to a much lesser degree in other
muscular dystrophies. The intracellular accumulation of calcium appears to
be the prelude to the breakdown and death (necrosis) of the muscle fibre.

At this early stage in the disease process, *regenerating* fibres are also

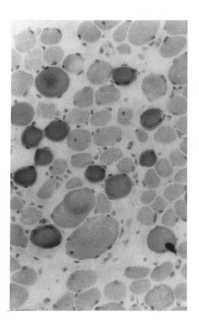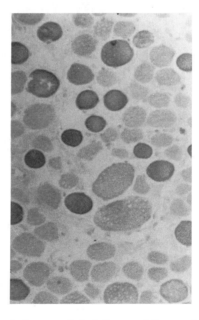

Fig. 4.8 Serial sections of gastrocnemius muscle in a preclinical (2-year-old) case of
Duchenne muscular dystrophy, stained with (*left*) haematoxylin and eosin, and
(*right*) alizarin red S. Note the numerous eosinophilic/calcium-positive fibres, but no
evidence of muscle fibre necrosis.

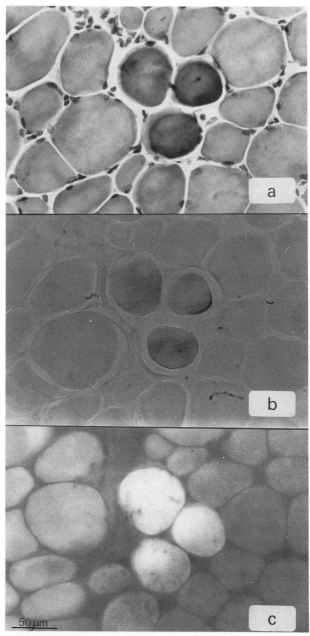

Fig. 4.9 Serial sections of muscle from an early case of Duchenne muscular dystrophy stained with (*a*) haematoxylin and eosin (note 3 centrally placed dark-staining eosinophilic fibres); (*b*) alizarin red S; and (*c*) fluorescent Morin. (From Emery and Burt 1980, with permission.)

Table 4.3 *Proportion (%) of eosinophilic and calcium-positive fibres in crysotat sections of gastrocnemius muscle biopsy samples from boys with no neuromuscular disorder and boys with Duchenne muscular dystrophy (unpublished data)*

	Age (years)	Eosinophilic fibres	Calcium-positive fibres
Controls			
($N = 7$)	5–12	<0.2	<0.1
DMD			
B103	10	6.0	5.8
B110	9	1.4	1.8
B115	7	3.0	2.9
B111	6	2.7	4.4
B106	5	4.1	6.5
B117*	3	3.7	5.3
B159*	2	15.3	18.3

* Preclinical cases.

commonly found. They are recognized by their smaller size in cross-section, basophilic cytoplasm, high concentration of ribonucleic acid (RNA), large pale vesicular nuclei with prominent nucleoli (Mauro 1979). However, such fibres become less frequent as the disease progresses and as fibres undergoing necrosis become more obvious. For reasons which are not yet clear, muscle fibres of smaller diameter seem more resistant to necrosis (Karpati and Carpenter 1986).

Later stages

The changes which take place as a muscle fibre undergoes necrosis are complex. As the intracellular structures are destroyed the fibre is invaded by phagocytic cells. In fact the '. . . most unequivocal evidence of necrosis is the presence of phagocytic cells within a disordered fibre' (Cullen and Mastaglia 1980). This is illustrated in Fig. 4.10.

As the necrotic fibres are phagocytosed they are replaced by fat and connective tissue so that eventually only small islands of muscle tissue remain.

Possible differences in muscle pathology between Duchenne and Becker types of muscular dystrophy have been described (Bradley *et al.* 1978). It seems unlikely, however, that any such differences point to any fundamental differences but are more likely to be reflections of the differing tempo in the two disorders.

The histological changes in muscular dystrophy are in general different from spinal muscular atrophy. In the latter group of disorders all those muscle fibres associated with the defective neurone gradually atrophy. This

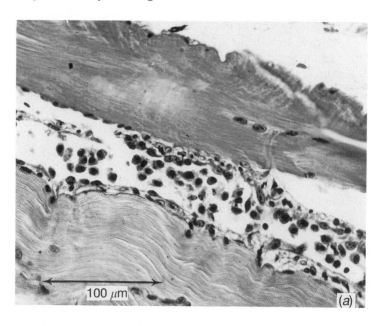

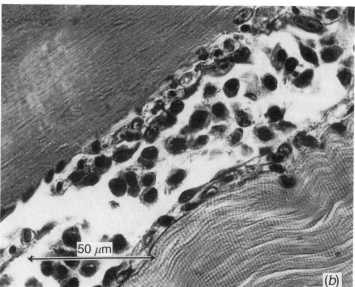

Fig. 4.10 Longitudinal sections of gastrocnemius muscle from a manifesting female carrier of Duchenne muscular dystrophy. (*a*) The upper fibre has lost most of the cross-striations which are still well defined in the lower fibre. Between the two fibres are the remains of a necrotic fibre which is undergoing phagocytosis. (*b*) Higher power magnification (haematoxylin and eosin).

produces the classical picture of group atrophy and is pathognomonic of spinal muscular atrophy (Fig. 4.11). The atrophy may be so profound as to present the appearance of 'nuclear clumps'. In spinal muscular atrophy, affected fibres undergo atrophy and tend to be grouped together. In contrast, in muscular dystrophy, affected fibres undergo structural changes and these occur in individual fibres at random. However, especially in the more chronic forms of neurogenic atrophy, muscle fibres adjacent to groups of atrophic fibres, may undergo changes similar to those seen in muscular dystrophy; variation in fibre size, central nuclei, and even occasionally fibre necrosis and phagocytosis. It is possible that such changes result from faulty attempts at reinnervation: the metabolism of these abnormally innervated fibres is disturbed in some way which then results in the structural changes usually associated with muscular dystrophy. In their detailed and elegant studies Bradley and his colleagues (1978) noted in some biopsy specimens from cases of Becker muscular dystrophy, changes which can be associated with denervation. However, there are limits in attempting to define pathogenesis purely on the basis of morphological appearances. As these investigators pointed out there can be problems in interpretation:

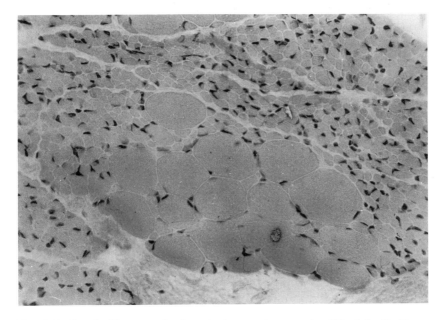

Fig. 4.11 Muscle fibre atrophy in spinal muscular atrophy (Werdnig–Hoffmann disease). Note large groups of atrophic fibres (haematoxylin and eosin).

... small, angular fibers can derive from fiber splitting, which can be the result of either a chronic myopathy, denervation, or tenotomy. Small groups of atrophic fibers can result from splitting or regeneration after necrosis. The changes described as characteristic of myopathy have been reported in biopsies from muscles affected by chronic denervation.   (Brådley *et al.* 1978)

In polymyositis there can also be muscle fibre necrosis and regeneration, but the distinctive pathological feature in this disorder is the infiltration of muscle tissue by inflammatory cells (mainly lymphocytes and plasma cells). This is usually focal and occurs in connective tissue, around blood vessels and within muscle fibres; a reaction which is not seen in Duchenne muscular dystrophy or cases of spinal muscular atrophy occurring in childhood. However, as Schmalbruch (1982) has emphasized, the distinction between groups of phagocytes engaged in phagocytosis, and perivascular infiltrates of lymphocytes and plasma cells is not always clear. Furthermore, in childhood polymyositis/dermatomyositis muscle histology may show only minimal changes or practically no significant changes at all. For this reason some advocate open biopsy in suspected polymyositis to ensure that as much tissue as possible can be examined. Dubowitz (1985) in fact suggests that in a suspected case of polymyositis in whom the muscle histology appears normal, a trial of therapy with steroids is advised because a positive response would be diagnostic, and also delay in treating this condition can seriously influence the prognosis.

Muscle histochemistry

On the basis of physiological experiments in animals, and biochemical and histochemical studies on muscle tissue, it is possible to classify human skeletal muscle fibres into three distinct types which are designated as 1, 2A,

Table 4.4 *Some characteristics of various fibre types in human skeletal muscle*

	Type 1	Type 2A	Type 2B
Speed of contraction	Slow	Intermediate	Fast
Appearance			
(myoglobin content)	Dark	Dark	Pale
Size	Small	Intermediate	Large
Enzyme activities			
1. ATPase pH 9.4	+	+ + +	+ + +
2. ATPase pH 4.3	+ + +	+	+
3. Oxidative*	+ + +	+ +	+
4. Phosphorylase	+	+ +	+ + +

* NADH-tetrazolium reductase, succinic dehydrogenase.

and 2B (Brooke and Kaiser 1970). Some of the differences between these fibre types are summarized in Table 4.4.

Animal experiments have shown that muscle fibres innervated by a single motor neurone possess similar physiological properties and identical histochemical characteristics. Thus there would appear to be at least three types of motor neurones. Figure 4.12 shows the effects of denervation as it occurs in spinal muscular atrophy. If this is rapidly progressive there may be little time for reinnervation. However, if reinnervation occurs, from nerve fibres from another neurone, this will lead eventually to groups of atrophic fibres being of the same histochemical type.

The appearance of fibre type atrophy in a case of Werdnig–Hoffmann disease is given in Fig. 4.13 in which type 2 fibres are predominantly affected.

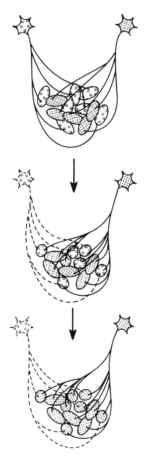

Fig. 4.12 Diagrammatic representation of the possible effects of denervation followed by reinnervation. For simplicity only two types of fibres are illustrated.

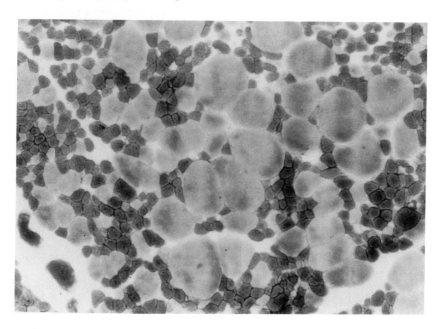

Fig. 4.13 Fibre type atrophy in a case of Werdnig–Hoffmann disease (ATPase pH 9.4).

However, both fibre types can atrophy after denervation though most larger fibres tend to be of type 1. In muscular dystrophy and polymyositis no particular fibre type is predominantly affected and there is no grouping of fibre types (Brumback and Leech 1984).

The reason why certain groups of muscles are especially affected early in the course of muscular dystrophy (p. 31) is not at all clear. This presumably reflects some difference in their biochemical/physiological properties compared with muscles affected to a lesser degree and only in the later stages of the disease. Johnson *et al.* (1973) approached this problem by considering the proportions of type 1 and type 2 fibres in normal skeletal muscles which in Duchenne muscular dystrophy are either severely affected or relatively unaffected. They found that there was a tendency for the proportion of type 2 fibres to be higher in muscles which are more *severely* affected, but there was no simple correlation between fibre type composition of individual muscles and their being affected or spared in the disease. Using their extensive data, there would also appear to be a slight excess of type 2 (or deficiency of type 1) fibres in those muscles affected *early* in the disease, but there is considerable variation, and the difference from those muscles affected later in the course of the disease is not statistically significant (Table 4.5). What-

Table 4.5 *Mean proportion (%) of type 1 and type 2 fibres in various normal human muscles (Johnson* et al. *1973) divided into those muscles clinically affected early or late in the course of Duchenne muscular dystrophy*

		Type 1	Type 2
Affected early			
Sternomastoid		35.2	64.8
Pectoralis major			
(sterno-costal)		43.1	56.9
Triceps			
(surface)		32.5	67.5
(deep)		32.7	67.3
Brachioradialis		39.8	60.2
Extensor digitorum		47.3	52.7
Extensor digitorum brevis		45.3	54.7
Latissimus dorsi		50.5	49.5
Iliopsoas		49.2	50.8
Gluteus maximus		52.4	47.6
Vastus medialis			
(surface)		43.7	56.3
(deep)		61.5	38.5
Rectus femoris			
(lat. head surface)		29.5	70.5
(lat. head deep)		42.0	58.0
(medial head)		42.8	57.2
Tibialis anterior			
(surface)		73.4	26.6
(deep)		72.7	27.3
	Mean	46.68	53.32
	s.d.	—	12.74
Affected later			
Trapezius		53.7	46.3
Pectoralis major			
(clavicular)		42.3	57.7
Biceps brachii			
(surface)		42.3	57.7
(deep)		50.5	49.5
Biceps femoris		66.9	33.1
Flexor digitorum brevis		44.5	55.5
Flexor digitorum profundis		47.3	52.7
Gastrocnemius			
(lat. head surface)		43.5	56.5
(lat. head deep)		50.3	49.7
(medial head)		50.8	49.2
Soleus			
(surface)		86.4	13.6
(deep)		89.0	11.0
	Mean	55.63	44.37
	s.d.	—	16.42

ever may be responsible for the differential involvement of muscles in Duchenne muscular dystrophy, this is not a simple matter of histochemical fibre type.

Muscle innervation

A most useful technique for diagnosing neurogenic atrophy is the intra-vital or supravital staining of motor nerve filaments and end-plates with methylene blue (Coërs and Woolf 1959). The motor end-plate is a complex structure at the site where excitation is transmitted from the motor nerve to the muscle fibre (Fig. 4.14).

In spinal muscular atrophy there is branching of subterminal intra-muscular nerve fibres (Fig. 4.15) with collateral reinnervation, and degeneration of motor end-plates (Pearce and Harriman 1966; Hausmanowa-Petrusewicz *et al.* 1968*a*).

Branching of nerve fibres in this way is found in all forms of spinal muscular atrophy, but is very rarely seen in normal or dystrophic muscle.

Electronmicroscopy

Electronmicroscopy of muscle has provided details of the ultrastructural changes which take place in muscular dystrophy and spinal muscular atrophy (Mair and Tomé 1972; Cullen *et al.* 1988). In Duchenne muscular dystrophy these changes include distention of the sarcoplasmic reticulum, Z band degeneration ('streaming') and disruption and loss of myofilaments, followed later by complete disarray of the band structure (Fig. 4.16). These

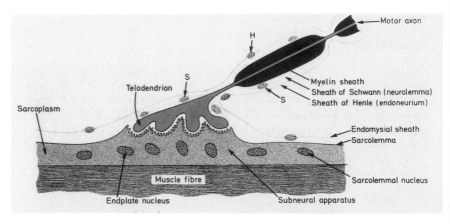

Fig. 4.14 The structure of the normal human motor end-plate. (H, nucleus of sheath of Henle; S, nucleus of sheath of Schwann.)

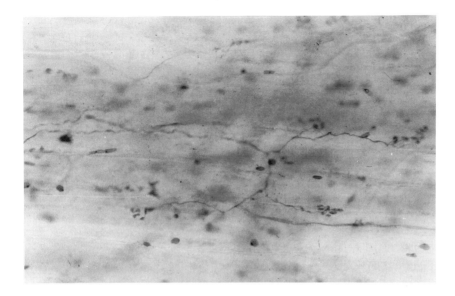

Fig. 4.15 Branching of subterminal intramuscular nerve fibres in a case of Wohlfart–Kugelberg–Welander spinal muscular atrophy (supravital staining with methylene blue).

changes however are not specific to Duchenne muscular dystrophy but occur in other forms of dystrophy. Various alterations in the sarcolemma have also been described early in the course of the disease (Cullen and Mastaglia 1980; Carpenter and Karpati 1984), and include defects in the plasma membrane and reduplication of the basement membrane.

DNA and dystrophin studies

The approach to the diagnosis of Duchenne and Becker muscular dystrophies has been revolutionized by the introduction of gene markers and dystrophin studies. It is now arguable whether there is a place for any diagnostic investigations other than a serum creatine kinase test (Zatz *et al.* 1991*a*) (because of its simplicity, cheapness, and relative specificity), and DNA and dystrophin studies. In fact DNA analysis is now essential for the diagnosis of muscle disease (Rowland 1988; Hoffman 1991).

DNA studies on peripheral blood

As will be discussed in greater detail later, the gene locus for Duchenne and Becker muscular dystrophies has been located on the short arm of the X

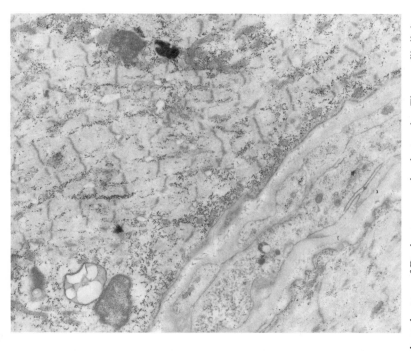

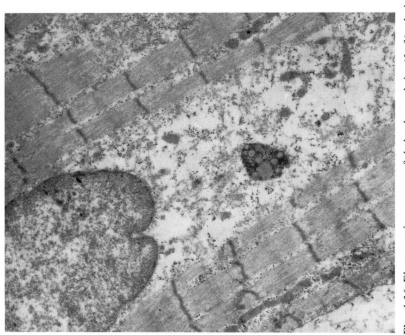

Fig. 4.16 Electronmiscroscopy of skeletal muscle in: (*Left*) relatively early stage of Duchenne muscular dystrophy. The myofibrils have lost some myofilaments with widening of the intermyofibrillar space which contains a lysosome (phosphotungstic acid × 14 000). (*Right*) later stage showing disorganization of the band structure (2% uranyl acetate and lead citrate × 7000). (Reproduced by kind permission of Dr J. Trevor Hughes and Lloyd-Luke, publishers.)

chromosome (at Xp21). So-called restriction fragment length polymorphisms (RFLPs) are available which are close to the gene (extragenic) or
actually within the gene (intragenic). In affected families such linked RFLPs
can be used for diagnosis using DNA obtained from peripheral blood
samples (p. 175). Unfortunately because the gene is so large (2400 kilobases)
not unexpectedly markers even within the gene may show recombination
(cross-over) with a particular mutation and could therefore lead to
misdiagnosis.

It has been shown, for example, that polymorphic markers which lie at the
two extremities of the dystrophin locus show a recombination frequency of
0.12 or 12 per cent (Abbs *et al*. 1990). Using extragenic markers the error rate
can be even greater. This has therefore to be taken into account when using
linked markers for diagnosis and the use of informative *flanking* markers is
therefore recommended (p. 178, 234).

Another approach, which does not require other affected members in the
family in order to determine the so-called phase (p. 229) of a DNA marker,
is to use a gene specific (cDNA) probe. By using such a probe(s) it is possible
to determine if there is a gene *deletion* or *duplication* at Xp21. Roughly 70
per cent of cases have a deletion or a duplication which can be detected on
a Southern blot in this way or by the simpler and quicker method of blot
hybridization (Konno *et al*. 1989).

An interesting finding is that deletions tend to be clustered around two
'hot-spot' regions (Fig. 4.17). Thus the majority of deletions can be detected
by examining only a subset of exons within the gene. This is possible using
a method developed by Chamberlain *et al*. (1988). This is referred to as the
'multiplex method' in which a number of regions (which are deletion susceptible) are simultaneously analysed by amplifying these regions using the
polymerase chain reaction (PCR). Details of this important technique,
particularly in regard to Duchenne muscular dystrophy, have been reviewed
by Chamberlain *et al*. (1991). It involves amplifying very small amounts of
DNA such that eventually there is sufficient to visualize on a gel by
fluorescence when stained with ethidium bromide. Particular regions of the
DNA (in this case exonic regions most likely to be deleted) are amplified by
PCR using primers which specifically flank these regions. The results of the
multiplex method are shown in Figure 4.18.

Thus in family 1 the affected boy (B) has a deletion of exon *f* (as does a
fetus (F) at risk in the same family); in family 2 the deletion is more extensive
and involves exons *a–e* inclusive; in family 3 there is a deletion of exon *a*
only. This is an extremely rapid method for screening for deletions and by
using two mixtures of primers, each of which amplifies nine exons, over 98
per cent of detectable deletions can be identified in this way (Beggs and
Kunkel 1990; Abbs *et al*. 1991).

In a recent multicentre study involving no less than 745 unrelated patients

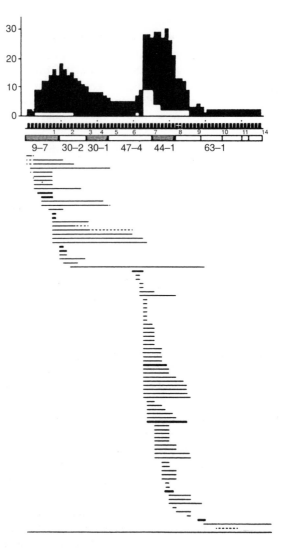

Fig. 4.17 Distribution and extent of gene deletions and duplications in Duchenne (solid) and Becker (open) muscular dystrophies. (Reproduced by kind permission of Dr E. Bakker, from *Genetics of neuromuscular disorders*, (ed. C. S. Bartsocas). Copyright © 1989 Wiley-Liss, a division of John Wiley and Sons, Inc.)

with Duchenne or Becker muscular dystrophy, multiplex PCR gave accurate results in all but one of the cases examined (Chamberlain *et al.* 1992). As the authors conclude, multiplex PCR is a reliable and accurate method for detecting deletions. It requires only one day for analysis, with experience is

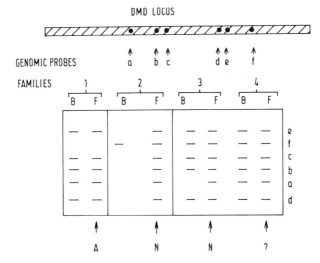

Fig. 4.18 Diagram of the results of the multiplex method used to simultaneously detect deletions in exons *a–f* in four families. (B, boy; F, fetus; A, affected; N, normal.)

easy to perform and, unlike Southern blot analysis, does not require radio-active probes. The method of course cannot be used unless the patient being tested is related to an individual already known to carry a deletion detectable by the system. If, as in family 4 in Figure 4.18, there is no detectable deletion with this method then resort has to be made to Southern blot analysis with full length cDNA probes. But in roughly 30 per cent of cases even with this detailed analysis no deletion or duplication can be found, and in these cases the cause is a point mutation within the promoter region of the dystrophin gene or more likely within the gene itself. Roberts and colleagues (1992) have developed an ingenious technique for detecting such point mutations within the gene. The method is complicated but essentially involves preparing total RNA from peripheral blood lymphocytes which is then reverse-transcribed to cDNA and the relevant region corresponding to the Duchenne locus is amplified by PCR (Roberts *et al.* 1991). The products are hybridized with normal cDNA and any mismatches identified from chemical modification of mismatched residues.

Thus by these various methods it is possible to detect deletions, duplications, and point mutations in the dystrophin gene and thus make a precise molecular diagnosis of both Duchenne and Becker muscular dystrophies. These methods also make carrier detection and prenatal diagnosis possible as will be discussed later.

Dystrophin studies on muscle biopsy material

The diagnosis of Xp21 myopathies, as Duchenne, Becker, and related muscle diseases are sometimes referred to, can also be established on the basis of studies of the gene product (dystrophin) in muscle biopsies. This is possible either by Western blot analysis or immunohistochemistry. The former involves separating proteins from a muscle extract on one-dimensional electrophoresis which is then 'blot probed' with various monoclonal antibodies to dystrophin. Using molecular weight markers, any difference from normal dystrophin (molecular weight 427 kDa) can be noted and the amount present semiquantified (Ho-Kim *et al.* 1991).

The results of such studies using various antibodies reveal a complete absence or only trace amounts of dystrophin in Duchenne muscular dystrophy. In Becker muscular dystrophy on the other hand, dystrophin is present but in reduced amounts. Furthermore, in the latter disorder the dystrophin molecule is often of abnormal size, usually with a reduced molecular weight but occasionally with an increased molecular weight (Nicholson *et al*, 1989*a*,1990; Voit *et al.* 1991*a*).

Immunohistochemistry of cryostat sections of muscle provides another way of studying muscle dystrophin. In this method monoclonal antibodies to various parts of the dystrophin molecule (for example, the N-terminal region, central rod region, and C-terminal region of the molecule) are raised in an appropriate animal and then labelled with a suitable marker (for example, peroxidase or fluorescent marker). This technique has revealed that in normal muscle, dystrophin is located close to the sarcolemma, and ultrastructural studies indicate that it forms a lattice-like network adjacent to the membrane (Cullen *et al.* 1991). The appearance on cryostat sections is shown in Figure 4.19. This illustrates that in normal muscle, dystrophin is clearly localized at the periphery of muscle fibres. In Duchenne muscular dystrophy however, the majority of fibres *fail to show any staining at all*. These observations were first made in 1988 by Sugita and by Zubrzycka-Gaarn and their colleagues and have since been confirmed by many others. In Becker muscular dystrophy most fibres do show some staining but this varies in intensity both between and within fibres (Nicholson *et al.* 1989*b*,1990; Vainzof *et al.* 1990; Slater and Nicholson 1991).

However, though most fibres in Duchenne muscular dystrophy show no staining at all, occasional fibres may show some labelling around the periphery (Fanin *et al.* 1992). These positive fibres usually occur singularly but may be arranged in clusters, and are found in both familial and non-familial cases. Furthermore, using a panel of antibodies which span the entire dystrophin molecule, in patients with deletions the positive fibres only stain with antibodies raised to polypeptide sequences outside the deletion and not those within the deletion. These dystrophin-positive fibres are

Normal   BMD

DMD   DMD

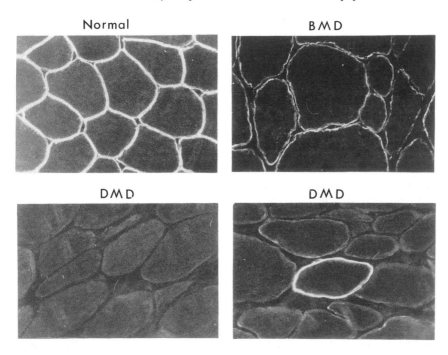

Fig. 4.19 Cryostat sections of muscle from a control and from patients with Duchenne muscular dystrophy (DMD) and Becker muscular dystrophy (BMD) labelled with anti-dystrophin monoclonal antibody using a fluorescent marker. (Reproduced by kind permission of Dr Louise Nicholson and *The Journal of the Neurological Sciences.*)

therefore most likely to be due a second site in-frame mutation which restores the reading frame (Klein *et al.* 1992). If the mutation occurred in a particular myoblast which was approaching its terminal division, so that its resultant daughter cells which ultimately unite to form a single multinucleate muscle fibre would all carry this second mutation, this would result in an *isolated* positive fibre. By the same token an occasional negative fibre might be expected in normal muscle. On the other hand, if such a mutation occurred a little earlier in myoblast development then this would account for occasional clustering of positive fibres. But whatever the mechanism, the ocurrence of occasional dystrophin-positive fibres under normal conditions in Duchenne muscular dystrophy must be taken into account in assessing any possible beneficial effects of, say, myoblast transfer (p. 290).

A protein similar to dystrophin and referred to as dystrophin-like protein ('utrophin') has been identified and is synthesized by a gene on chromosome 6 (Love *et al.* 1989). This protein is concentrated in the region of neuromuscular junctions (Fardeau *et al*. 1990), myotendinous junctions, peripheral nerves, and vasculature of skeletal muscle as well as the sarcolemma (Khurana *et al*. 1991). However, unlike dystrophin, this protein is expressed in normal abundance, size, and distribution in Duchenne and Becker muscular dystrophies and therefore would seem unlikely to play a significant role in the pathogenesis of these disorders. It is apparently normal, as is dystrophin, in autosomal recessive muscular dystrophy of childhood (p. 91).

From a practical point of view it is important that antibodies to dystrophin used for diagnostic purposes *must* be very carefully characterized and cross reaction to dystrophin-like protein(s) excluded (Voit *et al*. 1991*a*).

In summarizing this section on dystrophin, the use of Western blot and immunohistochemistry on muscle tissue are important techniques for diagnosing a suspected case of Xp21 myopathy. In general, these two techniques complement each other (Nicholson *et al*. 1989*b*; Voit *et al*. 1991*b*). If the size and abundance of dystrophin on Western blot and its distribution on immunohistochemistry are normal, then this excludes an Xp21 myopathy. A young patient with significant weakness and a muscle biopsy consistent with muscular dystrophy but *normal* dystrophin is very likely to have autosomal recessive muscular dystrophy of childhood.

The results of these investigations can also provide valuable information of *prognostic* value. According to Beggs and Kunkel (1990) the probability of Duchenne muscular dystrophy exceeds 99 per cent if there is a com-

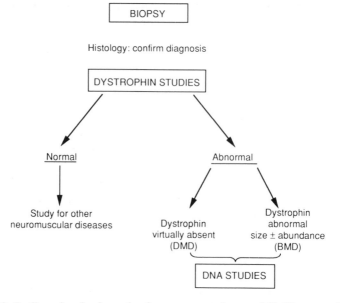

Fig. 4.20 Outline plan for investigating a suspected case of Xp21 myopathy.

plete absence of dystrophin, whereas the probability of Becker muscular dystrophy exceeds 95 per cent if dystrophin is present but of abnormal size (larger or smaller) and/or reduced abundance. Patients with less than 20 per cent of normal levels of dystrophin tend to have an intermediate phenotype, becoming wheelchair-bound between the ages of 13 and 20 years. Dystrophin of reduced size has also been reported in a case of very mild, late onset dystrophy as well as in a boy with myoglobinuria in the same family (Lucci *et al.* 1990). Also, a smaller than normal dystrophin (due to a single in-frame exon deletion) has even been reported in a healthy individual (Nordenskjöld *et al.* 1990). Such an abnormality may, in fact, not be infrequent among those who are very mildly affected or even asymptomatic (Beggs *et al.* 1991), thus widening the spectrum of expression of defects at Xp21 (p. 185).

The use of dystrophin studies in assessing prognosis and in differential diagnosis will be discussed in more detail in Chapter 5. An outline plan for investigating a suspected case of Xp21 myopathy is summarized in Figure 4.20.

Other investigations

The diagnosis of Duchenne muscular dystrophy can be established in all cases on the basis of the clinical findings, SCK level, EMG examination, and muscle biopsy for histology and dystrophin studies. However, additional investigations may be useful in helping to differentiate the disorder from other conditions. Thus nerve conduction studies will be important if a neuropathy is suspected since this will be associated with a reduced nerve conduction velocity. Electrocardiography (p. 111) may help to distinguish between autosomal recessive and X-linked recessive forms of childhood dystrophy (Skyring and McKusick 1961; Emery 1972).

Ultrasound (Heckmatt *et al.* 1982) and computed tomography (CT scanning) (Kawai *et al.* 1985; Heckmatt *et al.* 1989), have been used to demonstrate and localize muscle loss by showing areas of changed density (Fig. 4.21). They have the advantage of being non-invasive, and CT scanning seems sufficiently sensitive to detect significant abnormalities in a proportion of carriers (Rott and Rödl 1985; Stern *et al.* 1985; de Visser and Verbeeten 1985*a*, *b*). It also offers a method of assessing inaccessible muscles such as the psoas and erector spinae (Smith *et al.* 1986). These techniques, however, are unlikely to replace more conventional methods of establishing a diagnosis of muscular dystrophy.

Summary and conclusions

In the case of an otherwise healthy little boy who presents with evidence of proximal limb girdle muscle weakness and who has a grossly elevated SCK

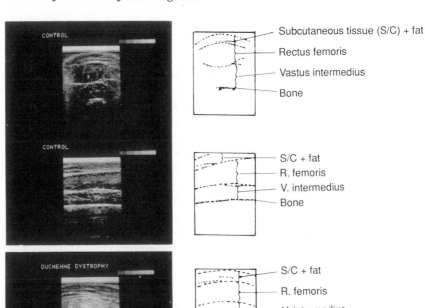

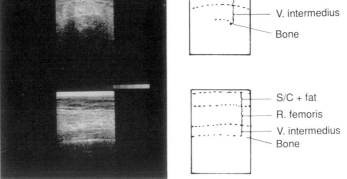

Fig. 4.21 Ultrasonogram of transverse (*above*) and longitudinal (*below*) sections of the thigh in a 7-year-old healthy boy and a boy with Duchenne muscular dystrophy of the same age. In the latter there is increased echogenicity throughout all the muscles. (Reproduced by kind permission of Dr Adnan Manzur and Professor Victor Dubowitz.)

level (50–100 times normal), the diagnosis of Duchenne muscular dystrophy is almost certain. However, because of the importance of not missing poly-myositis which is treatable, and the need to exclude other disorders which can be inherited differently, electromyography, and certainly a muscle biopsy, is indicated in all cases. This is best carried out using a biopsy needle under local anaesthesia. The characteristic features of muscle histology are necrosis and phagocytosis of scattered individual muscle fibres in muscular dystrophy, muscle fibre group atrophy in spinal muscular atrophy, and infiltration with inflammatory cells (mainly lymphocytes and plasma cells) in polymyositis.

A significant feature of Duchenne muscular dystrophy is the presence of prominent, rounded fibres which stain densely with eosin, so-called eosinophilic fibres, which contain increased intracellular calcium.

Other investigations, such as muscle histochemistry, motor end-plate and muscle innervation studies, electronmicroscopy, electrocardiography, and computed tomography can all provide useful additional information. But a definitive diagnosis of Duchenne muscular dystrophy can only be made by demonstrating a significant defect in the dystrophin gene and a virtual absence of muscle dystrophin. The *essential* laboratory investigations are therefore a serum creatine kinase estimation and muscle histology (to establish the diagnosis of muscular dystrophy), and DNA and muscle dystrophin studies (to establish the specific diagnosis of Duchenne muscular dystrophy).

5 Differential diagnosis

Disorders which could possibly be confused with Duchenne muscular dystrophy include polymyositis, which must always be considered because it is treatable, other forms of muscular dystrophy which may present in early childhood, various congenital myopathies, and spinal muscular atrophy.

The congenital muscular dystrophies

This is a relatively ill-defined group of disorders which is clearly very heterogeneous. In all cases the disorder is evident at birth or in the neonatal period, with hypotonia and muscle weakness (Fig. 3.1, p. 26). The muscle weakness is generalized and may affect the face but never the extraocular muscles. Tendon reflexes are usually reduced and joint contractures may be present at birth or develop later in childhood. Intelligence is usually unimpaired and the disorder is inherited as an autosomal recessive trait (Topaloglu *et al.* 1989). In some instances progression is rapid and death occurs in infancy or early childhood. In other cases the disease is either non-progressive or only slowly progressive. However, the distinction between severe and benign forms may not be entirely justified, and it is often difficult to predict at the time the diagnosis is first made what the ultimate prognosis may be (McMenamin *et al.* 1982). Congenital muscular dystrophy, including the Fukuyama type, is commoner in Japan than elsewhere (Nakagawa *et al.* 1991).

Relatively slowly progressive forms of congenital muscular dystrophy have been described in association with infantile cataracts and hypogonadism (Bassöe 1956), CNS malformations (Kamoshita *et al.* 1976), congenital heart disease (Lebenthal *et al.* 1970), and certain dysmorphic features associated with hyperhidrosis and recurrent upper respiratory tract infections (Furukawa and Toyokura 1977). Since some of these associations have been described in multiple affected sibs, they may well represent different rare autosomal recessive forms of congenital muscular dystrophy. Lewis and Besant (1962) have also described a rapidly progressive form of the disease in sibs in which the dystrophic process was almost entirely limited to the diaphragm.

The SCK level in congenital muscular dystrophy may occasionally be comparable to levels found in Duchenne muscular dystrophy (Donner *et al.* 1975; Topaloglu *et al.* 1989). But why in many cases the SCK level is normal or only slightly elevated yet the muscle histology appears to be no different from other cases of congenital muscular dystrophy and Duchenne muscular dystrophy in which the SCK level is grossly elevated, is not at all clear.

The Fukuyama type of congenital muscular dystrophy merits special mention because of its relatively high birth incidence in Japan of 6.9–11.9 × 10^{-5} (Fukuyama *et al.* 1960, 1981). It differs from Duchenne muscular dystrophy because hypotonia and weakness date from birth or early infancy, patients never walk well, and mental retardation is profound. This condition is inherited as an autosomal recessive trait, and yet in 3 of 23 affected males a deficiency of muscle dystrophin has been found by Beggs and colleagues (1992). These investigators consider the most likely explanation is that these cases are heterozygous for Fukuyama dystrophy as well as hemizygous for Duchenne dystrophy (one did have a deletion in the Xp21 locus).

Congenital myopathies

In recent years useful reviews of this heterogeneous group of disorders have been given by Heckmatt and Dubowitz (1990), Bundey (1992), and Baraitser (1985), who consider their differential diagnosis in detail and provide extensive bibliographies. Some of the more important types are listed in Table 5.1.

None of these myopathies however is likely to be confused with a case of Duchenne muscular dystrophy because most, but not all, present at birth or in the neonatal period with hypotonia and generalized muscle weakness, often associated with respiratory problems and feeding difficulties. Facial features may be dysmorphic (nemaline myopathy, myotubular myopathy), and marked fatiguability (mitochondrial myopathy), or muscle cramps

Table 5.1 *Some defined congenital myopathies and their suggested modes of inheritance*

	AR	AD	XR
Central core disease		+	
Nemaline myopathy	+	+	
Centronuclear myopathy	+	+	+
Minicore (multicore) disease	+		
Congenital fibre type disproportion	+	+	
Mitochondrial myopathies	Mt		
Kearn–Sayre syndrome	Mt		
Muscle carnitine deficiency	Mt		
Carnitine palmityltransferase deficiency	Mt		
Muscle glycogenoses (II, III, IV, V, VII)	+		

AR, autosomal recessive; AD, autosomal dominant; XR, X-linked recessive; Mt, mitochondrial.

(glycogenoses, carnitine palmityltransferase deficiency) may be important features. Serum enzyme levels are usually normal and a specific diagnosis is based on muscle histology with special stains or electronmicroscopy.

Centronuclear (myotubular) mycopathy derives its name from the preponderance of centrally placed nuclei in muscle tissue. The X-linked form of the disease, the locus for which is at Xq28 (Liechti-Gallati *et al.* 1991), is unlikely to be confused with the X-linked forms of dystrophy because there is severe generalized hypotonia and muscle weakness from birth, and affected boys rarely survive early childhood because of respiratory failure. There appears to be a defect in cytoskeletal proteins but not in dystrophin (van der Ven *et al.* 1991).

Other X-linked muscular dystrophies

Over the years several other X-linked muscular dystrophies have been recognized, all relatively more benign than Duchenne muscular dystrophy. The commonest of these is Becker muscular dystrophy which occasionally presents in childhood when it can then be confused with Duchenne muscular dystrophy.

Becker type muscular dystrophy

This disease was first clearly delineated by Becker some thirty years ago (Becker and Kiener 1955; Becker 1962) since when there have been many reports of affected families. The condition has been extensively reviewed by Rotthauwe and Kowalewski (1966), Zellweger and Hanson (1967*a*), Heyck and Laudahn (1969), Shaw and Dreifuss (1969), Markand *et al.* (1969), Conomy (1970), and more recently by Emery and Skinner (1976), Ringel *et al.* (1977), Bradley *et al.* (1978), and Bushby and Gardner-Medwin (1992). In contrast to Duchenne muscular dystrophy, Becker muscular dystrophy displays a wide range of clinical expression. Such variation often occurs within the same family, the cause of which is unknown, though one possibility may be the occasional association with Klinefelter's syndrome (Suthers *et al.* 1989). It is less common than Duchenne muscular dystrophy (Mostacciuolo *et al.* 1987), but using cDNA probes and dystrophin studies in non-familial cases suspected of having the disease as well as in familial cases, the birth incidence is at least 54×10^{-6}, indicating that the disorder is more common than previously thought (Bushby *et al.* 1991*a*).

The distribution of muscle wasting and weakness is very similar to Duchenne muscular dystrophy and like this latter disorder the hip flexors and quadriceps muscles tend to be affected early in the lower limbs, while in the upper limbs the serrati, pectoralis, biceps, brachioradialis, and triceps muscles are usually affected first (Fig. 5.1).

Although weakness almost always begins in the lower limbs, eventually the

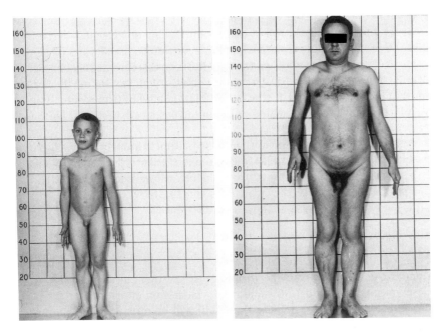

Fig. 5.1 A 6-year-old boy with preclinical Becker muscular dystrophy (note the enlarged calves) and his affected 26-year-old uncle.

upper limb musculature becomes affected. Calf enlargement is invariably present and contractures are a late development. Cardiac involvement, if it occurs, is usually a late manifestation, although not always (Kuhn *et al.* 1979; Lazzeroni *et al.* 1989). A proportion, as yet not precisely determined, have some impairment of intellect (Bushby and Gardner-Medwin 1992). The SCK level is substantially raised, especially in the early stages and gradually falls as the disease progresses. In the preclinical stage of the disease, which may last 10 years or more, when the only abnormality is calf enlargement and there is no apparent muscle weakness, the SCK level is grossly elevated to levels comparable to those found in boys with Duchenne muscular dystrophy of the same age but who are clinically affected. Why in Becker muscular dystrophy there should be this lag period before the onset of muscle weakness remains unexplained.

In Duchenne muscular dystrophy SCK levels are maximal between 1–6 years and thereafter decline by 0.18 units per year, compared with Becker muscular dystrophy where SKC levels are maximal between 10–15 years and thereafter decline by 0.06 units per year, changes which reflect different rates of muscle degeneration in the two diseases (Zatz *et al.* 1991*a*).

Because of the very high SCK levels early in the course of Becker muscular dystrophy and overlap in age in onset with Duchenne muscular dystrophy, this can present a diagnostic dilemma in an isolated case. Points of clinical value in distinguishing between the two disorders are revealed by comparing details of the course of the disease in the two disorders. Excluding index cases (probands) the course of the disease in 10 large families (Emery and Skinner 1976) has been compared with the findings in cases of established Duchenne muscular dystrophy.

Penrose (1951) has shown that if two approximately normal curves overlap the point of overlap (x), measured in standard deviation units from either mean, can be determined from the means (m_1 and m_2) and standard deviations (s_1 and s_2) of the two curves (Fig. 5.2):

$$x = \frac{m_1 - m_2}{s_1 + s_2}$$

Thus, if the point where two curves overlapped corresponded to 1.96 standard deviations from the means of either then, since 95 per cent of observations lie within 1.96 standard deviations on either side of the mean of a normal curve, 2.5 per cent (one-tail) will lie outside and therefore be misclassified.

By calculating the point of overlap (x) in terms of the number of standard deviations from the mean, it is possible to determine the percentage misclassification from appropriate tables of the normal probability integral (Fisher and Yates 1967). When this is applied to data for Duchenne and Becker types of muscular dystrophy, the value of x and the percentage misclassification (in parentheses) for age at onset is 1.182 (11.9 per cent), for age at becoming chairbound is 1.753 (4.0 per cent), and for age at death is 1.533

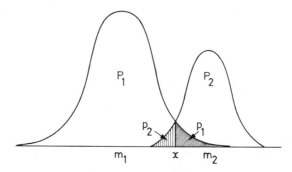

Fig. 5.2 Method for calculating the point of overlap in two normally distributed curves. The point of overlap (x) is such that $p_1/P_1 = p_2/P_2$. (From Emery (1986) with permission.)

(6.3 per cent). Thus in (100–11.9) or 88.1 per cent of boys with Duchenne muscular dystrophy onset is before the age of 3.3 + (1.182) (1.7) or 5.3 years, whereas in 88.1 per cent of males with Becker muscular dystrophy, symptoms develop *after* the age of 5.3 years. Similarly, (100–4.0) or 96.0 per cent of boys with Duchenne muscular dystrophy become chairbound before the age of 9.4 + (1.753) (1.7) or 12.4 years, whereas 96.0 per cent of males with Becker muscular dystrophy become chairbound *after* the age of 12.4 years. Finally, (100–6.3) or 93.7 per cent of boys with Duchenne muscular dystrophy die before the age of 16.3 + (1.533) (3.1) or 21.1 years, whereas 93.7 per cent of males with Becker muscular dystrophy die *after* the age of 21.1 years (Table 5.2). These calculations however are based on familial cases of Becker muscular dystrophy who might be expected, on average, to be less severely affected than some sporadic cases. Reproductive fitness in familial cases has been estimated to be 0.67 (Emery and Skinner 1976) compared with 0.82 in sporadic cases (Bushy and Gardiner-Medwin 1992).

The two disorders are best distinguished on the age at becoming confined to a wheelchair, and further help may be afforded by electrocardiography. Whereas there is electrocardiographic evidence of right ventricular preponderance in most boys with Duchenne muscular dystrophy (*see* p. 111) we have found no significant difference in the algebraic sum of $|R-S|$ in V_1 between 102 healthy males and 19 males with Becker muscular dystrophy (Emery and Skinner 1976). Thus, if an affected boy with no family history is still walking at the age of 12 and there is also no electrocardiographic evidence of right ventricular preponderance (but see p. 114), he is more likely to have Becker muscular dystrophy than Duchenne muscular dystrophy, and the prognosis is therefore much better.

If other relatives are affected, then usually the diagnosis will be easier to make. But manifesting female carriers in a family of X-linked Becker muscular dystrophy may give the appearance of dominant inheritance which could then cause some confusion in establishing a diagnosis (Aguilar *et al.* 1978) but this appears to be an uncommon occurrence. Although usually inherited as an autosomal recessive trait, limb girdle muscular dystrophy of adult onset may occasionally be inherited as an autosomal dominant trait, and in some such families can sometimes be limited to males. However, this latter form of muscular dystrophy is unlikely to prove a serious diagnostic problem because it appears to be very rare, having so far been described in only three families (De Coster *et al.* 1974; Hastings *et al.* 1980). Autosomal recessive limb girdle muscular dystrophy of adult onset however is not uncommon and is clinically indistinguishable from Becker muscular dsytrophy (Passos-Bueno *et al.* 1991). However the two disorders can be differentiated by muscle dystrophin and dystrophin cDNA probes which reveal abnormalities only in Becker dystrophy (Norman *et al.* 1989*a*).

Table 5.2 *Clinical course in Duchenne and Becker types of muscular dystrophy*

	Onset			Chairbound			Death		
	No.	Mean age (yrs)	s.d.	No.	Mean age (yrs)	s.d.	No.	Mean age (yrs)	s.d.
Duchenne	144	3.3	1.7	120	9.4	1.7	129	16.3	3.1
Becker	27	11.1	4.9	9	27.1	8.4	10	42.2	13.8
P		$P < 0.001$			$P < 0.001$			$P < 0.001$	
'χ'		1.182			1.753			1.533	
Misclassification (%)		11.9			4.0			6.3	

Apparent Duchenne and Becker muscular dystrophies in the same family

For many years a distinction between Duchenne and more benign X-linked forms of muscular dystrophy was questioned. It was really only when several large families were described in which all affected males had a consistently benign disease did the concept become accepted. Nevertheless, there have been occasional reports in recent years in which cases of presumed Duchenne and Becker muscular dystrophy occurred in the same family (Robert and Vignon 1972; Jackson *et al.* 1974; Furukawa and Peter 1977; Hausmanowa-Petrusewicz and Borkowska 1978; Gardner-Medwin 1982*b*; Spiegler *et al.* 1987). Since there is considerable clinical variation in both these disorders it is perhaps to be expected that occasional families may be found in which affected males at opposite ends of the spectrum of severity may occur.

Perhaps it is more helpful to consider that we are in fact dealing with a *spectrum of disability* with Duchenne muscular dystrophy at one end of the spectrum, through so-called 'outliers' to frank Becker muscular dystrophy, and eventually very mild disease and even normality (p. 185). Such a spectrum would reflect different types of mutation at the Xp21 locus, their effects on dystrophin synthesis and the cellular concentration of any truncated protein, together with the possible interplay of other (? autosomal) genes and perhaps environmental factors.

Dystrophin in Becker muscular dystrophy

In 1988, Monaco and colleagues proposed that the milder Becker muscular dystrophy resulted from mutations at Xp21 which maintained the translational reading frame (in-frame mutations), resulting in an abnormal, but partially functional dystrophin, whereas in Duchenne muscular dystrophy the mutations shifted the reading frame (frame-shift mutations) so that virtually no dystrophin was produced (Monaco *et al.* 1988). This 'reading frame' hypothesis holds up in 90 per cent of cases and is of diagnostic and prognostic significance (Gillard *et al.* 1989; Koenig *et al.* 1989)

These molecular approaches to diagnosis and prognosis will become increasingly refined with time. Meanwhile an approach involving muscle immunohistochemistry can also provide valuable information. We have seen already that with this technique, as well as Western blotting, in Duchenne muscular dystrophy there is a virtual absence of dystrophin whereas in Becker muscular dystrophy dystrophin is present but of abnormal size and/or abundance (p. 74).

A further refinement is the use of antibodies *specific* to the C- (carboxy-) terminal region of dystrophin. Using such antibodies, immunohistochemistry reveals that the C-terminal region is almost always absent in Duchenne but invariably present in Becker muscular dystrophy (Arahata *et al.* 1991), a finding also confirmed by Western blotting (Bulman *et al.* 1991). Thus when this region of the molecule is missing, a more severe phenotype is

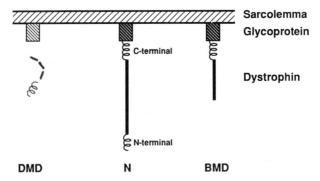

Fig. 5.3 The possible consequences of a deficiency of the C-terminal region of the dystrophin molecule.

likely. Such truncated dystrophins have also been found in male fetuses with Duchenne muscular dystrophy (Ginjaar *et al*. 1991*a*). In these studies however it is essential that the antibodies used are carefully characterized and are specific for the C-terminal region of dystrophin (Ellis *et al*. 1990).

Since the dystrophin molecule is believed to be attached by its C-terminal region (via a glycoprotein) to the sarcolemma, it is feasible that if this region is missing the resultant truncated dystrophin will fail to become attached to the membrane and subsequently undergo degradation (Fig. 5.3). However this may be an oversimplification and may not fit all cases. For example, a mentally handicapped boy with severe Duchenne muscular dystrophy has been described in whom the C-terminal region was lacking yet the resultant dystrophin was associated with the plasma membrane and was *not* degraded (Hoffman *et al*. 1991). Nevertheless, this case as well confirms that a deficiency of the C-terminal region is associated with a more severe disease.

Mabry type muscular dystrophy

In 1965 Mabry and his colleagues described a large family from Kentucky with an X-linked muscular dystrophy with prolonged survival and associated with relatively severe disability and myocardial involvement. However, there appears to have been no further reports of any families with exactly this clinical picture.

X-linked muscular dystrophy with early contractures and cardiomyopathy (Emery–Dreifuss type)

In 1961, Dreifuss and Hogan described a large family in Virginia in the United States with an X-linked form of muscular dystrophy which they considered at the time to be a benign type of Duchenne muscular dystrophy. However, on reinvestigating the family a few years later, this seemed to the author to be a very different disease from either Duchenne or Becker muscular dystrophy and a report setting out the differences was published in 1966 (Emery and Dreifuss 1966). This same disorder may well have been first described by Cestan and Lejonne in 1902 in two affected brothers, and has been reviewed more recently (Emery 1987, 1989*a, b*). The onset is in early childhood and is marked by progressive muscle wasting and weakness which, in the beginning, affects the lower limbs more than the upper limbs. The progression is relatively slow and most affected individuals survive into

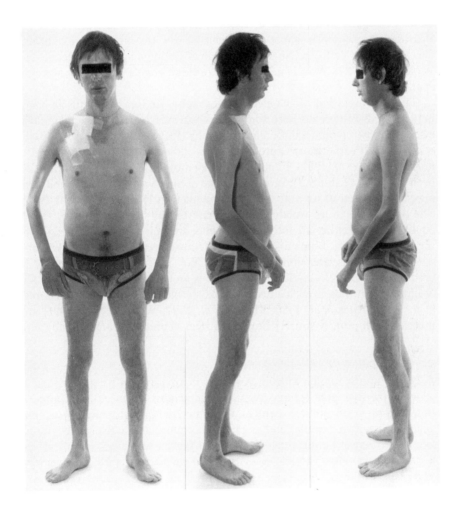

Fig. 5.4 A 17-year-old boy with X-linked muscular dystrophy with early contractures and cardiomyopathy. Note the flexion contractures of the elbows, and wasting of the lower legs. A cardiac pacemaker has been inserted.

middle age with varying degrees of incapacity. There does not appear to be any intellectual impairment. The SCK level is usually slightly raised but even in the early stages never approaches the grossly elevated levels found in Duchenne muscular dystrophy. The distinctive features of this disorder are as follows. Firstly, *early* contractures of the elbows and Achilles tendons and later the posterior cervical muscles. Secondly, muscle weakness is more proximal (scapulo-humeral) in the upper limbs and distal (anterior tibial and peroneal muscles) in the lower limbs, at least in the beginning. Thirdly, there is no calf pseudohypertrophy. Fourthly, myocardial involvement with cardiac conduction defects is a frequent and important feature (Fig. 5.4). Provided the diagnosis is made sufficiently early, the insertion of a cardiac pacemaker can be life-saving. Cardiological findings have been detailed in Wyse *et al.* (1987), Voit *et al.* (1988), Yoshioka *et al.* (1989), and Merchut *et al.* (1990).

The interpretation of the electromyographic findings and muscle histology in the disorder have been somewhat controversial, but the accumulated evidence most favours a muscular dystrophy (Rowland *et al.* 1979; Hopkins *et al.* 1981). Furthermore, autopsy studies indicate that the spinal cord is normal (Hara *et al.* 1987). Finally, although most cases described so far have been X-linked (Table 5.3), rare, somewhat similar variants of the syndrome may be inherited as an autosomal dominant trait (Sood and Goyal 1969). The occurrence in an isolated female reported by Takamoto *et al.* (1984) could represent either an autosomal form or the heterozygous expression of the X-linked form. Some distinguishing features between the X-linked and autosomal forms are summarized in Table 5.4, but the differences in predominant muscle involvement may be more apparent than real. The X-linked form has been located at Xq28 (Hodgson *et al.* 1986*b*; Thomas *et al.* 1986; Yates *et al.* 1986; Müller *et al.* 1991; Wehnert *et al.* 1991) and muscle dystrophin is entirely normal in size, abundance, and distribution.

X-linked myopathy with autophagy

A large Finnish family with an X-linked myopathy has been described in which excessive authophagy was a conspicuous feature. The latter is observed on electronmicroscopy and charaterized by autophagic lysosomal vacuoles in which granular and membranous material is actively exocytosed. Clinically there is a mild, slowly progressive muscle weakness, mainly affecting the lower limbs. There is no evidence of cardiac or neural involvement. The responsible gene has been assigned to distal Xq (Saviranta *et al.* 1988).

Quadriceps myopathy

It is now very doubtful whether weakness which only affects the quadriceps muscles represents a separate disease entity. Abnormalities of muscle dystrophin have been found in many instances which indicates that these cases at least represent an early stage of Becker muscular dystrophy.

X-linked scapulo-peroneal muscular dystrophy

This has previously been considered a possible separate disease entity. However, reports of the condition by Rotthauwe *et al.* (1972) and Thomas *et al.* (1972) have been considered by others (Rowland *et al.* 1979; Hopkins *et al.* 1981) to be cases of X-linked muscular dystrophy with early contractures and cardiomyopathy. Two further families (Waters *et al.* 1975) previously considered to have X-linked scapulo-peroneal muscular dystrophy were subsequently restudied by one of the authors who then decided that these too represented the form with early contractures and cardiomyopathy (Hopkins *et al.* 1981). Some confusion may have arisen because in the original report of Emery and Dreifuss (1966) weakness of the anterior tibial muscles was not emphasized. However, a scapulo-peroneal syndrome clearly exists which is inherited as an autosomal dominant trait and can be either neurogenic (Kaeser 1965) or myopathic (Thomas *et al.* 1975) in origin. However, in these cases onset is in adult life (a rare recessive neurogenic form may begin in childhood) and *early* contractures and cardiac conduction defects are *not* associated features. The myopathic form can be confused with facioscapulohumeral muscular dystrophy (Kazakov *et al.* 1976).

Autosomal recessive limb girdle muscular dystrophy of childhood

Two of Duchenne's original 13 cases of muscular dystrophy were in fact girls; and there have been many similar reports since. However, in the past many cases of girls with purported muscular dystrophy may well have had some other cause for their muscle weakness, such as a congenital myopathy or spinal muscular atrophy (Penn *et al.* 1970). Nevertheless, with improvements in diagnostic techniques it is now clear that muscular dystrophy can occur in young girls, for which there are several possible explanations. This may be a manifestation of X-linked Duchenne muscular dystrophy. Firstly, she may be homozygous for the mutant gene, her mother being a carrier and a new mutation having occurred on her paternally derived X-chromosome. Such a perturbation, although theoretically possible, would be extremely rare depending on the mutation rate in sperm. Secondly, she may be a manifesting carrier of the disease as a result of random X-inactivation (p. 97). Thirdly, she may have a sex chromosomal abnormality or an X/autosome translocation (p. 170). These possibilities will be discussed later. However, apart from in some way manifesting X-linked Duchenne muscular dystrophy, there is now clear evidence that an autosomal recessive form of a clinically similar disorder exists. This accounts for the disease in isolated affected girls, and families with affected sisters, or brothers and

Table 5.3 *More recent reports of X-linked muscular dystrophy associated with early contractures and cardiomyopathy (Emery-Dreifuss type) (+, present, in at least some; –, absent in all; NR, not recorded.)*

Reference	Number		Onset	Contractures (early)			Calf pseudo-hypertrophy	Muscle weakness		Cardiac involvement	Comments
	Families	Total cases		Elbows	Tendo achilles	Post-cervical muscles		Proximal (UL)	Distal (LL)		
Emery and Dreifuss (1966)	1	8	4–5	+	+	NR	–	+	?	+	
Rothauwe et al. (1972)	1	17	<10	+	+	+	–	+	+	+	See text
Thomas et al. (1972)	1	5 (6)	<5	+	+	+ (1)	–	+	+	+	See text
Mawatari and Katayama (1973)	1	5	7–10	NR	+	+	NR	+	+	+	Considered to be SMA (but see Rowland et al. 1979)
Cammann et al. (1974)	1	8	7–11	+	+	NR	–	+	+	?+	
Waters et al. (1975)/ Hopkins et al. (1981)	2	37/35	2–15	+ (late)	+	+	–	+	+	+	
Wadia et al. (1976)	1	5	10–?32	+ (late)	+ (late)	NR	+3/4	+	–	+	Possibly a different disorder
Hassan et al. (1979)	1	12	childhood	+	+	NR	–	+	+	+	
Rowland et al. (1979)	1	1	7	+	+	+	NR	+	+	+	
Tomelleri et al. (1980)	1	2 (brothers)	Early childhood	+	NR	+	–	+	+	+	Considered to be possibly neurogenic
Serratrice et al. (1982)	1	10	2–10	+	+	Limited extension	NR	+	+	+	

Fowler and Nayak (1983)	1	2	Early childhood	+	+	+	+	−		+	+	
Dickey et al. (1984)	2	6 (1 isolated)	1-5	+	+	+	+	NR	+	+	+	
Dominici et al. (1984)	1	5	Childhood	+	+	+	NR	NR	+	NR	+	See Dominici et al. 1984
Dubowitz (1985) (pp. 341–2)	1	3	11-12	+	+	?+	NR	NR	NR	NR	+	
Merlini et al. (1986)	1	5	Early childhood	+	+	+	+	−	+	+	+	
Johnston and McKay (1986)	1	3	Early childhood	+	+	+	−		+	+	+	
Oswald et al. (1987)	1	8	Early childhood	+	+	+	+	NR	+	+	+	
Goto et al. (1986)	2	3	Childhood	+	+	+	+	NR	+	+	+	
Petty et al. (1986)	1	4	Childhood	+	+	+	+	−	+	+	−	
Serratrice et al. (1988)	1	8	Childhood	+	+	+	+	NR	+	+	+	Also proximal weakness in LL
Voit et al. (1988)	4	6	<20	+	+	+	+	−	+	+	+	
Turpin et al. (1989)	1	1	Early childhood	+	+	+	+	−	+	+	+	

Table 5.4 *Some distinguishing features between the X-linked and autosomal forms of muscular dystrophy with early contractures and cardiomyopathy (Emery–Dreifuss type)*

| Inheritance | Childhood onset | Course | Contractures | | | Calf pseudo hypertrophy | Predominant muscle weakness | Cardio myopathy | Reference |
			Elbows	Tendo achilles	Cervical				
XR	+	Slow	+	+	+	−	Scapulo-humero-peroneal	+	—
AD	+	Rapid (mostly)	+	+	+	−	Scapulo-peroneal	+	Chakrabarti and Pearce (1981)
AD	+	Slow	−	+	+/−	−	Humero-pelvic	+	Fenichel *et al.* (1982)
Isolated female	+	Slow	+	+	+	?	Humero-pelvic	+	Takamoto *et al.* (1984)
AD	+	Slow	+	+	+	+	Humero-peroneal	+	Miller, R. G. *et al.* (1985)
AD	+	Slow	+	+	+	?	Humero-peroneal	+	Gilchrist and Leshner (1986)
AD	+	Slow	+	+	+	?	Scapulo-humero-pelvo-peroneal	+	Serratrice and Pouget (1986)

									Reference
AD	+	Slow	+	+	+	–	Humero-peroneal	+	Galassi *et al.* (1986)
AD	+	Slow (mostly)	+	+	+	?	Humero-pelvo peroneal	+/–	Krendel and Jannun (1987)
AD	variable	Slow	+	+	+	NR	Humero-peroneal	+	Baur *et al.* (1987) Witt *et al.* (1988)
Isolated female	+	Slow	+	+	+ (also other joints)	NR	Humero-pelvo peroneal	–	Riggs *et al.* (1988)
Isolated female	<3	Slow	+	+	?	NR	Scapulo peroneal	+	Voit *et al.* (1988)
AD	+	Slow	+	+	+	–	Scapulo humero pelvo peroneal	+	Tanaka *et al.* (1989)
Isolated female	+	moderate	+	+	+	NR	Humero peroneal	+	Merchut *et al.* (1990)
AD	late childhood	Slow	+	+	+	NR	Humero peroneal	+/–	Ørstavik *et al.* (1990)
AD	+	Slow	?	+	+	–	Humero pelvic	+	Michaels *et al.* (1991)

sisters; and presumably also a proportion of isolated cases of affected boys or families with only affected brothers. Very rarely a limb girdle type myopathy *limited to females* may be inherited as an autosomal dominant trait (Henson *et al.* 1967; Yoshioka *et al.* 1986).

One of the earliest and most detailed accounts of the autosomal recessive condition was given by Dubowitz in 1960, since when there have been many reports of the disorder which have been reviewed (Gardner-Medwin and Johnston 1984; Somer *et al.* 1985; Yoshioka *et al.* 1986). Gardner-Medwin and Johnston (1984) considered that although the X-linked and autosomal recessive forms were very similar, some points might be helpful in differentiation: in the autosomal recessive form toe walking is a prominent early feature before significant difficulties in walking occur, the course of the disease is relatively milder, affected children often not becoming confined to a wheelchair until their early teens or even later, the deltoids are relatively more affected than the biceps or triceps muscles, and intelligence is usually normal. Calf enlargement is often present and SCK levels are about the same in both disorders for individuals of the same age.

To these clinical differences it should be added that although most boys with X-linked Duchenne muscular dystrophy have significantly taller R waves in the right praecordial lead of the electrocardiogram (p. 112), at least after the age of 6, this is never found in the autosomal recessive form (Skyring and McKusick 1961; Emery 1972). Furthermore, the changes in muscle pathology have been reported to be perhaps more 'focal' than in X-linked Duchenne muscular dystrophy (Gardner-Medwin and Johnston 1984).

The distinction between the two disorders, however, is often not at all clear in the individual case (Somer *et al.* 1985). If a brother and sister are affected and the parents are cousins, then the autosomal recessive form would seem most likely. However, in Britain and North America, the X-linked form would seem to be at least 20 times commoner than the autosomal recessive form (Emery 1964*a*). So in these countries it is probably better to assume that the X-linked form is more likely until proved otherwise. Certainly any affected girl should be fully karyotyped and all affected boys and girls should have an ECG examination for evidence of right ventricular preponderance. The situation in some other countries, however, may well be different. The autosomal recessive form seems common and may be more severe in certain Arabic communities in Tunisia (Ben Hamida *et al.* 1983), and the Sudan (Salih *et al.* 1983). Interestingly, those inbred communities in North America in which cases of the autosomal recessive form have been reported (Jackson and Strehler 1968; Shokeir and Kobrinsky 1976; Shokeir and Rozdilsky 1985) originated from Switzerland where this form of muscular dystrophy seems to be particularly common (Moser *et al.* 1966). This so called Amish form of autosomal recessive muscular dystrophy, as well as the disease on the Isle of La Réunion in the Indian Ocean, map to chromosome 15 (Beckmann *et al.* 1991). The gene for one form of rare autosomal dominant limb girdle dystrophy is located on chromosome 5 (Speer *et al.* 1992).

It is of course disturbing that Duchenne muscular dystrophy and limb girdle muscular dystrophy of childhood are clinically so similar because confusion between the two will lead to some normal sisters of isolated affected brothers being given inappropriate genetic advice. However dystrophin and gene studies have now shown that in this form of dystrophy, dystrophin is of normal size on Western blot analysis (Norman *et al.* 1989*b*), and shows normal immunostaining in muscle (Tachi *et al.* 1990; Vainzof *et al.* 1990) and there is no abnormality in the dystrophin gene itself (McGuire and Fischbeck 1991). Using these techniques Francke and her colleagues (1989) have clearly demonstrated genetic heterogenity in brother/sister pairs affected by early onset dystrophy: while the mutation involved the dystrophin gene in some families (i.e. an affected brother with X-linked disease with a manifesting heterozygous sister) in others it did not, and these latter therefore represent the autosomal recessive form. And based on such studies the latter disorder, at least in Brazil, may account for around 10 per cent of isolated affected boys diagnosed as having 'Duchenne muscular dystrophy' (Vainzof *et al.* 1991*a*).

In autosomal recessive limb girdle muscular dystrophy of childhood, though muscle dystrophin is normal there is a specific deficiency of 50K dystrophin-associated glycoprotein (Matsumura *et al.* 1992). In contrast, in Duchenne muscular dystrophy *all* dystrophin-associated glycoproteins are greatly reduced and dystrophin is virtually absent. Immunohistochemical studies of these muscle proteins therefore provide a means of differentiating the two disorders. Furthermore, the 50K dystrophin-associated glycoprotein is a common factor in the pathogenesis of both disorders.

The manifesting carrier of Duchenne muscular dystrophy

Female relatives of boys with X-linked Duchenne muscular dystrophy may occasionally manifest certain features of the disease. This appears to have been first recognized by Kryschowa and Abowjan in 1934 who described a large family with the disease, one of the female carriers having noticeably enlarged calves. Later Sidler (1944) described a 23-year-old woman (case 4) who had increasing difficulty climbing stairs from the age of 19, and on examination her right quadriceps was found to be atrophied. She had a brother and three maternal uncles with Duchenne muscular dystrophy. There have been many similar reports since, manifestations of the disease ranging from calf enlargement, through varying degrees of muscle weakness, to occasionally severe incapacity (Fig. 5.5).

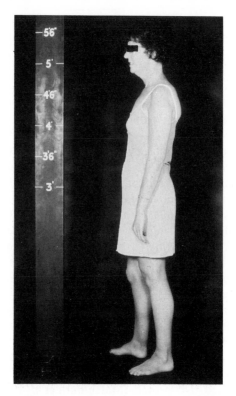

Fig. 5.5 A manifesting female carrier of Duchenne muscular dystrophy, aged 36, with lumbar lordosis, some enlargement of the calves, weakness of the anterior tibialis, quadriceps, and gluteal muscles, and to a lesser extent the shoulder girdle muscles. By age 47 weakness had progressed to such an extent that she became confined to a wheelchair.

Onset of weakness also varies considerably and may develop in childhood or may not become evident until adult life, and the weakness may be progressive or remain static. In many ways the distribution of weakness resembles that seen in adult limb girdle muscular dystrophy, but differs in that pseudohypertrophy is usually present, the weakness is often asymmetric, electrocardiographic abnormalities similar to those seen in affected boys can occur, and the SCK level is invariably very high and occasionally may even approach levels found in affected boys. On the other hand, some female carriers may have very high SCK levels yet have no muscle weakness at all (Fig. 5.6).

It is important to distinguish a manifesting adult female carrier from a woman with autosomal recessive limb girdle muscular dystrophy (Table 5.5)

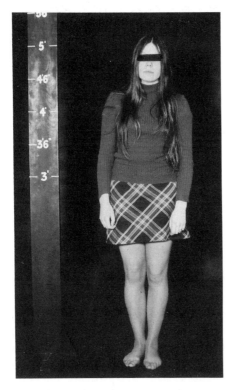

Fig. 5.6 A 19-year-old sister of a boy with Duchenne muscular dystrophy who has SCK levels in excess of 1500 iu, yet has no clinical manifestations of the disease.

both of which occur with very roughly the same frequency (Moser and Emery 1974; Yates and Emery 1985; Norman and Harper 1989), because genetic counselling in these two situations will be quite different. The risks to the sons of a manifesting carrier of X-linked Duchenne muscular dystrophy will be 50 per cent, but the risks to the offspring of a woman affected with autosomal recessive limb girdle muscular dystrophy will be negligible. So-called 'limb girdle dystrophy' can also be inherited as an autosomal dominant trait, but the nosology of this disorder remains unclear (Somer *et al*. 1991). Manifesting carriers of Becker dystrophy also occur, but are rare (Glass *et al*. 1992).

Such manifestations in heterozygous females can be explained in terms of random inactivation of the X chromosome: in those women with no clinical manifestations and a low SCK level, the active X chromosome in most cells is presumably the one bearing the normal gene, whereas in those women with manifestations of the disease and a high SCK level, the active X chromosome

Table 5.5 *Differentiation between a manifesting carrier of Duchenne muscular dystrophy (DMD) and a woman with limb girdle muscular dystrophy (LGMD)*

Symptom or sign	DMD carrier	LGMD
Pseudohypertrophy	> 80%	Rare
Muscle weakness	Often asymmetric	Rarely asymmetric
ECG abnormalities		
(R–S in V_1 increased)	5–10%	–
SCK level elevated	> 95%	< 50%
	Often very high	Rarely high
Muscle dystrophin	Mosaicism	Normal
Dystrophin DNA		
analysis	Abnormal	Normal

in most cells is presumably the one bearing the muscular dystrophy gene (Emery 1963, 1965*b*). Markers have now been identified on the X chromosome which can be used to prove this hypothesis (Curnutte *et al.* 1992). There is often familial concordance for such manifestations, mothers and daughters or sisters often being affected (Moser and Emery 1974). This would suggest that X-inactivation, at least in these women, may not be entirely random but is perhaps under genetic control (p. 219).

Bonilla and colleagues (1988*b*) and Arahata and colleagues (1989*a*) have shown, and this has been confirmed by many others, that there is mosaic expression of muscle dystrophin in symphomatic carriers of Duchenne muscular dystrophy. Such mosaicism however is rarely found in female carriers without symptoms. Mosaicism of dystrophin expression is believed to result from the formation of multinucleate muscle fibres from uninucleate myoblasts, in some of which the normal X chrosomes is active (and therefore dystrophin-positive) while in others the abnormal X chromosome is active (and therefore dystrophin-negative). But a simple mosaicism of positive and negative fibres would not be expected (p. 221) but rather variation in staining intensity, both within and between individual fibres (Emery 1990*b*). Presumably in non-manifesting carrier the proportion of abnormal nuclei is usually insufficient to produce any clearly observable evidence of mosaicism. Whatever the mechanism, mosaicism of muscle dsytrophin expression provides a good way of distinguising a manifesting carrier from a case of limb girdle dystrophy, in whom of course there will be no such mosaicism, all muscle fibres staining uniformly. A further way of distinguishing between these two conditions is by DNA analysis which will be discussed later (p. 238). The possibility that an isolated female with a myopathy, myopathic histopathology, and an SCK level greater than 1000 iu must seriously be considered as probably a manifesting carrier (Hoffman *et al.* 1992).

A particularly confusing situation arises if the manifesting female happens to be a young girl and the weakness is progressive (Aymé *et al.* 1979; Held *et al.* 1980; Olson and Fenichel 1982). If she is the only affected individual in the family or is the sister of an isolated case of Duchenne muscular dystrophy, this could be confused with autosomal recessive limb girdle muscular dystrophy of childhood (p. 91).

Heterozygous identical twins

Over the years a number of female *identical* (monozygotic, MZ) twins have been described who have been discordant for manifestations for various X-linked recessive disorders, most notably Duchenne muscular dystrophy (Table 5.6). The simplest explanation is that during the process of twinning, by chance the affected twin received a greater proportion of cells in which the active X chromosome was the one bearing the mutant gene. Certainly there is experimental evidence that in these cases the clinical expression of the disease in the affected twin is the consequence of the inactivation of the normal X chromosome in *most* of her cells as compared with the unaffected twin sister (Richards *et al.* 1990; Lupski *et al.* 1991). But why is the expression limited to only one twin of a pair and that concordant expression in MZ

Table 5.6 *Recorded examples of monozygotic female twins discordant for various X-linked recessive disorders*

Disorder	Author
Colour blindness	Philip *et al.* (1969)
Haemophilia B	Jørgensen *et al.* (1992)
G-6-P-D deficiency	Revesz *et al.* (1972)
Hunter's disease	Phelan *et al.* (1980)
Duchenne muscular dystrophy	Winchester *et al.* (1990)
	Fraser (1963)
	Gomez *et al.* (1977)
	Pena *et al.* (1982, 1987)
	Burn *et al.* (1986)
	Chutkow *et al.* (1987)
	Bonilla *et al.* (1990)
	Richards *et al.* (1990)
	Zneimer *et al.* (1990)
	Abbadi *et al.* (1991)
	Lupski *et al.* (1991)

heterozygous female twins is extremely uncommon? This may be because the twinning event occurs *after* X-inactivation and in these cases in some way non-random X-inactivation itself causes the twinning process (Burn *et al.* 1986; Nance 1990). But discordance in female MZ twins has also been reported in certain *autosomal* disorders. The situation is therefore not clear. Lubinsky and Hall (1991) suggest that genomic imprinting, monozygous twinning, and X-inactivation may all be somehow related and '. . . their interactions may provide important clues to the nature of early develop-mental processes'.

The spinal muscular atrophies

The spinal muscular atrophies may be defined as a group of inherited diseases in which there is degeneration of the anterior horn cells (lower motor neurones) of the spinal cord and often the bulbar motor nuclei, but with no evidence of pyramidal tract or peripheral nerve involvement (Emery 1971). There is therefore no evidence of spasticity or hyper-reflexia, the plantar response is flexor and there are no sensory changes or any reduction in the peripheral nerve conduction velocity. This group of diseases excludes motor neurone disease (progressive bulbar palsy, progressive muscular atrophy, and amyotrophic lateral sclerosis), and its variants, as well as the peripheral neuropathies. In any event motor neurone disease in childhood is excep-tionally rare and when it does occur is unlikely to be confused with muscular dystrophy because spasticity is usually the predominant clinical feature (Emery and Holloway 1982).

The spinal muscular atrophies are a very heterogeneous group of disorders and vary considerably in their clinical presentation and mode of inheritance. The clinical features and the relationships of these disorders have been much discussed in recent years (Russman *et al.* 1983; Hausmanowa-Petrusewicz *et al.* 1984; Serratrice *et al.* 1984; Zerres 1989; Pearn 1990; Dubowitz 1991*a*). A classification favoured by the author is given in Table 5.7.

Much of the controversy concerning the detailed nosology of this group of disorders will be resolved now that the gene locus for proximal spinal muscular atrophy of childhood has been located at 5q11–5q13 (Davies *et al.* 1991). In can be predicted that *at least* four different mutant alleles at this locus will determine the phenotypic variation seen in this disorder (Emery 1991*b*).

The only forms which might possibly be confused with Duchenne mus-cular dystrophy are those in which muscle weakness is predominantly *proximal* in distribution. This group is much commoner than the others. Whether it is possible to separate the so-called infantile and juvenile forms of proximal spinal muscular atrophy on clinical grounds has been hotly debated in the past. Much of the confusion arose because of overlap in the

Table 5.7 *A clinical and genetical classification of the spinal muscular atrophies (SMA)*

1. *Proximal SMA*
   (*a*) Infantile (type I)
   Autosomal recessive
       (*i*) Usual form (Werdnig–Hoffmann)
       (*ii*) With arthrogryposis multiplex congenita
   (*b*) Intermediate (type II)
   Autosomal recessive
   (*c*) Juvenile (type III)
   Autosomal recessive
       (*i*) Usual form (Wohlfart–Kugelberg–Welander)
       (*ii*) 'Ryukyuan' SMA
       (*iii*) With microcephaly and mental subnormality
   Autosomal dominant
   X-linked recessive (very rare)
   (*d*) Adult (type IV)
   Autosomal recessive
   Autosomal dominant
   X-linked recessive (Kennedy syndrome)
2. *Distal SMA*
   Autosomal recessive
   Autosomal dominant
3. *Juvenile Progressive Bulbar Palsy*
   Autosomal recessive
       (*i*) Usual form (Fazio–Londe)
       (*ii*) With nerve deafness (Van Laere)
4. *Scapulo-peroneal SMA*
   Autosomal recessive
   Autosomal dominant

age at onset which is notoriously difficult to assess accurately. If other features are also taken into account, such as the course of the disease and age at death, then it would seem quite legitimate to separate these disorders. The frequency of spontaneous activity on electromyography (Buchthal and Olsen 1970), and the degree of collateral reinnervation (Hausmanowa-Petrusewicz *et al.* 1968*a*), have also been found to differ in the infantile and juvenile forms. Features which can be used clinically to distinguish not only these two forms of proximal spinal muscular atrophy but also intermediate and adult forms are summarized in Table 5.8.

The severe infantile (type I, Werdnig–Hoffmann disease) and the intermediate (type II) forms are quite distinct from Duchenne muscular dystrophy because of the very marked hypotonia and weakness from an

Table 5.8 *Some distinguishing features of the various forms of proximal spinal muscular atrophy*

Type	Age (usual)		Ability to sit without support*	Muscle fasciculations	SCK
	Onset	Survival			
I (Infantile)	< 6 mths	< 2 yrs	Never	+/-	Normal
II (Intermediate)	< 18 mths	> 2 yrs	Usually	+/-	Usually normal
III (Juvenile)	> 18 mths	Adulthood	Always	+ +	Often raised
IV (Adult)	> 30 yrs	50 yrs +	Always	+ +	Often raised

*At some time during the course of the illness (*see Neuromusc. Disorders* **1**, 81 (1991)).

early age, the presence of fasciculations, and an SCK level which is rarely raised and then only slightly. However differentiation from the juvenile form (type III, Wohlfart–Kugelberg–Welander disease) on clinical grounds may not be so easy. In fact this was first regarded as pseudomyopathic because of its similarity with muscular dystrophy (Wohlfart *et al.* 1955; Kugelberg and Welander 1956). Furthermore, although usually inherited as an autosomal recessive, or less commonly as an autosomal dominant trait, males are more often affected than females (Emery *et al.* 1976*a, b*; Hausmanowa-Petrusewicz *et al.* 1984). This form of spinal muscular atrophy is more benign than Werdnig–Hoffmann disease with onset in early childhood and with survival into adulthood (Fig. 5.7).

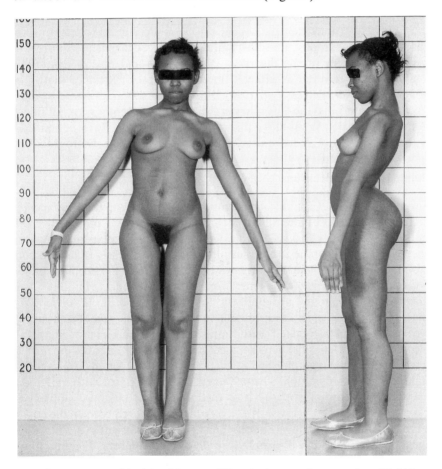

Fig. 5.7 A 17-year-old girl with type III spinal muscular atrophy (Wohlfart–Kugelberg–Welander disease). Note the marked lordosis and wasting of the left deltoid muscle. An older and two younger brothers were also affected.

The clinical presentation may closely resemble Duchenne muscular dystrophy: weakness first affects the pelvic girdle musculature and patients often present with a tendency to fall and a waddling gait. Later, the pectoral girdle, neck, trunk, and distal limb muscles also become affected. Interestingly muscle weakness, at least in the early stages, is often asymmetric which is unlike muscular dystrophy, pseudohypertrophy of the calf muscles is uncommon, and muscle fasciculations are often present and are a useful diagnostic sign. A fine tremor of the outstretched hands is common and *minipolymyoclonus*, intermittent and irregular movement which is sufficient to produce visible movement of the joints and head, may also be present. The progression of the disease is very variable, even within families, although the majority require a wheelchair in their twenties or thirties. The SCK level is very rarely grossly elevated, but it can be moderately elevated. In most cases electromyography, muscle histology, and histochemistry confirm the neurogenic nature of the disorder. DNA probes and muscle dystrophin studies will differentiate an affected male from a case of X-linked dystrophy (Lunt *et al.* 1989; Zerres *et al.* 1990). In X-linked spinal muscular atrophy (Kennedy syndrome) the defect lies in the androgen receptor gene but in any event on clinical grounds alone this rare disorder is unlikely to be confused with other forms of spinal muscular atrophy or muscular dystrophy.

Summary and conclusions

Several disorders can mimic Duchenne muscular dystrophy. They include certain other forms of muscular dystrophy which may present in early childhood, various congenital myopathies, and spinal muscular atrophy. Among the muscular dystrophies, the congenital forms are unlikely to lead to confusion because in general they are evident at birth or in the neonatal period with severe hypotonia and generalized muscle weakness. Similarly, the congenital myopathies are unlikely to pose a problem in differential diagnosis because most cases present in early life with generalized muscle weakness, often associated with respiratory problems and feeding difficulties, or may have distinctive clinical features, serum enzymes are normal and the diagnosis is established on muscle histology. Among the other X-linked muscular dystrophies, the benign form associated with early contractures and cardiomyopathy is so distinctive that this too is unlikely to cause confusion. But because of the very high SCK levels early in the course of the disease, overlap in age at onset and similar pattern of muscle involvement, Becker muscular dystrophy can present a diagnostic dilemma in the isolated case. However, an important point of distinction is that in the Becker form almost all affected males are still walking at 12. Furthermore, muscle dystrophin is virtually absent in Duchenne muscular dystrophy whereas in Becker muscular dystrophy dystrophin is present but abnormal.

A particularly difficult problem is posed by autosomal recessive limb girdle muscular dystrophy of childhood when only a boy is affected in the family. The disease is relatively more benign than Duchenne muscular dystrophy and there are reported to be some minor clinical differences, and whereas most boys with Duchenne muscular dystrophy have electrocardiographic evidence of right ventricular preponderance, this is not found in the autosomal recessive limb girdle form. But the distinction is often not at all clear, although *a priori* in Britain and North America a case is much more likely to be Duchenne muscular dystrophy since this is much the commoner of the two disorders. Furthermore, in this disorder in contrast to Duchenne muscular dystrophy, muscle dystrophin is of normal size and abundance and there is no abnormality in the dystrophin gene itself but there is a specific deficiency of 50K dystrophin-associated glycoprotein.

Finally, the only form of spinal muscular atrophy which might possibly be confused with Duchenne muscular dystrophy is the proximal juvenile form (type III, Wohlfart–Kugelberg–Welander disease). However, points which would suggest this disease rather than Duchenne muscular dystrophy would be some asymmetry of muscle involvement, absence of pseudohypertrophy, and evidence of muscle fasciculations. In most cases electromyography, muscle histology, and histochemistry will confirm the neurogenic nature of the disorder. And again DNA and muscle dystrophin studies will differentiate between these two disorders.

6 Involvement of tissues other than skeletal muscle

The muscular dystrophies have often been described as *primary* diseases of muscle. The term primary in this context could have two interpretations; either that muscle is the most obviously affected tissue which is certainly true, or that the fundamental molecular defect is expressed only in skeletal muscle, which is patently not true. In recent years it has been shown that significant abnormalities can be found in a variety of tissues quite apart from skeletal muscle. This is perhaps not unexpected since the abnormal gene is present in all cells of the body. However, why a particular gene is expressed in some tissues and not in others raises a fundamental question in molecular biology.

The variety of manifestations of a genetic disease can result from the pleiotropic effects of a single gene or, at the molecular level, either from the involvement of adjacent genes which control other phenotypic features or from different point mutations within the same gene.

Pleiotropy refers to the multiple effects that a gene mutation may have as a trail of consequences leading on from the basic defect. An excellent example of this is provided by sickle cell anaemia whereby the responsible gene mutation results in sickle cell haemoglobin which is less soluble than normal haemoglobin and therefore tends to crystallize out resulting in deformation of the red cell which becomes sickle shaped. These abnormal cells are then destroyed (haemolysed) resulting in anaemia. But at the same time they also tend to clump together, thereby obstructing small arteries, resulting in ischaemia of tissues with a variety of consequences including attacks of abdominal pain, splenic infarction, limb pains, osteomyelitis, cerebro-vascular accidents, haematuria, renal failure, 'pneumonic' episodes, and heart failure. The diversity of clinical manifestations in Duchenne muscular dystrophy can also be partly explained in terms of the pleiotropic effects of the responsible mutant gene.

An association of *different genetic disorders* in the same individual can occur purely by chance, such as the reported occurrence in Duchenne muscular dystrophy of haemophilia (Konagaya *et al*. 1982), trisomy-21 (Moser 1971) and even facioscapulohumeral muscular dystrophy (Lecky *et al*. 1991). However, very occasionally such an association may result from the deletion of genetic material involving adjacent genes which are responsible for different diseases. Thus, Francke and her colleagues (Francke *et al*.

1985) have described a boy with Duchenne muscular dystrophy who also had chronic granulomatous disease and seemingly retinitis pigmentosa. Cytogenetic studies revealed that he had a small but visible interstitial deletion of the short arm of his X chromosome (Xp21) which presumably involved the loss of genetic material from all three of the *adjacent* genes responsible for these different diseases (p. 173). In another case a smaller, but also visible deletion in the same region of the X chromosome was found in a boy with Duchenne muscular dystrophy, glycerol kinase deficiency, and adrenal insufficiency (Bartley *et al.* 1986). It is possible that the reported associations of Duchenne muscular dystrophy with retinitis pigmentosa (Marandian *et al.* 1977) or with chronic granulomatous disease (Kousseff 1981) *could* also be due to a similar mechanism. However, this sort of molecular abnormality is rare and very much the exception. Much more likely is that the variations in clinical manifestations of the disease in different families are due to differences in the site and extent of mutations *within* the dystrophin gene at Xp21.

Whatever the mechanism, it is important in patient management to appreciate that Duchenne muscular dystrophy is a multi-system disease and that a variety of tissues other than skeletal muscle can be affected. It is also important in genetic counselling to acquaint would-be parents with the possible consequences of the disease in an affected child so that they can better appreciate the full extent of the problem.

Smooth muscle

Circumstantial evidence that smooth muscle may be affected in Duchenne muscular dystrophy comes from the occasional occurrence of bladder paralysis, paralytic ileus, and gastric dilatation in affected boys (Robin and Falewski 1963; Stark *et al.* 1988). More direct evidence is provided by detailed autopsy studies such as those carried out by Bevans (1945), Huvos and Pruzanski (1967), Jedrzejowska-Kulakowska *et al.* (1968), Leon *et al.* (1986), and Barohn *et al.* (1988). These studies have shown that the smooth muscle of the gastrointestinal tract often shows variation in fibre size, atrophy and loss of muscle fibres, and areas of fibrosis. These changes are comparable in many ways to those seen in affected skeletal muscle and have occasionally been found in cases who did not have any relevant gastrointestinal symptoms in life. However, no lesions of the smooth muscle of the vascular system have so far been reported.

Cardiac muscle

There is overwhelming evidence from clinical, pathological, and physiological studies (Hunter 1980; Hunsaker *et al.* 1982) that cardiac muscle is involved in Duchenne muscular dystrophy.

From an early age there is very often a persistent sinus tachycardia, arrhythmias and non-specific murmurs are common. Clinically apparent cardiomyopathy however, first becomes evident usually after the age of 10 and increases in incidence with age thereafter (Nigro *et al.* 1990*a*). Mitral valve prolapse has been recorded in up to a quarter of affected boys, auscultatory evidence of which can be confirmed by echocardiography (Biddison *et al.* 1979). *Sudden* death may occur from cardiac causes, but progressive heart failure is rare (Gaffney *et al.* 1989). Plasma atrial natriuretic peptide levels have been suggested as a means of evaluating cardiac function in the disease (Kawai *et al.* 1990).

At autopsy microscopic studies of cardiac muscle reveal features which resemble those seen in skeletal muscle with variation in fibre size, fragmentation of muscle fibres, replacement by connective tissue, and some fatty infiltration (Bevans 1945; Gilroy *et al.* 1963; Perloff *et al.* 1966). Such changes have even been found in patients who did not necessarily have any symptoms of heart disease during life. Fibrosis appears to be a particularly important feature (Fig. 6.1). It begins in the outer myocardium involving the more postero-basal part of the outer-free wall of the left ventricle. At first

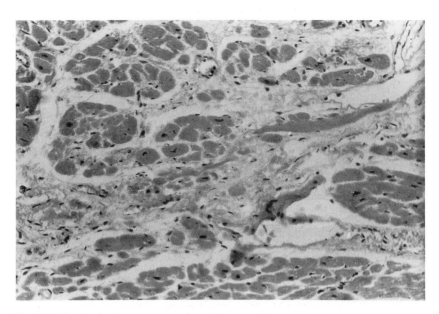

Fig. 6.1 Histological appearance of cardiac muscle from the left ventricle from a boy with Duchenne muscular dystrophy, age 21. Note the variation in fibre size and marked increase in connective tissue (haematoxylin and eosin).

fibrosis appears in discrete small areas, but eventually becomes more diffuse and involves most of the outer half of the ventricular wall. The right ventricle and atria are rarely involved and this pattern of myocardial fibrosis does not seem to occur in any other disease (Frankel and Rosser 1976) except perhaps Becker muscular dystrophy (p. 114).

Early in the course of the disease cardiac catheterization studies have shown few consistent abnormalities, but in severely affected boys approaching cardiac failure significantly elevated right atrial and right ventricular end-diastolic pressures have been recorded (Perloff *et al*. 1966, 1967; Demany and Zimmerman 1969). Non-invasive techniques such as ballistocardiography (Lowenstein *et al*. 1962), vectorcardiography (Ronan *et al*. 1972), echocardiography (Danilowicz *et al*. 1980), and particularly electrocardiography have all been used to study cardiac involvement in Duchenne muscular dystrophy, and to assess its extent and severity in the individual patient. Electrocardiography has proved particularly valuable and therefore merits some special consideration.

One of the earliest descriptions of electrocardiographic (ECG) abnormalities in muscular dystrophy was made by Schliephake in 1929. Since then a variety of ECG changes have been observed in Duchenne muscular dystrophy in particular, and these have been reviewed in detail (Lowenstein *et al*. 1962; Slucka 1968; Durnin *et al*. 1971; Jellett *et al*. 1974), and are listed in Table 6.1. Evidence of defective cardiac conduction has also been reported (Sanyal and Johnson 1982).

Numerous attempts have been made to determine if any particular ECG pattern is distinctive in Duchenne muscular dystrophy. Ishikawa and his colleagues in Japan have suggested that high frequency 'notches' on the QRS complexes can be used for estimating the extent and severity of cardiac involvement in Duchenne muscular dystrophy (Ishikawa *et al*. 1982), and Nigro *et al*. (1984) have found shortening of the PQ interval to be particularly valuable. These conclusions now await further evaluation. There is

Table 6.1 *ECG abnormalities arranged in decreasing order of frequency in Duchenne muscular dystrophy*

Tall R waves in V_1
R/S ratio ↑
$\|R{-}S\|$ ↑
Shortened P–R interval
Deep Q waves in V_{5-6}
Complex RSr[1], right bundle branch block
Altered T waves
Left axis deviation

however general agreement that tall R waves in V_1 is a particularly frequent and consistent abnormality in the disease (D'Orsogna *et al.* 1988). A useful measure of this is the algebraic sum of the R and S waves in this lead (i.e. $|R-S|$ in V_1) which is abnormal in over 80 per cent of affected boys (Fig. 6.2). It is particularly interesting that the same abnormality has also been found in up to 10 per cent of female carriers of the disease (p. 100). It is uncommon in other forms of muscular dystrophy and spinal muscular atrophy which may occur in childhood, and seems to be specific to Duchenne muscular dystrophy (Emery 1972). A variety of ECG abnormalities also occur in polymyositis but are different from those most commonly seen in muscular dystrophy (Stern *et al.* 1984).

The aetiology of the tall R waves in the right praecordial lead of the ECG is not clear. Various suggestions have been made including thoracic deformity, pulmonary hypertension, conduction defect due to myocardial

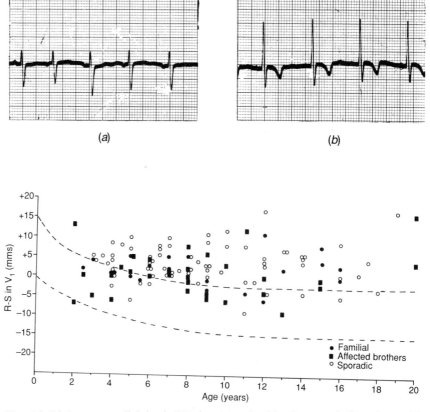

Fig. 6.2 Right praecordial lead (V_1) in: (*a*) a healthy boy, and (*b*) a boy with Duchenne muscular dystrophy, both age 10. Algebraic sum of R–S in V_1 for boys with Duchenne muscular dystrophy. Normal 90% confidence limits from Nadas (1963). (From Emery (1972) with permission.)

dystrophy, and ventricular septal hypertrophy. However none of these suggestions is entirely satisfactory. It seems (Perloff *et al.* 1967) that this anterior shift of the QRS complex is most likely due to the diffuse interstitial fibrosis in the postero-basal part of the left ventricle (Fig. 6.3). Involvement of the adjacent papillary muscle would account for mitral valve prolapse which can occur in the disease (Sanyal *et al.* 1980). Evidence supporting this idea comes from necropsy findings (Frankel and Rosser 1976) which have already been discussed, and also from echocardiography (Ahmad *et al.* 1978; Cattelaens *et al.* 1990; Miyoshi 1991). The latter has revealed contraction abnormalities of the left ventricle in most patients which is first noted in the posterior free wall behind the mitral valve (Goldberg *et al.* 1982). But why this portion of the myocardium should be so selectively involved in this particular disorder is not clear. Radionuclide imaging suggests a regional metabolic or blood flow alteration (Perloff *et al.* 1984).

It is now becoming clear that comparable cardiac abnormalities also occur

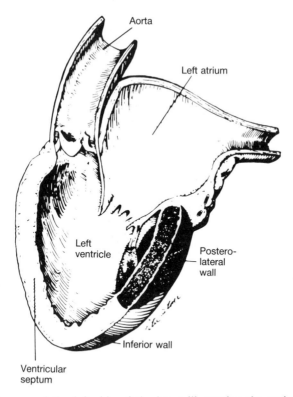

Fig. 6.3 Diagram of the left side of the heart illustrating the region of selective involvement in patients with Duchenne muscular dystrophy. (Reproduced by kind permission of Dr J. K. Perloff and the *American Journal of Medicine*.)

in Becker muscular dystrophy (Berlit and Stegaru-Hellring 1991) but are less marked, possibly reflecting the more benign nature of this disease in general. Interestingly some degree of right axis deviation and involvement of the left ventricle also occurs (Levin and Narahara 1985; Lazzeroni *et al.* 1989).

Vascular system

Trophic changes in the skin of the extremities of patients with Duchenne muscular dystrophy are common, especially in the lower limbs and in the later stages of the disease. These changes include coldness and cyanotic mottling, and on occasions even scleroderma-like changes. Such changes most likely stem from inactivity, although Duchenne himself even raised the possibility that muscular dystrophy might have a vascular aetiology. This idea was diligently pursued some twenty years ago by Démos and colleagues in Paris, and later by King Engel in the United States.

Studies which have been designed to determine if the vascular system is involved in Duchenne muscular dystrophy focused, perhaps understandably, on muscle vasculature. Démos and colleagues measured the circulation time in patients in two ways: arm-to-arm using fluorescein as a marker and arm-to-tongue using sodium dehydrocholate. By subtraction the 'peripheral circulation time' in the upper limb was determined. This they found in boys with Duchenne muscular dystrophy to be above or below the 95 per cent range for normal children of comparable age, and to be significantly reduced in some female carriers (Démos 1961; Démos and Maroteaux 1961; Démos *et al.* 1962). However, there is no defect in the capillary nail bed (Dudley and Gibson 1964) and using venous occlusion plethysmography we failed to detect any significant changes in limb blood flow in affected boys at different stages of the disease or in carrier females (Emery and Schelling 1965).

However, since these early observations, more sophisticated methods have been developed for measuring blood flow, notably tracer clearance (^{133}Xe, ^{85}Kr, ^{125}I-antipyrine) and hydrogen electrode techniques (Moxley 1984). Using the ^{133}Xe clearance method, Paulson *et al.* (1974) and Bradley *et al.* (1975*b*) found no significant difference in limb blood flow in affected boys compared with normal boys. However, in younger (less than 10 years old) affected boys though the number of capillaries per unit of muscle fibre area remains unchanged, capillary size is significantly increased (Jerusalem *et al.* 1974), and this would account for the slight increase in capillary diffusion capacity observed by Paulson *et al.* (1974). However, no structural abnormalities of the small arterial vessels or capillaries of the muscle have been detected with either light or electron-microscopy (Musch *et al.* 1975). More recently Mechler and colleagues, (1980) used the ^{133}Xe method to study blood flow in the tibialis anterior muscle in Becker muscular dystrophy. They found that whereas adrenergic beta-receptor responses of vascular smooth muscle to stimulation by adrenaline and blocking by propranolol was normal, there appeared to be some abnormality of alpha-receptor response to blocking by phentolamine which was not found in spinal muscular atrophy or polymyositis. The significance of this finding, however, is not clear.

The general consensus of both pathological and physiological studies seems to be that in the early stages of the disease there are no significant abnormalities in muscle vasculature apart from some slight increase in capillary size. Later any changes which do occur, such as diminution in capillary bed, are due to muscle replacement by fat and connective tissue which is relatively avascular, and are therefore secondary events.

Central nervous system

For some time there was, perhaps understandably, some reluctance to accept that boys with Duchenne muscular dystrophy could also be mentally handicapped. After all this was yet another misfortune for the affected child and his parents to bear. However, much research in the 1960s and 1970s confirmed the suspicion of many of the association, first noted in fact by Duchenne, that a proportion of affected boys can have some degree of mental handicap and that on occasions this can be severe. We have not systematically measured IQ in our patients although in one study we selected a group of boys who were *severely* mentally handicapped, some of them being ineducable (Emery *et al.* 1979*b*), and at least two of our patients are highly intelligent having been accepted for university degree courses.

Apart from some degree of intellectual impairment, a deficit of memory has also been reported (Whelan 1987) and behavioural problems occur (Smith *et al.* 1990*a*).

IQ of affected boys

There have been a great many studies of IQ in affected boys, the results of which are summarized in Table 6.2. There is considerable variation from those who are severely handicapped to a few with IQs above 130. The overall mean IQ is however about one standard deviation below the normal mean. Roughly 20 per cent have IQs below 70, and 3 per cent have IQs below 50.

This reduction in IQ is not due to any lack of educational opportunity as a result of their physical disability because it is not found in other diseases with comparable disability, such as juvenile spinal muscular atrophy. Furthermore, poor educational performance in Duchenne muscular dystrophy is often observed early in life when muscle weakness is relatively slight. Whatever causes the intellectual impairment must also operate at an early stage in development for it is not progressive and does not correlate with duration or severity of the disease. Though one study does

Table 6.2 *Studies of IQ in boys with Duchenne muscular dystrophy. Only the most recent or most detailed data included for any one centre*

Reference	No.	Mean	Range	≤70	≤50
Allen and Rodgin (1960)	30	82	14–117	9	5
Worden and Vignos (1962)	38	83	46–134	10	1
Schorer (1964)	28	79	–	–	–
Dubowitz (1965)	27	68	42–118	17	3
Zellweger and Niedermeyer (1965)	42	83	42–131	–	3
Cohen *et al.* (1968)	108	86	< 50–> 120	21	3
Desai *et al.* (1969)	28	79	42–115	16	2
Prosser *et al.* (1969)	52	87	51–113	–	–
Kozicka *et al.* (1971)	52	76	35–114	21	3
				(≤67)	(≤51)
Michal (1972)	74	85	39–122	–	–
Black (1973)	25	82	45–128	–	–
Marsh and Munsat (1974)	34	89	60–118	6	0
Florek and Karolak (1977)	129	79	30–127	27	–
				(<68)	
Leibowitz and Dubowitz (1981)	54	86	47–132	10	1
Total	*721*	*82*	–	*137*	*21*
				(19%)	(3%)

suggest some possible relationship with age (Sollee *et al.* 1985) others have not found this (Smith *et al.* 1990*a*). The fact that there is no difference in IQ of affected boys born to carrier mothers and those who are presumed to be the result of new mutations, excludes a maternal factor from being responsible for depressing the IQ.

The most likely explanation is that the depression in IQ is yet another pleiotropic effect of the mutant gene. This is supported by the fact that unaffected sibs have normal intellect, and there is often a good correlation between affected brothers (Kozicka *et al.* 1971; Ogasawara 1989). Cohen *et al.* (1968) found a high concordance ($P < 0.001$) for intellectual function in 37 of 39 families and in the two apparent exceptions there were reasonable explanations for their being discordant, and Bortolini and Zatz (1986) found mental capacity to be concordant in 16 out of 22 (73 per cent) families they studied. Furthermore, we have found that whenever an index case is *severely*

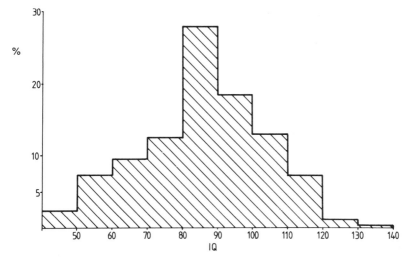

Fig. 6.4 Percentage distribution of IQ in Duchenne muscular dystrophy. (Data abstracted from Cohen *et al.* (1968); Marsh and Munsat (1974); Vignos (1977*a*); Leibowitz and Dubowitz (1981).)

mentally handicapped (IQ < 50) and has an affected brother, the latter is very often also severely mentally handicapped (Emery *et al.* 1979*b*; Emery 1984). The possibility that there might be bimodality in the distribution of IQ in affected boys was suggested by some earlier studies. But analysis of more recent and extensive data (from Cohen *et al.* 1968; Marsh and Munsat 1974; Vignos 1977*a*; Leibowitz and Dubowitz 1981) makes this seem unlikely (Fig. 6.4).

Perhaps because the mean depression of IQ in affected boys is relatively moderate, the majority of female carriers have normal IQs (Prosser *et al.* 1969). However, Murphy *et al.* (1965) and Bortolini and Zatz (1986) indicate that mental impairment may very occasionally be present in those with clinical manifestations and/or a very high SCK level.

Partition of IQ

Following the work of Sherwin and McCully in 1961, attempts have been made to determine what aspect of intellect may be especially affected in Duchenne muscular dystrophy by comparing performance and verbal IQs (Table 6.3). With one exception (Black 1973), verbal IQ is more affected, the overall difference from performance IQ being about 7 or 8 points. There is no suggestion of bimodality in the distribution of the *differences* between performance and verbal IQs (Table 6.4).

The impairment of verbal ability seems to be due to a defect in memory

Table 6.3 *Performance and verbal IQ in boys with Duchenne muscular dystrophy calculated from data given in various studies*

Reference	No.	Performance (P) Mean	s.d.	Verbal (V) Mean	s.d.	(P–V)
Zellweger and Niedermeyer (1965)	23	97.3	18.2	89.4	17.8	+7.9
Prosser *et al.* (1969)	39	88.0	14.2	87.1	16.5	+0.9
Black (1973)	25	80.2	22.4	84.8	19.1	−4.6
Marsh and Munsat (1974)	34	93.4	16.7	86.5	13.3	+6.9
Karagan and Zellweger (1978)	53	88.1	15.6	80.7	11.8	+7.4
Leibowitz and Dubowitz (1981)	54	91.5	16.0	83.7	19.3	+7.8
Appleton *et al.* (1991)	47	92.0	15.1	82.9	16.5	+9.1
Billard *et al.* (1991)	24	94.7	−	86.6	−	+8.1

for patterns, numbers, and verbal labels, implying a particular deficit, in memory function (Karagan *et al.* 1980). Some depression of verbal IQ has also been found in Becker muscular dystrophy but not in limb girdle or facioscapulohumeral muscular dystrophy (Karagan and Sorensen 1981). Interestingly, it seems that those boys with Duchenne muscular dystrophy who survive longest may have the least depression of verbal IQ (Miller, G. *et al.* 1985).

Behaviour and emotional disturbances

Behaviour and emotional disturbances have been commented upon by a number of investigators (Schorer 1964; Cohen *et al.* 1968; Leibowitz and Dubowitz 1981; Pullen 1984; Smith *et al.* 1990*a*). This seems likely to stem from a sense of failure, frustration, and distress generated by the progressive physical disability. However, in view of the nature of the disorder it is per- haps surprising that the majority of boys are not emotionally disturbed, and yet they are not. Nevertheless, allowing for age and IQ, boys with Duchenne muscular dystrophy do have a higher incidence of emotional disturbances than other physically handicapped children without cerebral involvement (Leibowitz and Dubowitz 1981), and it is just possible that this too could represent part of the disease. Epilepsy is not particularly frequent in Duchenne muscular dystrophy and visual and hearing acuity are normal (Allen 1973).

Neurological investigations

The failure to relate the impaired mental ability to any clear social or func- tional factors has led to the search for an organic explanation. Head cir-

Table 6.4 *Distribution of the differences between performance and verbal IQs (P–V)*

39 to 30	29 to 20	19 to 10	9 to 0	−1 to −10	−11 to −20	−21 to −30	Reference
0	5	9	14	3	2	1	Marsh and Munsat (1974)
2	5	17	13	12	4	0	Karagan and Zellweger (1978)
2	11	12	16	4	7	2	Leibowitz and Dubowitz (1981)
4	*21*	*38*	*43*	*19*	*13*	*3*	*Total*
2.8	*14.9*	*27.0*	*30.5*	*13.5*	*9.2*	*2.1*	*Percentage*

cumference appears to be significantly *greater* than normal but there is no correlation between head size and intellectual performance (Appleton *et al.* 1991). Electroencephalography (EEG) has been reported as normal in a carefully controlled and blind study by Barwick *et al.* (1965). In some other studies, however, up to a half of the records have been considered abnormal in some non-specific way (Zellweger and Niedermeyer 1965; Cohen *et al.* 1968; Kozicka *et al.* 1971; Black 1973; Florek and Karolak 1977). But many patients with apparently abnormal EEGs have had normal IQs. Whatever, no specific EEG abnormality has been detected in the disease.

Ventricular enlargement on pneumoencephalography has been reported in two cases (Hovstad *et al.* 1976). More recently the non-invasive technique of computerized tomography (CT) has been used to study central nervous system involvement. Yoshioka and colleagues (1980) found evidence of slight cerebral atrophy in two-thirds of the 30 cases they examined, and the older the patient the more severe was the atrophy. There were many with a low IQ in those with cerebral atrophy, but in those with apparently normal CT findings only three had a low IQ. Abnormal CT findings therefore seem to be associated with low IQ. Magnetic resonance imaging (MRI) has revealed no significant abnormality apart from mild cerebral atrophy in some cases (Al-Qudah *et al.* 1990).

Finally, Rosman and Kakulas (1966) examined the brains of seven cases of Duchenne muscular dystrophy (two at least of these could have been Becker muscular dystrophy). In all cases with mental defect they found microscopic heterotopias in the cerebral cortex. However, in a more extensive study of 21 cases of classical Duchenne muscular dystrophy, Dubowitz and Crome (1969) could detect no gross pathological abnormality. Detailed microscopic studies however have revealed abnormal dendritic development and arborization, at least in some cases, and the authors speculate that this may underlie the intellectual impairment (Jagadha and Becker 1988).

Skeletal system

A number of skeletal changes have been observed in Duchenne muscular dystrophy. They include progressive narrowing of the shafts of the long bones due to a reduction in the size of the medullary cavity and later thinning of the cortices. Since at the same time the head remains more or less the same size, the long bones assume a characteristic 'dumb bell' appearance (Fig. 6.5). There is often impaired development of the pelvic bones and scapulae, and various skeletal deformities occur including lumbar lordosis, scoliosis, and coxa valga. The bones themselves undergo progressive rarefaction and decalcification beginning at the ends of the long bones.

For a long time these changes were thought to be a direct consequence of a genetic defect, and such terms as 'bone dystrophy' and 'osteomyopathy'

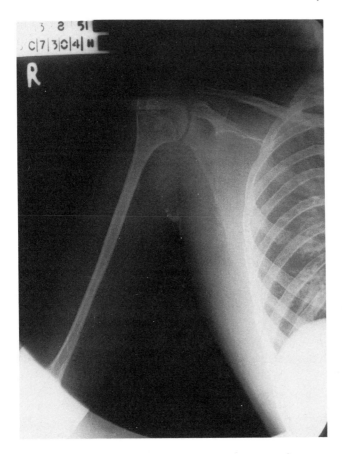

Fig. 6.5 Atrophy of the humerus in an advanced case of Duchenne muscular dystrophy. (Reproduced by kind permission of Lord Walton.)

were used. However, Walton and Warrick (1954) showed quite clearly that these same changes can occur in any disorder associated with prolonged immobility. They are not due to an associated genetic factor but to disuse: to the absence of the normal stresses and strains imposed by muscular attachments, and to the adoption of abnormal postures of the body and positions of the limbs as a consequence of muscle weakness and contractures.

Gastrointestinal system

Apart from manifestations of smooth muscle involvement affecting motility of the gastrointestinal tract which has been mentioned already (p. 109),

Bevans (1945) and Huvos and Pruzanski (1967) in reviewing the early literature referred to reports of recurrent diarrhoea and malabsorption in muscular dystrophy. Patterson *et al.* (1964) also furnished some evidence of
intestinal malabsorption but this work does not seem to have been repeated
or pursued further (Nowak *et al.* 1982). Clinically there is evidence of
oropharyngeal, oesophageal, and gastric dysfunction in the disease (Jaffe
et al. 1990), and gastric emptying is significantly delayed (Barohn *et al.*
1988), as is colonic transit (Gottrand *et al.* 1991). Constipation and halitosis
are frequent symptoms.

Other manifestations

Thymus hyperplasia has been noted in some cases (Bevans 1945; Huvos and
Pruzanski 1967), the relevance of which is not at all clear. Puberty can be
delayed, hyperoestrogenaemia occurs (Usuki *et al.* 1985), and obesity is frequent. There is no evidence of pancreatic dysfunction and an early report of
abnormal hepatic tests in some patients with muscular dystrophy (Morrell
1959) is difficult to interpret because no clear distinction was made between
Duchenne muscular dystrophy and other forms of dystrophy occurring later
in life.

However, apart from the study of skeletal muscle, cardiac muscle, and the
central nervous system, it has to be admitted that there have been few recent

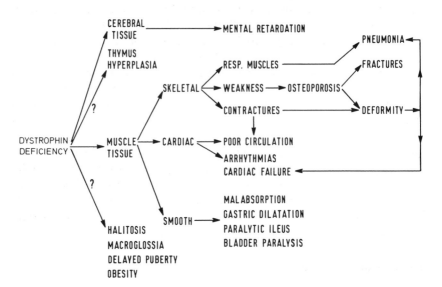

Fig. 6.6 Pleiotropic effects of the Duchenne gene. (From Emery (1990) with
permission.)

(Weiller 1985) systematic investigations of other systems, organs, or tissues.

With what is known so far, it is possible to construct a simple diagram of the pleiotropic effects of the Duchenne gene (Fig. 6.6). Some of the abnormalities found in the disease relate directly to skeletal, cardiac, and smooth muscle involvement. Others are at present more difficult to relate to the primary protein (dystrophin) defect in the disease.

Dystrophin synthesis and phenotype

Dystrophin mRNA represents less than 1 per cent of the total mRNA in skeletal muscle, yet its absence in Duchenne muscular dystrophy leads to a serious multisystem disease. The involvement of various organs and tissues can be explained by the fact that dystrophin transcripts are normally found not only in skeletal muscle, but also in cardiac muscle, smooth muscle of the gastrointestinal tract, and the brain as well as in various other tissues (Chelly *et al.* 1988). Its absence from these various tissues would explain their clinical involvement in the disease process. In the brain, for example, dystrophin is normally localized in the cortical synapses and its absence in Duchenne muscular dystrophy might account for central nervous system dysfuntion in the disease (Lidov *et al.* 1990). The situation however may not be quite so simple. It is now clear that muscle and brain dystrophin transcripts (and their encoded products) differ slightly in their structure and are controlled by different muscle and brain promoters (Nudel *et al.* 1989; Chelly *et al.* 1990*b*). It could be that the various clinical manifestations of the disease result from different levels of transcription of slightly different mRNAs in different tissues. There is also the possibility that the site and extent of mutations within the dystrophin gene itself may be related to the resultant phenotype. Several relatively small studies however have failed to find any correlation between the location and extent of dystrophin deletions and mental retardation. But Rapaport and her colleagues (1991*b*) in an extensive and detailed study of 66 patients with mental retardation found that almost twice as many were likely to have a deletion involving exon 52 than elsewhere in the dystrophin gene. But rather astonishingly two cases of Duchenne muscular dystrophy with normal intellect have been reported in whom the muscle-specific promoter as well as the brain-specific promoter (which lies 5′ of the former) were both deleted (Den Dunnen *et al.* 1991; Rapaport *et al.* 1992)! There is clearly scope for much further research in relating the multisystem involvement to the molecular basis of the disease.

Retinal neurotransmission

Though affected boys have normal visual acuity, electroretinography has revealed significant defects in most cases (Pillers *et al.* 1992). Furthermore, dystrophin has been localized to the outer plexiform layer of the normal retina (Bulman *et al*. 1992), and a defect in the retinal isoform in Duchenne muscular dystrophy may account for the observed retinographic changes and also indicates that dystrophin may well play a role in retinal neurotransmission.

Summary and conclusions

Most of the clinical features of Duchenne muscular dystrophy stem from involvement of skeletal muscle. However, there is increasing evidence that other tissues may also be directly affected by the disease.

Smooth muscle of the gastrointestinal tract and perhaps the bladder may be affected, and there is overwhelming evidence of cardiac muscle involvement, myocardial fibrosis being an important feature. This particularly affects the postero-basal portion of the left ventricle and accounts for the ECG changes of tall R waves in the right praecordial lead. They are evident from around the age of 6, and can be useful in the differentiation of Duchenne muscular dystrophy from other forms of motor disability in childhood. The vascular system does not appear to be affected and no consistent abnormalities in limb blood flow have been found.

There is clear evidence of a defect in cerebral function which is a direct consequence of the genetic defect most obviously expressed in a lowered IQ which on average is roughly one standard deviation below the normal mean, verbal IQ being more affected than performance IQ. Occasional behavioural and emotional disturbances may be associated with the disease.

The skeletal system is only secondarily affected by disuse atrophy, and so far there is no convincing evidence that any other tissues or organs are directly affected by the genetic defect.

The various clinical manifestations of Duchenne muscular dystrophy are now beginning to be related to the structure and functioning of the dystrophin gene in different tissues. There is much scope for research in relating the phenotype to molecular events in this disease.

7 Biochemistry of Duchenne muscular dystrophy

The literature on the biochemistry of muscular dystrophy is overwhelming and many biochemical abnormalities have been reported. It could be argued that now the primary defect has been identified in Duchenne muscular dystrophy and shown to be a deficiency of muscle dystrophin (Chapter 9), it is irrelevant to approach an understanding of pathogenesis through the findings of conventional biochemistry. I do not share this view but feel that molecular and biochemical studies could complement each other. What has been learned so far concerning biochemical changes in dystrophic muscle and how these relate to the deficiency of dystrophin will doubtless fill in details of how the disease process starts and progresses, and why it affects some muscles more than others. It is also conceivable that the more we know of the detailed pathogenesis of Duchenne muscular dystrophy the more we may understand these processes in other muscular dystrophies. And with such detail it may be possible to better consider a rational approach to any drug therapy.

Selection of material, patients, and controls

One important problem is the selection of appropriate material for study. Muscle is clearly the obvious choice but there is then the problem of assessing the significance of any changes which could be secondary to the disease process. There is also the very serious practical problem of obtaining material for study. In the past this was a major restraint. Investigators were forced to store material against the day when it might be used for a particular study, but there was then the possibility of changes taking place during the period of storage. The use of needle biopsy technique (p. 56) avoids these difficulties to some extent because it can be repeated, though even this is not a procedure to be undertaken lightly in a small boy. The stage of the disease is also important for clearly abnormalities found early in the course of the disease are more likely to be closer to the basic biochemical defect. It is for this latter reason that studies have sometimes been extended to healthy female carriers in the belief that any abnormalities found in such individuals are more likely to be meaningful. But in carriers there is also the problem of X-inactivation, and some may be expected to exhibit no abnormalities at all if the majority of their active X chromosomes are those bearing the normal gene.

It is a *sine qua non* that diagnosis in the affected individual has first to be clearly established, and of course material removed at biopsy can be used for both diagnostic histology and dystrophin studies as well as biochemical research. Unfortunately, all too often in the past Duchenne muscular dystrophy has not been differentiated from other forms of dystrophy or even from spinal muscular atrophy.

The choice of appropriate controls is also a problem for the diagnosis is usually established in an affected boy around the age of 3 to 5 years of age. Appropriate muscle tissue, usually the gastrocnemius, from a normal boy of this age is not too easily acquired. It is easier to obtain specimens of rectus abdominis muscle at laparotomy for example, but some would question whether it is valid to compare findings in this muscle with gastrocnemius muscle. Nor does it seem justified to use for comparisons only muscle tissue from other neuromuscular disorders such as spinal muscular atrophy or polymyositis, although such studies may later be necessary in order to establish whether or not any abnormality is specific to Duchenne muscular dystrophy.

Molecular basis

When the gene responsible for a particular disorder can be isolated and cloned, it is possible to see what the gene synthesizes. The product can then be compared with normal and in this way the biochemical basis of the disease can be identified. This has sometimes been referred to as 'reverse genetics' for, in the past, it was necessary to start by identifying the product of the defective gene, but now it is possible to identify the mutant gene first and then determine its product. This has been successfully achieved in Duchenne muscular dystrophy where the primary genetic defect has been shown to be a deficiency of dystrophin (p. 187).

Muscle tissue

There have been many excellent reviews of earlier reported biochemical abnormalities in Duchenne muscular destrophy, some of the most valuable and penetrating being provided by Ellis (1978), Rowland (1980), Lucy (1980), Pennington (1980, 1988), and Armstrong and Appel (1981). It would be impossible to review all the abnormal findings which have been reported, nor would this be valuable. Instead, the discussion will concentrate on those which have been found in *early* cases of the disease and preferably have been confirmed in several different laboratories.

It should be pointed out from the beginning that no consistent abnormality has ever been found in any of the obvious muscle proteins such as myoglobin, actin, myosin, tropomyosin, and troponin (Pennington 1988).

The various biochemical changes which have been observed in affected muscle can be conveniently considered as being the result of wasting, invasion by other tissue elements, and 'dedifferentiation'.

Muscle wasting

As the disease progresses so functioning muscle tissue degenerates, and is gradually replaced by fat and connective tissue. If the results are expressed in terms of *total* muscle weight then particular constituents may appear to be reduced when in fact the levels in *functioning* muscle tissue may be normal. A solution to this problem is to express results in terms of some specific reference base. In the past this has been total protein or better still non-collagen protein which corresponds to that fraction of the total muscle protein which is soluble in dilute alkali (Lilienthal *et al.* 1950; Pennington and Robinson 1968). In health the amount of non-collagen protein (expressed as non-collagen nitrogen) is roughly the same in different skeletal muscles (Table 7.1) and at least in later childhood and young adulthood it is not significantly affected by age or sex. Non-collagen protein represents over 90 per cent of the total protein of normal muscle but it may be less than 50 per cent in severely affected dystrophic muscle (Horvath and Proctor 1960).

Myosin or some similar contractile protein has also been recommended as a reference base (Samaha *et al.* 1981). Whereas fibroblasts, macrophages, lipocytes, and other cells present in dystrophic tissue might contribute to non-collagen protein, they would not affect the myosin content. As would

Table 7.1 *Non-collagen nitrogen (NCN) expressed as mg. (g wet weight)$^{-1}$, in various normal human skeletal muscles (unpublished data)*

Muscle	No.	NCN Mean	NCN s.d.
Rectus abdominis	20	23.3	6.2
Gastrocnemius	8	26.7	5.5
Deltoid	6	20.7	2.7
Pectoralis major	10	23.9	5.6
Miscellaneous*	9	24.0	3.6
Total	53	23.7	5.3

* Quadriceps (3); sternomastoid (2); sartorius (1); transversalis (1); diaphragm (1); latissimus dorsi (1).

be expected, and known for a long time (Vignos and Lefkowitz 1959), as dystrophic muscle degenerates so its myosin content decreases. When levels of ATP and creatine phosphate are expressed in terms of myosin they are no different from normal (Samaha *et al*. 1981). This result is in stark contrast to several earlier studies which reported reduced levels using non-collagen protein as the reference base. Normal levels of ATP have also been confirmed by the technique of nuclear magnetic resonance (NMR) by Griffiths *et al*. (1985). That ATP levels are normal has important implications. It means that energy stores for muscle contraction are adequate, at least early

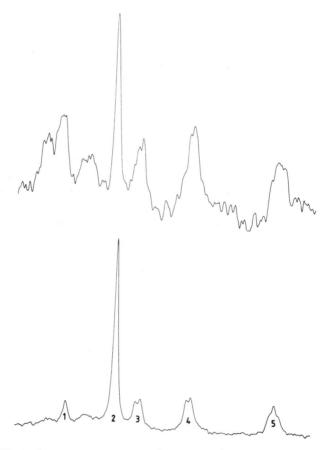

Fig. 7.1 Magnetic resonance spectrum of gastrocnemius muscle in a control (*below*), and a 15-year-old boy with Duchenne muscular dystrophy (*above*). In the affected boy there is a significant increase in intracellular pH (normal 7.01, affected 7.28) and an apparent reduction in the ratio of creatine phosphate to inorganic phosphate (1, inorganic phosphate; 2, creatine phosphate; 3–5, ATP peaks). (Reproduced by kind permission of Dr S. P. Frostick.)

in the course of the disease, and therefore this is *not* the cause of muscle weakness (Edwards 1977). The latter seems more likely to be a reflection of the loss of muscle fibres due to their degeneration. However, studies using nuclear magnetic resonance (now referred to as magnetic resonance spectroscopy) seem to indicate (S. O. Frostick, personal communication, 1986) that creatine phosphate may be reduced (Fig. 7.1).

As the amount of functioning muscle tissue decreases, this has several other consequences. Occasionally the glucose tolerance curve may be mildly abnormal, due to an inadequate disposal of glucose associated with the reduced muscle mass (Haymond *et al*. 1978), and plasma free fatty acids may be raised (Takagi *et al*. 1970). Glucose and lipid metabolism have been studied in detail by Nishio *et al*. (1990) and the abnormal energy metabolism they observed is atributed to either calorie shortage or, more likely, muscle degeneration. More importantly, changes occur in creatine and creatinine metabolism, changes which have also been recognized for many years (Levene and Kristeller 1909). Creatine is largely synthesized in the liver and is delivered to the skeletal muscle where it is converted to creatinine which readily diffuses into the circulation and is excreted in the urine. In fact the amount of creatinine excreted each day by any individual is remarkably constant and is roughly proportional to the total body muscle mass.

In general terms as muscle wastes from whatever cause, so the level of creatine in the plasma and especially the urine will increase, and the amount of creatinine in the urine will decrease. These changes however appear to be somewhat removed from the basic defect in dystrophy, not only because they are not specific, but also because no abnormalities in creatine and creatinine excretion occur in female carriers of the disease unless they have significant

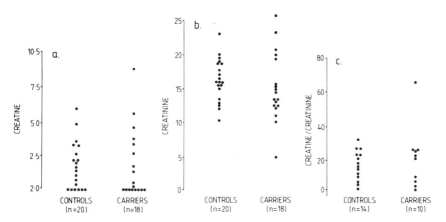

Fig. 7.2 The urinary excretion of (*a*) creatine, (*b*) creatinine (mg kg^{-1} 24 h^{-1}), and (*c*) ratio of creatine/creatinine (×100) in healthy women and carriers of Duchenne muscular dystrophy. (Unpublished data.)

muscle weakness (Emery 1963). Of 10 female carriers investigated, in only one who was a manifesting carrier with marked muscle weakness, was the creatine/creatinine ratio abnormally high (Fig. 7.2).

As skeletal muscle degenerates various breakdown products will be released and appear in the urine. For example, 3-methylhistidine is a known constituent of both actin and myosin, and as muscle breaks down the concentration in muscle decreases, and when expressed in terms of creatinine the urinary excretion increases (Ballard *et al.* 1979). In fact the urinary excretion of 3-methylhistidine is an excellent measurement of myofibrillar protein catabolism (Mussini *et al.* 1984). Thus, while creatinine excretion may be taken as an index of total muscle mass, 3-methylhistidine excretion is an index of muscle breakdown.

Carnitine is largely synthesized in the liver and kidneys and is subsequently taken up by cardiac and skeletal muscle. As muscle breaks down so carnitine is released and concentrations in dystrophic muscle are significantly reduced (Berthillier *et al.* 1982). Since carnitine is an important co-factor in fatty acid oxidation, the reduction in muscle carnitine might also explain the accumulation of long-chain fatty acid derivatives in this tissue (Carroll *et al.* 1983).

Ionasescu and colleagues have reported increased muscle ribosomal protein synthesis and collagen synthesis *in vitro* not only in affected boys but also in some carriers (Ionasescu and Ionasescu 1982). The idea that this increased protein synthesis may reflect attempted regeneration is attractive.

The loss of contractile muscle protein in Duchenne muscular dystrophy could result from a reduced rate of synthesis, an abnormally high rate of degradation or a combination of both. *In vivo* protein synthesis has been measured by the intravenous infusion of labelled leucine, the incorporation of which into skeletal muscle is subsequently determined in needle biopsy specimens. These experiments have suggested that *total* muscle protein synthesis may actually be reduced in Duchenne muscular dystrophy (Rennie *et al.* 1982). However, these observations were made on boys aged 12 to 18 years when any attempts at regeneration are clearly failing. It would certainly be valuable to know what happens to *in vivo* protein synthesis in the very early stages of the disease.

Finally, although there is no doubt that many proteins are lost from dystrophic muscle, there is also evidence that some substances may actually *enter* affected muscle fibres. Experimentally, ingress of horseradish peroxidase (MW 40 000 Da) (Mokri and Engel 1975), and Procion yellow (MW 674 Da) (Bradley and Fulthorpe 1978) have been demonstrated, and evidence suggests that calcium (p. 199), IgG and complement (Engel and Biesecker 1982), and albumin (Cornelio and Dones 1984) enter affected muscle fibres.

Of particular interest is the finding that calcium and albumin enter fibres lacking dystrophin in female carriers of X-linked dystrophy (Morandi *et al.*

1990). This has important implications for pathogenesis and will be discussed later (p. 199).

Enzyme changes in dystrophic muscle

There is general agreement that glycolysis as well as the activities of most individual glycolytic enzymes are reduced in muscle from patients with Duchenne muscular dystrophy as well as several other dystrophies (Ronzoni *et al.* 1960). Ellis' detailed studies indicate that in dystrophic muscle fructose is incorporated into the glycogen pathway at the expense of glucose and this results in increased lipogenesis (Ellis 1980). Fatty acid oxidation is also reduced but again this is not specific to Duchenne muscular dystrophy (Shumate *et al.* 1982).

A great many individual enzymes have been studied in muscle tissue from patients with Duchenne muscular dystrophy. (For example, Dreyfus *et al.* 1956; Vignos and Lefkowitz 1959; Heyck *et al.* 1963; DiMauro *et al.* 1967; Pennington 1962, 1977*a*, 1988; Kar and Pearson 1980.) In those instances where enzyme levels have been expressed in terms of non-collagen protein and studies made specifically on Duchenne muscular dystrophy, some general conclusions can be made. The level of activity of some enzymes appears to be normal, at least in the early stages of the disease (Table 7.2).

Other enzymes however have reduced activity (Table 7.3), in some cases even from very early on in the disease process as in the case of AMP deaminase (Kar and Pearson 1973). Interestingly, a deficiency of the

Table 7.2 *Enzymes with* normal *activity in skeletal muscle tissue in Duchenne muscular dystrophy*

Aminotransferases (GPT, GOT)
Succinic dehydrogenase
Hexokinase
Phosphohexose isomerase
Aconitase
Cytochrome oxidase
Alkaline phosphatase
Acyl phosphatase
Fructose 1,6-diphosphatase
Lysolecithin phospholipase
Superoxide dismutase
Methylthioadenosine nucleosidase
Adenylosuccinase
Monamine oxidase
Glyoxalase II

Table 7.3 *Enzymes with* reduced *activity
in skeletal muscle tissue in
Duchenne muscular dystrophy*

Phosphoglucomutase
Phosphofructokinase
Aldolase
Triosephosphate isomerase
Phosphoglyceraldehyde dehydrogenase
Phosphoglycerate kinase
Enolase
Pyruvate kinase
Lactate dehydrogenase
Fumarase
Glycogen phosphorylase
Glycogen synthetase
Creatine kinase
AMP deaminase
Adenylate kinase

erythrocyte form of phosphofructokinase is not associated with muscle disease but results is a non-spherocytic haemolytic anaemia (Etiemble *et al.* 1976).

The reduced activity of these various enzymes is probably largely the result of efflux from diseased muscle fibres though this cannot be the entire story. Thus, adenylate kinase, which has a relatively low molecular weight (21 000 Da), is reduced in affected muscle but is not increased in serum (p. 49) and this is also true of AMP deaminase. On the other hand, the aminotransferases are not significantly reduced in affected muscle but are increased in serum. Finally, acyl phosphatase is one of the smallest enzyme molecules known (9400 Da) and is abundant in skeletal muscle, largely in the soluble sarcoplasm, yet there is apparently normal activity in affected muscle (Kar and Pearson 1972*a*, but see Nassi *et al.* 1985). The explanation for these apparent contradictions may lie in the relative rates of synthesis (perhaps influenced to some extent by physical activity) versus destruction of different enzymes in affected muscle fibres, as well as their clearance rates from plasma. So far, however, very little is known of the relative importance of these different factors for individual enzymes (Pennington 1988).

Finally, and perhaps more interestingly, the activity of some enzymes is actually *increased* in Duchenne muscular dystrophy (Table 7.4). These changes are attributable to the invasion of affected muscle by macrophages and fibroblasts, as well as to the necrosis of affected muscle fibres. Macrophages and fibroblasts are known to contain several NADP-linked dehydrogenases (glucose-6-phosphate dehydrogenase, 6-phosphogluconate

Table 7.4 *Enzymes with* increased *activity
in skeletal muscle tissue in
Duchenne muscular dystrophy*

Glucose-6-phosphate dehydrogenase
6-Phosphogluconate dehydrogenase
Isocitrate dehydrogenase
Malate dehydrogenase
5'-Nucleotidase
Ribonuclease
Glutathione reductase
Prote(in)ases
Carnitine palmityltransferase
Lipid peroxidation
Phosphodiesterases

dehydrogenase, isocitrate dehydrogenase, and malate dehydrogenase), and other enzymes such as 5'-nucleotidase and ribonuclease. These cells also contain a number of proteases, including cathepsins, lysosomal acid hydrolases, and calcium activated proteases, which are all increased in dystrophic muscle (Pennington 1977b; Kar and Pearson 1972b, 1977). These enzymes attack and break down muscle protein and their increase is probably also an adaptive response of the muscle fibre to its degeneration and necrosis (Pennington 1988).

It should be noted, however, that this division into enzymes which are normal, reduced, or increased in dystrophic muscle though convenient is somewhat arbitrary because it often depends at what stage in the disease process the assays are carried out. In almost all cases activity is normal at the beginning and abnormally low or high levels are found only later in the course of the disease. But some, such as acyl phosphatase, seem to remain at more or less normal levels right until the very late stages of the disease.

Membrane enzymes

Many muscle enzymes are free in the sarcoplasm but some are attached to membranes, such as the sarcoplasmic reticulum. The latter include adenylate cyclase, guanylate cyclase, and Ca^{2+}, $(Na^+ + K^+)$, and Mg^{2+}-ATPases. Until fairly recently enzyme studies have been limited to whole muscle homogenates which, at least later, are contaminated by extraneous adipose and connective tissue. It has therefore not been possible to study the activity in isolation of those enzymes which are attached specifically to muscle membranes. To circumvent this problem minimally affected muscle should be studied, and the technique of using 'skinned fibres' has been developed, largely by Takagi and colleagues in Japan (Takagi and Nonaka 1981; Takagi

1984). In these preparations the surface membrane of the muscle fibre is removed mechanically or disrupted chemically. Using these techniques it seems that in the *early* stages of the disease the sarcoplasmic reticulum and contractile protein functions are normal (Wood 1984) as is calcium uptake by the sarcoplasmic reticulum (Takagi 1984). The study of skinned fibres has also shown that in Duchenne muscular dystrophy, despite the deficiency of dystrophin, these contract normally and therefore the myofibrils must themselves be intrinsically normal (Horowitz *et al.* 1990).

'Dedifferentiation'

A number of observations indicate that in many ways dystrophic muscle resembles fetal muscle for which the term 'dedifferentiation' has sometimes been used. Firstly, it is less easy to distinguish different histochemical fibre types in dystrophic muscle (W. K. Engel 1970) which is also a feature of fetal muscle (Fig. 7.3), even at term (Toop 1975). Secondly, certain phospholipid changes in dystrophic muscle (more sphingomyelin, less lecithin plus choline plasmalogen, and more total cholesterol) are very similar to those found in fetal muscle (Hughes 1972). Thirdly, fetal myosins are found in muscle from patients with Duchenne muscular dystrophy and spinal muscular atrophy (Fitzsimons and Hoh 1981). Fourthly, another fetal isoform of muscle protein re-expressed in regenerating muscle is cardiac troponin-T (Gorza *et al.* 1991). Finally, and most intriguingly, the isoenzyme patterns of dystrophic muscle resemble fetal muscle rather than adult muscle. This was first shown in the case of lactate dehydrogenase (LDH) (Dreyfus *et al.* 1962; Wieme and

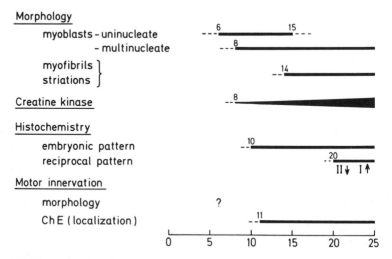

Fig. 7.3 Times (weeks of gestation) at which various aspects of muscle development become apparent. Ch E, choline esterase. (Data from various sources.)

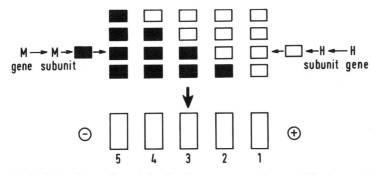

Fig. 7.4 The formation of the five isoenzymes of lactate dehydrogenase.

Herpol 1962). This enzyme is composed of five isoenzymes, each being formed by the tetrameric association of two sub-units, synthesized by two separate genes, referred to as M and H (Fig. 7.4). The M sub-unit predominates in adult skeletal muscle and the H sub-unit in cardiac muscle. On electrophoresis the most rapidly migrating isoenzyme LDH-1 has the composition H_4, LDH-2 = H_3M, LDH-3 = H_2M_2, LDH-4 = HM_3, and LDH-5 = M_4. The amounts and proportions of the M and H sub-units (LDH-M, LDH-H) can be determined in a number of ways including preferential inhibition by urea (Emery 1967*a*). The proportions of LDH-M and LDH-H in some normal skeletal muscles are given in Table 7.5.

Although there are some variations in different skeletal muscles, LDH-M clearly predominates. However, in fetal skeletal muscle LDH-H predominates, and the isoenzyme pattern resembles that seen in Duchenne muscular dystrophy even in the preclinical phase (Fig. 7.5). It may be that the normal adult pattern is never attained, in which case the term

Table 7.5 *Proportions (%) of LDH-M and LDH-H in various normal skeletal muscles (unpublished data)*

Muscle	No.	LDH–M	LDH–H
Rectus abdominis	5	87.0	13.0
Diaphragm	1	89.2	10.8
Gastrocnemius	3	86.7	13.3
Quadriceps	1	89.6	10.4
Latissimus dorsi	1	87.4	12.6
Pectoralis major	6	87.9	12.1
Deltoid	2	95.6	4.4
Soleus	2	67.1	32.9

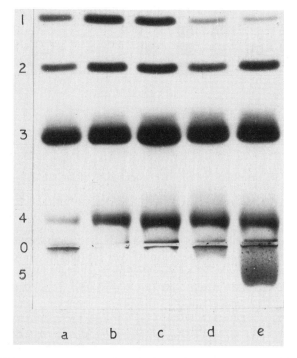

Fig. 7.5 LDH isoenzyme patterns in muscle extracts from: (*a*) 3-year-old boy with preclinical Duchenne muscular dystrophy, (*b*) 400 g fetus, (*c*) 7-month stillbirth, (*d*) neonate, (*e*) 3-month-old normal infant. O is the origin and the anode is at the top.

'dedifferentiation' is hardly appropriate. Incidentally, there does not appear to be a complete absence of LDH-5 in all cases of Duchenne muscular dystrophy. A reduction in LDH-M is also found in some female carriers (Emery 1964*b*) but the change is not specific to Duchenne muscular dystrophy but is also found in a number of other neuromuscular disorders (Emery 1968).

Analogous changes in isoenzyme patterns have since been reported for creatine kinase, aldolase, isocitrate dehydrogenase, malate dehydrogenase, adenylate kinase, and enolase (reviewed by Ellis 1978).

The implication of these various findings is that dystrophic muscle synthesizes polypeptides not normally produced postnatally and that these changes are presumably a result of regenerative activity: newly synthesized peptides reflecting the activity of genes normally active only during fetal development. The enzyme hypoxanthine–guanine phosphoribosyltransferase is significantly increased in muscle in patients with Duchenne muscular dystrophy even from the age of 2, and this has been interpreted as being a means of enhancing increased protein synthesis and regenerative activity (Neerunjun *et al.* 1979). Finally, using immunohistochemical techniques, the re-expression of fetal-specific myosins has now in fact been localized to regenerating fibres in Duchenne muscular dystrophy (Schiaffino *et al.* 1986).

Cultured myoblasts

The study of myoblasts in tissue culture, free from all the possible confounding effects of extraneous factors, would seem to offer the ideal system for investigating Duchenne muscular dystrophy. Unfortunately, it soon became clear that there were serious technical difficulties to be overcome in this approach, not least of which was the presence of other cell types (mostly fibroblasts) which 'contaminate' such cultures. This was particularly a problem with primary explants where the biopsy material is first freed of any obvious fat and connective tissue, and then small fragments, about 1 mm in size, are grown in culture vessels with appropriate nutrient medium, usually enriched with chick embryo extract or fetal calf serum. To avoid problems of possible contamination with fibroblasts, cellular outgrowths from explants can be dissociated and the dissociated cells then transferred to secondary monolayer cultures, a procedure which can be repeated. In this way we chose to study fetal muscle in which fibroblast contamination is minimal in any event (Fig. 7.6). A dissociation technique coupled with special culture conditions can also be used which ensures that growth of myoblasts is encouraged at the expense of other cell types (Yasin *et al.* 1977).

As a further refinement *clonal* cultures can be set up whereby the progeny of single myoblasts can be studied. Finally, muscle–nerve co-cultures (e.g. Duchenne muscular dystrophy muscle and rodent spinal cord) can be used to study the possible effects of innervation *in vitro* (Askanas *et al.* 1985; Peterson *et al.* 1986).

Whether muscle is cultured aneurally or innervated, no *gross* morphological abnormalities are evident in Duchenne muscular dystrophy (Askanas *et al.* 1987). Detailed scanning electron microscopic studies, however, have revealed changes in cell surface morphology, which could explain the low adhesiveness and delayed fusion of dystrophic myoblasts in culture, and these abnormalities are expressed maximally *after* myoblast fusion (Delaporte *et al.* 1990). Some reported biochemical abnormalities have been interpreted by Miranda and Mongini (1984) as indicating that dystrophic muscle in culture reaches a lesser degree of maturity than normal muscle. For example, in dystrophic muscle culture creatine kinase BB isoenzyme is significantly increased (and the CK MM decreased), although this is not specific to Duchenne muscular dystrophy (Franklin *et al.* 1981). Protein degradation rate in cultured Duchenne muscle cells is normal which

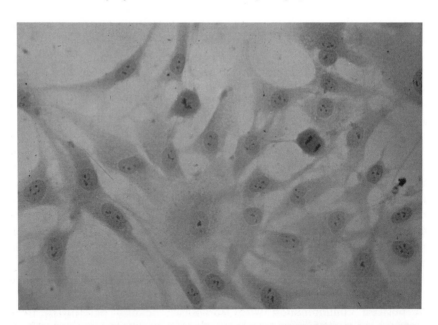

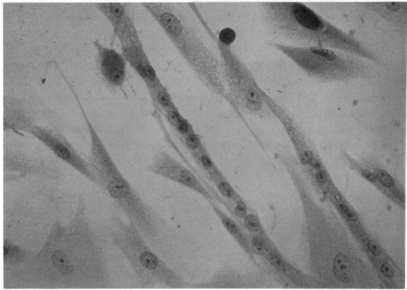

Fig. 7.6 Fetal muscle in tissue culture. (*Above*) dividing uninucleate myoblasts. (*Below*) fusion of myoblasts to form multinucleate myotubes.

supports the idea (p. 130) that the loss of contractile muscle proteins in the disease is largely the result of reduced synthesis rather than increased degradation (Neville and Harrold 1985).

With regard to the expression of dystrophin in cultured muscle, normally it is not demonstrable in undifferentiated myoblasts but appears only after myoblast fusion to form myotubes (Lev *et al.* 1987; Scott *et al.* 1988). At first it appears in circumscribed areas in the sarcoplasm but later in more mature myotubes it appears predominantly at the sarcolemma. Since these observations have been made with cultured aneural muscle and in the absence of 'trophic' nerve factors, the expression of dystrophin *per se* does not require innervation. But muscle contractile activity induced by innervation does play an important role in determining the *continuous* and *even distribution* of dystrophin in the sarcolemma (Park *et al.* 1991). Thus the sequence of changes in the distribution of dystrophin in developing muscle *in vitro* is not very dissimilar from that which occurs during the development of fetal muscle *in vivo* (Wessels *et al.* 1991).

In cultured Duchenne muscle, dystrophin is virtually absent, even in mature myotubes (Miranda *et al.* 1988). Furthermore, in clonal myogenic cell cultures from heterozygous female carriers, as might be expected, some clones express dystrophin whereas others do not (Hurko *et al.* 1989). Cultured Becker muscle expresses dystrophin with an expected abnormal molecular weight (Sklar *et al.* 1990).

What light do these various studies throw on the pathogenesis of Duchenne dystrophy? Perhaps one of the most interesting findings is an increase in intracellular calcium in aneurally cultured dystrophic muscle at a time when dystrophin would be expressed in normal tissue (Mongini *et al.* 1988; Fong *et al.* 1990). However the relationship between innervation, the expression of dystrophin, and subsequent intracellular events is complex. Muscle development (Kelly and Blau, 1992) both *in vitro* and *in vivo* involves the interplay of a number of myogenic factors as well as innervation (Fig. 7.7).

The interactions between these factors and dystrophin expression might be crucial in determining the full expression of dystrophy in cultured cells. As Valerie Askanas (personal communication, 1991) has postulated '. . . even

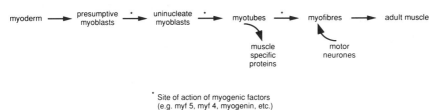

Site of action of myogenic factors
(e.g. myf 5, myf 4, myogenin, etc.)

Fig. 7.7 The site of action of myogenic factors during muscle development.

though there is dystrophin deficiency in cultured Duchenne muscle, only some aspects of the abnormal phenotype, namely calcium accumulation (aneural cultures) and decreased CK–MM (innervated cultures), are expressed. It is possible that more advanced maturation of muscle is require for the full expression of an abnormal phenotype in Duchenne muscle in culture, which would be similar to the situation occurring *in vivo* . . .'.

Cultured fibroblasts

The growth, behaviour, morphology, and biochemistry of skin fibroblasts in tissue culture from patients with Duchenne muscular dystrophy have been studied intensely in recent years. Unfortunately, some earlier observations have either not been corroborated subsequently, or have not been repeated and it is often difficult to assess the relevance of an isolated finding.

Recent reports seem to substantiate some earlier indications that though the cells grow in size and divide normally (Hirsch-Kauffmann *et al.* 1985), intercellular adhesiveness may be reduced, although there is much overlap with controls (Jones and Witkowski 1983), and muscle cell motility *in vitro* is not significantly different from normal (Witkowski and Dubowitz 1985). Ribosomal protein synthesis has been reported to be reduced (Pöche and Schulze 1985).

However emphasis has now turned to what is termed 'illegitimate' transcription of dystrophin in skin fibroblasts. The amounts of transcript synthesized are of course very small and for their study they need to be amplified by PCR (p. 73). The use of skin fibroblasts in this way does provide a very useful tool for investigating pathological transcripts in easily accessible material (Chelly *et al.* 1989).

Peripheral blood leucocytes

There have so far been few studies directed toward studying the metabolism of peripheral blood leucocytes in Duchenne muscular dystrophy. Yet in many ways this provides an ideal tissue for such studies.

Several individual enzymes, including phosphorylases, appear to have normal activity in leucocytes from patients with Duchenne muscular dystrophy (Scholte and Busch 1980). Our own studies of leucocytes in short-term culture have revealed no defect in glycolysis or the tricarboxylic acid cycle and electron transport chain (Emery *et al.* 1971). Furthermore there appears to be no *major* defect in fatty acid oxidation (β-oxidation) either (King and Emery 1973). 'Illegitimate' transcription of dystrophin in peripheral blood leucocytes provides yet another approach to studying defective transcription in Duchenne muscular dystrophy.

Serum

Most studies have concentrated on the levels of various muscle enzymes in the serum of patients with Duchenne muscular dystrophy. Elevated levels of most enzymes can be accounted for by their relative abundance in muscle tissue as compared with serum, and their release from dystrophic muscle into the circulation (p. 49). It has been suggested that enzymes may also be released from other organs, including the liver (Kleine 1970), but the evidence is not very convincing. Certainly the characteristic liver enzymes, γ-glutamyltransferase and sorbitol dehydrogenase, are normal.

Whatever the mechanism of muscle enzyme release, this is not a significant factor in producing muscle weakness because serum levels are highest when muscle weakness is least, and drugs such as thyroid hormones, diethylstilboestrol, and lithium carbonate when given orally for some time are associated with a decrease in serum enzyme activity in boys with Duchenne muscular dystrophy but there is no marked effect on muscle strength. How these diverse compounds affect enzyme release is not known (Rowland 1980).

Other serum proteins which are raised to varying degrees in the serum of patients with Duchenne muscular dystrophy include: α_2-globulin, myoglobin, and haemopexin which binds myoglobin and other haem compounds. However, all these various proteins also occur in normal serum, albeit often at very low levels. No abnormal metabolite has yet been detected in serum in Duchenne muscular dystrophy.

'Toxic plasma factor'

Although it seems most likely that the release of muscle proteins into the circulation is the result of muscle necrosis and/or the molecular defect in the muscle membrane, there is also the possibility that some circulating 'toxin' might affect the membrane and further increase its permeability. Evidence on this point is scanty. Sugita and Tyler (1963) incubated rat intact peroneus longus muscles in Krebs–Ringer-bicarbonate-glucose buffer to which they added fresh serum from controls and boys with Duchenne muscular dystrophy in the proportion of 1 ml to 30 ml of buffer. In the controls there was little creatine kinase activity in the buffer solution, but with serum from affected boys, creatine kinase activity progressively increased over a two hour incubation period. These interesting observations however do not seem to have been repeated.

The effects of dystrophic serum on normal erythrocyte ATPase activity have been studied by Peter *et al.* (1969) and Lloyd and Emery (1981). These investigators found that $(Na^+ + K^+)$ATPase activity in erythrocyte ghosts is inhibited by ouabain in normal controls but stimulated in Duchenne muscular dystrophy. However, if normal ghosts were incubated in Duchenne serum then their activity also became stimulated by ouabain. The serum 'factor' responsible for this effect was rendered inactive by deproteination. Peter *et al.* (1969) have suggested that one possible explanation for these findings is that an autoimmune process may be involved whereby damaged muscle membranes induce an antibody response to membranes in general, but at present there is no experimental evidence for this interesting idea (but see p. 203).

Finally, a number of investigators have noted some increase in SCK activity when serum is diluted before assay, and it has therefore been postulated that there may be an inhibitor of the enzyme in plasma. However since the effect is observed in serum samples from normal women as well as carriers of Duchenne muscular dystrophy (Simpson *et al.* 1979) it is unlikely to be related to dystrophy *per se*.

Urine

As in the case of serum, no abnormal metabolites have been detected in urine specifically in Duchenne muscular dystrophy. The changes in urinary composition which have been observed can all be explained on the basis of the release of various breakdown products from degenerating muscle into the circulation and then excretion in the urine. As described previously (p. 129), the urinary excretion of creatine is increased, whereas the excretion of creatinine is decreased so that the ratio of creatine to creatinine in the urine is significantly increased.

Breakdown products excreted in increased amounts in urine, when expressed in terms of creatinine, include carnitine (DiMauro and Rowland 1976), various amino acids (Bank *et al.* 1971; Emery *et al.* 1979*b*), and 3-methylhistidine (p. 130). The aminoaciduria in Duchenne muscular dystrophy is generalized with no consistent pattern (plasma amino acid levels are normal). Our own results determined by ion-exchange chromatography using a single-column gradient elution technique are given in Table 7.6. Frank myoglobinuria is not associated with Duchenne muscular dystrophy (Rowland 1984).

None of these changes in urinary composition are specific to Duchenne muscular dystrophy but may be found in any neuromuscular disorder in which muscle breakdown occurs. The increased urinary excretion of dimethylarginines in muscular dystrophy however has a different origin (Inoue *et al.* 1979; Lou 1979; Hirano *et al.* 1983). N^G, N^G-Dimethylarginine is mainly located in cell nuclei as a component of non-histone nuclear protein and its increased excretion reflects myosin turnover in muscle regenerating from satellite cells. It is therefore an index of regenerative activity and could be a useful parameter for assessing the value of any proposed therapy.

Table 7.6 *Urinary excretion of amino acids (mg.100 mg.α-amino N$_2^-$'24 h^{-1}) in boys with Duchenne muscular dystrophy and severe mental handicap (+MH, N = 12) and normal intelligence (−MH, N = 7), and healthy boys of the same age (N = 6) (unpublished data)*

	+MH		−MH		Controls	
Amino acid	Mean*	s.d.	Mean*	s.d.	Mean	s.d.
Taurine	*59.1*	55.6	23.3	10.8	19.8	10.0
Hydroxyproline	0.0	0.0	*0.6*	1.5	0.0	0.0
Aspartic acid	1.3	1.9	1.5	1.3	2.3	3.0
Threonine	9.4	5.8	7.4	4.0	6.7	1.5
Serine	*23.6*	17.0	9.9	6.8	11.9	3.0
Glutamine	*47.9*	52.0	24.5	7.9	26.7	6.8
Asparagine	0.3	0.9	0.3	0.5	0.7	0.9
Glutamic acid	*5.2*	9.0	*3.9*	5.1	0.9	0.4
Proline	0.0	0.0	0.5	0.8	0.1	0.2
Glycine	*92.8*	86.8	*33.0*	12.6	24.5	4.1
Alanine	*23.9*	22.7	9.9	4.6	11.1	2.7
Cystine	7.7	10.3	2.0	2.3	2.6	3.4
Valine	*4.9*	3.9	*5.6*	10.8	1.8	0.8
Methionine	0.3	0.5	0.8	0.3	1.1	0.4
Isoleucine	*1.2*	1.5	*1.1*	0.9	0.5	0.1
Leucine	0.8	1.0	3.6	2.9	4.4	1.8
Tyrosine	11.6	8.8	6.4	3.3	6.4	3.7
Phenylalanine	*7.0*	5.0	3.5	1.8	3.1	0.9
β-Amino isobutyric acid	10.7	18.7	3.2	2.9	4.7	4.0
Ethanolamine	12.2	9.3	3.0	1.2	6.2	4.1
Ornithine	*4.5*	2.7	1.0	0.5	1.7	0.9
Lysine	7.9	5.4	6.3	4.5	4.5	2.7
Histidine	*93.3*	61.4	46.4	18.1	43.7	11.9
Tryptophan	5.1	9.6	4.5	2.5	2.5	1.6
Carnosine	6.9	12.9	6.4	3.1	8.0	0.9
Arginine	1.6	1.5	1.4	0.5	1.1	0.3

* Mean values exceeding the normal range (mean + 2 s.d.) are italicized.

Animal models

Various neuromuscular disorders have been described in many animals including mink, sheep, duck, cow, hamster, and chicken (Harris 1979; Averill 1980; Cosmos *et al.* 1980; Harris and Slater 1980; Bradley *et al.* 1988). But none of these has proved to be strictly analogous to human muscular dystrophy.

Muscular dystrophy in the mouse

In 1955, Michelson, then a student working at the Jackson Memorial Research Laboratory, Bar Harbor, Maine, identified a spontaneous mouse mutant with a myopathy in the inbred strain 129 (Michelson *et al.* 1955). This discovery was heralded with great enthusiasm by all workers in the field because a good mouse analogue of the human disease could conceivably provide an excellent model for investigating pathogenesis and even possible treatment (Fig. 7.8). But there were many problems to be overcome. It proved to be an autosomal recessive trait, and it was very difficult to maintain stocks of affected animals by breeding from homozygous affected parents. Furthermore, it gradually became clear that in the disease in this mutant (*dy*) as well as in two different milder allelic mutants (*dy^{2J}* and *dy^{K}*), there were morphological, functional, and electrophysiological abnormalities in the *nervous* system (Mendell *et al.* 1979; Bradley *et al.* 1988).

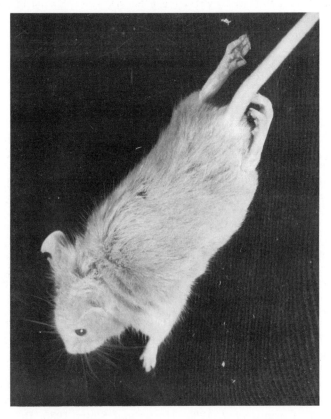

Fig. 7.8 Mouse mutant (Bar Harbor 129/ReJ *dy/dy*) with myopathy. Note the paralysed hind limbs and hunched forequarters.

However, a more recently identified mouse mutant in the C57BL/10 inbred strain, referred to as *mdx*, seems more like the human disease (Bulfield *et al*. 1984). The genetics and phenotype of this *mdx* mouse have been reviewed by Miller (1990). Points of similarity with Duchenne muscular dystrophy are the X-linked mode of inheritance, elevated serum levels of creatine kinase and pyruvate kinase, primary involvement of skeletal muscle, and an absence of muscle dystrophin (human and mouse dystrophins are very similar). The *mdx* mutant maps to the mouse dystrophin gene. But there are significant differences from the human disease. The muscle histology is different because though muscle degeneration is evident early on, subsequently regeneration occurs, the regenerated fibres remaining centrally nucleated (Fig. 7.9). The diaphragm on the other hand does undergo progressive degeneration (Stedman *et al*. 1991). Furthermore, there is no evidence of fibre loss or progressive fibrosis as there is in the human disease (Torres and Duchen 1987). But the most important difference is that in *mdx* mice after a period of muscle degeneration at 2–3 weeks of age, the muscles apparently recover (Dangain and Vrbova 1984). Thereafter affected mice remain essentially normal with no obvious weakness and a normal life span. Thus, though this mutant provides a good model for some aspects of Duchenne muscular dystrophy, the most intriguing question it poses is why,

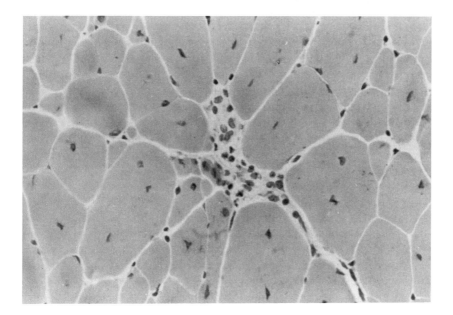

Fig. 7.9 Muscle histology in mouse mutant *mdx*. Note the variation in fibre size and preponderance of central nuclei (haematoxylin and eosin).

when there is a deficiency of dystrophin, is the weakness not only non-progressive but actually recovers in time? An answer to this question could be of considerable significance in understanding the cause of the *progressive* weakness in the human disease.

Muscular dystrophy in the cat

Dystrophin deficiency has also been described in male cats (Gaschen *et al.* 1992). in which the histopathology is remarkable and shows muscle hypertrophy with progressive accumulation of calcium. Clinically it seems unique in that diaphragmatic and glossal hypertrophy are predominant features, though the latter is not uncommon in Duchenne muscular dystrophy.

In the dystrophic cat, like the *mdx* mouse but unlike the human disease and the dystrophic dog, there is no progressive loss of muscle fibres, no progressive fibrosis and no progressive weakness despite the deficiency of dystrophin (Hoffman and Gorospe 1991). Perhaps the study of the reasons for these species differences could be very revealing and help our understanding of the pathogenesis of the human disorder.

Muscular dystrophy in the dog

Breeds of dog with an X-linked muscular dystrophy associated with an absence of dystrophin (which in the dog is identical to that in humans) have been found in the golden retriever (Valentine *et al.* 1986; 1992; Cooper *et al.* 1988) and wire-haired fox terrier (Gorospe *et al.* 1991). In many ways these are more comparable to Duchenne muscular dystrophy because the muscle pathology is more-or-less identical to the human disease, and muscle weakness is progressive with the later development of limb contractures. In the retriever, but not the fox terrier, occasional dystrophin-positive fibres occur as in Duchenne muscular dystrophy (p. 74). So far these breeds of dog are the best animal models of the human disease and could provide excellent subjects for studying the effects of any therapeutic approaches to the disease.

Summary and conclusions

Many biochemical abnormalities have been found in Duchenne muscular dystrophy. Abnormal findings are likely to be relevant to pathogenesis only when they relate specifically to Duchenne muscular dystrophy and occur in the very early stages of the disease process before there is any significant muscle wasting and weakness.

Muscle tissue has been studied the most, and the observed biochemical changes are conveniently considered as being the consequence of three main processes. Firstly, there are those changes which result from wasting and degeneration, and these include the reduction in muscle myosin, carnitine, and most glycolytic enzymes. Secondly, there are changes attributable to the invasion of affected muscle by macrophages and fibroblasts as well as to the necrosis of affected muscle fibres. These include the increase in enzymes present in fibroblasts and macrophages (such as NADP-linked dehydrogenases) and proteases (cathepsins, lysosomal acid hydrolases, and calcium-activated proteases). Thirdly, in many ways dystrophic muscle resembles fetal muscle (histochemically, and lipid, myosin, and isoenzyme patterns) for which the term 'dedifferentiation' has sometimes been used. The balance of evidence indicates that mitochondrial oxidation, sarcoplasmic reticulum and contractile protein functions are essentially normal, at least in the early stages of the disease. The results of studies on cultured dystrophic myoblasts have shown that there is a deficiency of dystrophin but only some aspects of the abnormal phenotype are expressed by these cells in culture.

Studies on peripheral blood leucocytes suggest that there is no defect in glycolysis, the tricarboxylic acid cycle or electron transport chain, or fatty acid oxidation. No abnormal metabolites have yet been found in plasma or urine, and most of the changes which have been observed can be explained in terms of efflux from dystrophic muscle fibres.

So far the best animal models of Duchenne muscular dystrophy are the *mdx* mouse and certain breeds of golden retriever and fox terrier. In all these models the disease is X-linked and associated with a deficiency of muscle dystrophin. However the disease is only progressive in the dog models which could therefore provide the best subjects for therapeutic trials.

8   Genetics

The familial nature of Duchenne muscular dystrophy was noted very early on by both Meryon (1852, 1864) and Gowers (1879*b*). In fact, as we have seen (p. 19), Gowers recognized that the disorder was limited to males and transmitted by healthy females, a mode of inheritance now recognized to be that of an X-linked recessive trait (Fig. 8.1).

Mode of inheritance

Evidence of X-linked recessive inheritance includes not only the typical pedigree pattern but also occasional female heterozygous carriers have had affected sons by different husbands. However, neither of these observations excludes the possibility that the disorder could be inherited as an autosomal dominant trait which is expressed only in males, so-called sex-limitation. But two lines of evidence refute this. First, the disorder has been recorded in females with XO Turner's syndrome (Walton 1957; Chelly *et al.* 1986), XO mosaicism (Ferrier *et al.* 1965; Jalbert *et al.* 1966; Averyanov *et al.* 1977; Bortolini *et al.* 1986)), or with a structurally abnormal X chromosome (Berg and Conte 1974) or an XY chromosome constitution (Wulfsberg and Skoglund 1986). Secondly, statistical evidence indicates that the proportion of cases due to new mutations more closely resembles that expected for an

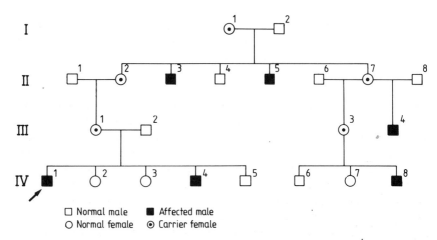

Fig. 8.1 Pedigree of a family with Duchenne muscular dystrophy.

X-linked recessive trait than for an autosomal dominant trait with male limitation (Morton and Chung 1959). However, until relatively recently the disease locus did not appear to be within measurable distance of other known X-linked loci. But, using DNA probes as well as other information, the disease locus has now been shown to be located on the short arm of the X chromosome at position Xp21 (p. 170).

Paternal inheritance

Thompson and her colleagues (1962) described two large families with Duchenne muscular dystrophy in which the gene appeared to be non-penetrant in certain males. In one family described in detail, a healthy brother of a known carrier had a daughter with an affected son. However, it is possible that the affected boy's mother was not a carrier and that her son was the result of a new mutation. Recently there have been other reports of the ocurrence of the disease in paternal lineages, molecular studies revealing more than one mutation in each of the families concerned (Zatz *et al.* 1991*b*; Miciak *et al.* 1992). Two different mutations have also been reported in the *same* maternal lineage of a family (Laing *et al.* 1992; Kakulas *et al.* 1992 [pp. 78–9]). There is also a suggestion that in the very extensive family first described by Sidler (1944), which can be traced to the fifteenth century, different branches may harbour different mutations (H. Moser, personal communication, 1992). It has been argued that the occurrence of more than one mutation within the same family could be accounted for by chance alone (Hunter 1992; ten Kate and van Essen 1992). But there is also the possibility that in these unique families either the dystrophin gene is particularly prone to mutation, or a particular transposon is involved which disrupts the gene. For obvious reasons most studies have concentrated on maternal lineages in affected families. Perhaps studies should now be extended to paternal relatives as well, and even to the nature of the mutation in affected individuals in different branches of the same family. After all, geneticists have often 'cherished their exceptions' with rewarding results.

Penetrance

There have been reports of minor abnormalities in muscle histology, electromyography, total body potassium, and urinary amino acids in some *unaffected male relatives* of affected boys. However, many of these findings were non-specific and based on few results, and they are therefore of doubtful significance. More importantly, several early studies indicated that a proportion of clinically unaffected male relatives of affected boys had slightly elevated SCK levels (reviewed in Emery and Spikesman 1970*a,b*), raising the possibility that these might represent subclinical cases of the disease. Unfortunately, in most of these studies very few relatives were investigated and⁻ information on control values was rarely given. We investigated the problem in detail by studying 101 first degree male relatives of patients with Duchenne and Becker types of muscular dystrophy and in an equal number of age-matched healthy male controls. We found that around the same proportion of males in both groups had *slightly* elevated SCK levels. We concluded that an elevated SCK level in a male relative (excluding preclinical cases) is unrelated to muscular dystrophy. It should be remembered however, that a defect in the dystrophin gene has been reported in occasional males with a raised SCK level who are otherwise normal (p. 185).

Complex segregation analysis in a large number of families with the disease indicates that the gene for Duchenne muscular dystrophy is always fully penetrant (Williams *et al.* 1983).

Heterozygous advantage and fetal loss

Of theoretical importance in Duchenne muscular dystrophy is whether heterozygous carriers exhibit increased reproductive fitness, and if there is increased prenatal or perinatal mortality which might be a reflection of an early manifestation of the disease. Evidence on both these points is still scanty and largely anecdotal.

With regard to the possibility that carriers might have larger families than normal, Danieli *et al.* (1980) found in their study that the mean family size of carriers was 5.38 ± 0.30 compared with 3.98 ± 0.24 in normal women (on the paternal side of the carriers' families), a difference which was statistically significant. However, in such studies there is always a problem of ascertainment: that at least some women may not have been designated as carriers until they had had at least one son who was affected. There are also theoretical reasons for doubting that significant heterozygous advantage occurs in any X-linked recessive disorder which is highly deleterious (Skolnick *et al.* 1977).

Danieli and colleagues (1980) in their extensive studies in Venetia (Italy) have suggested that the spontaneous abortion and male stillbirth rates in families with Duchenne muscular dystrophy may be increased. An apparent excess of male infant deaths was also observed by Lane *et al.* (1983). These interesting observations await further confirmation in other large population studies.

Incidence

In order to determine the frequency of the responsible gene and its rate of mutation it is necessary to determine the population frequency of the disorder. This information is also essential in order to determine if various preventive measures are being effective, and to help in the planning of adequate resources and welfare services for affected families.

Incidence refers to the number of *new* cases per unit of population. Prevalence on the other hand refers to *all* cases present in the population, either within a given period (so-called period prevalence rate) or at a particular point in time (so-called point prevalence rate) per unit of population at-risk at that time. In the case of Duchenne muscular dystrophy prevalence, particularly after early childhood, would be less than the true incidence at birth because of increasing mortality.

Since the disorder is not clinically recognizable at birth, birth incidence is usually derived from knowing the number of normal boys born in the same years that affected boys were born. However, a small proportion of normal boys may die by the age affected boys are diagnosed. It has therefore been argued that incidence should perhaps be related not to the number of normal live births but rather to the number of normal children who survive to the age affected boys are diagnosed. But some affected boys may also die before clinical manifestations become evident. The best compromise seems to be to calculate incidence from the assumed frequency at birth as a proportion of all births.

Incidence may also be derived from prevalence by taking into account the probability of ascertaining affected individuals in the population and the probability of an individual developing the disease by a given age (Morton and Chung 1959; Yasuda and Kondo 1980).

Some estimates of incidence and prevalence in various countries are given in Table 8.1. The estimates vary considerably. There are differences between different countries and even within a single country such as the United Kingdom or Italy. In Israel there appears to be a considerable difference in

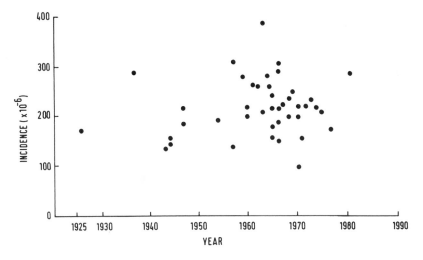

Fig. 8.2 Incidence of Duchenne muscular dystrophy and the mean year of study.

Table 8.1 Duchenne muscular dystrophy: prevalence in the population and incidence in live male births (LMB)

Country	Prevalence				Incidence				Reference
	Year	Affected	Total	x 10^{-6}	Years	Affected	Total (LMB)	x10^{-6}	
Australia									
N.S.W.	—	—	—	—	1960–71	99	532 302	186	Cowan et al. (1980)
Victoria	—	—	—	—	1957–63	49	223 330	219	Lawrence et al. (1973)
Western	—	—	—	—	1950–69	35	173 126	202	Hurse and Kakulas (1974), Kakulas and Hurse (1977)
Canada									
Alberta	1979	94	989 100	95.0**	1950–74	110	420 374	262	Monckton et al. (1982)
Ontario	—	—	—	—	1956–76	—	—	292	Williams et al. (1983)
Denmark	1965	—	—	69.4**	1965–75	—	—	222	Leth et al. (1985)
Finland									
Helsinki	—	—	—	—	1965–80	29	122 595	237	Lang et al. (1989)
Germany									
Dresden	—	—	—	—	1960–69	26	145 990	178	Kunath (1983)
Dresden	—	—	—	—	1970–79	25	117 650	213	Kunath (1983), see also Lössner and Wagner (1987)
Erfurt	—	—	—	—	1958–73	51	165 898	307	Spiegler and Herrmann (1983)
Magdeburg	—	—	—	—	1964–76	24	119 624	201	Szibor and Steinbicker (1983)
Sudbaden	—	—	—	—	1918–32	21	125 000	168	Becker (1980), reported originally in 1955
Wurzburg (Unterfranken)	1976	36	1 192 631	30.2	1965–79	28	125 538	223	Höhn (1987)

		Year	Population	Rate	Period		Population		Reference
Iceland	11	1963	187 200	58.8	—	—	—	—	Gudmundsson (1968)
Israel									
Ashkenazi	9	1973	353 382	25.5***	—	—	—	—	Kott et al. (1973)
Non-Ashkenazi	39	1973	655 840	59.5***	—	—	—	—	Kott et al. (1973)
*Italy**									
Campania	—	—	—	—	1960–71	156	721 163	216	Nigro et al. (1983)
Emilia	28	1975	403 730	69.3	1951–75	24	61 470	390	Lucci (1980)
Friuli	—	—	—	—	1962–78	9	92 631	97	Nigris (1984)
Piedmont	—	—	—	—	1955–74	73	301 283	242	Schiffer et al. (1981)
Puglia	126	1975	3 771 329	33.4	1956–75	121	805 335	150	Ferrari et al. (1980)
Sud Tyrol	—	—	—	—	1960–75	8	39 980	200	Danieli (1984)
Veneto	85	1970	2 498 422	34.0	1959–68	66	234 369	282	Danieli et al. (1977)
Veneto	106	1980	3 335 577	31.8	1959–68	76	292 637	260	Mostacciulo et al. (1987)
Japan									
Chiba	46	1965	1 343 167	49.9** ($\pi = 0.686$)	—	—	—	217	Yasuda and Kondo (1980)
Fukuoka	—	—	—	—	1949–58	9	46 465	194	Kuroiwa and Miyazaki (1967)
Kumamoto	31	1983	1 800 000	17.2	—	—	—	—	Araki et al. (1987)
Okinawa	43	1989	603 392	71.3**	1957–85	49	311 433	157	Nakagawa et al. (1991)
Shimane	32	1975	768 876	41.6	1956–70	19	91 157	208	Takeshita et al. (1977)
'Pooled data'	384	1979–82	8 508 000	67.1** ($\pi = 0.673$)	—	—	—	292	Kanamori et al. (1987)
Libya	—	1985	—	60.0**	—	—	—	—	Radhakrishnan et al. (1987)
Netherlands									
Groningen	384	1983	7 102 598	54.0**	1961–74	397	1 673 791	237	van Essen et al. (1992a)
Norway	32	1983	293 833	108.9***	—	—	—	—	Tangsrud and Halvorsen (1988)

Table 8.1 *Contd.*

Country	Prevalence				Incidence				Reference
	Year	Affected	Total	$\times 10^{-6}$	Years	Affected	Total (LMB)	$\times 10^{-6}$	
Poland									
Warsaw	–	–	–	19.5**	1953–60	46	328 110	140	Prot (1971)
Rumania	–	–	–	–	1961–68	214	1 387 694	154	Radu and Sarközi (1978)
Switzerland									
Bern	–	–	–	–	1939–54	26	119 395	218	Moser *et al.* (1964)
United Kingdom									
England (NE)	1968	136	3 300 000	41.2	1940–46	18	138 403	130	Walton (1955)
England (NE)	1979	113	3 130 000	36.1	1952–61	86	275 990	311	Gardner-Medwin and
	1988	71	3 070 000	23.1	1962–71	65	290 017	224	Sharples
					1972–81	37	207 873	178	(1989)

England (Midlands)									
Leeds	—	—	—	—	1939–49	7	46 210	151	Blyth and Pugh (1959)
West Riding	—	—	—	—	1939–49	15	105 310	142	Blyth and Pugh (1959)
England (Midlands)	1976	27	110 434	244.5***	—	—	—	—	Bundey (1981)
N. Ireland	—	—	—	—	1942–51	28	153 692	182	Stevenson (1958)
Scotland (SE)	—	—	—	—	1953–68	47	177 413	265	Brooks and Emery (1977)
U.S.A.									
Colorado	—	—	—	—	—	51	—	220	Lubs (1974)
Minnesota	1955	1	14 942	66.9**	—	—	—	—	Kurland (1958)
Utah	—	—	—	—	1931–41	18	63 000	286	Stephens and Tyler (1951)
Wisconsin	1959	51	1 850 000	65.8** ($\pi = 0.419$)	—	—	—	276	Morton and Chung (1959)
Yugoslavia									
Ljubljana	1990	71	1 000 000	71.0**	—	—	—	—	Zidar (1990),[a] *see also* Faganel *et al.* (1977)
Total (mean ± SE)	1956	—	46 282 453	42 ± 1	—	2111	10 236 248	206 ± 4	—

* Estimates for other regions given in Nigro *et al.* (1983) and Danieli (1984).
** Prevalence in total male population.
*** Prevalence in boys.
π Ascertainment probability.
[a] Personal communication to the author.

frequency between non-Ashkenazis and Ashkenazis (Kott *et al.* 1973).

Despite increasing awareness of the disease in recent years there has been no significant increase in reported incidences (Fig. 8.2). It could be that in the past any inflation by the inclusion of other forms of dystrophy and perhaps even spinal muscular atrophy, has been balanced in more recent studies by improved ascertainment of true cases. The overall incidence based on over 10 million live male births is $206 \pm 4 \times 10^{-6}$, or one case in 4854. But this figure includes some seemingly abnormally low estimates. In several more recent and exhaustive studies birth incidence approaches 300×10^{-6} or roughly 1 in 3500 male births (Emery 1991*a*).

The birth incidence of the disease can also be determined by screening for a raised SCK level in the neonatal period and subsequently confirming the diagnosis by muscle biopsy (Guibaud *et al.* 1981) and dystrophin studies (Greenberg *et al.* 1991). These screening programmes first began in the 1970s with subsequent reports from New Zealand (Drummond 1979), Scotland (Skinner *et al.* 1982), France (Dellamonica *et al.* 1983), and Germany (Scheuerbrandt *et al.* 1986). Since then there have been a number of technological improvements and current results from several extensive studies are summarized in Table 8.2, from which the overall incidence is $199 \pm 14 \times 10^{-6}$.

At present it is really not possible to say if there are any significant differences within countries or even between different countries because of the confounding effects of variations in ascertainment. Certainly the incidences in two Japanese studies are roughly the same as values obtained in several European countries. In certain communities reproductive compensation, whereby families reproduce until they have a healthy male offspring, could conceivably lead to an increase in incidence (Templeton and Yokoyama 1980). On the other hand, preventive measures, such as family limitation and prenatal diagnosis, might be expected to lead to a reduction in incidence. Otherwise incidence will depend on the rate at which new mutations occur, and this is likely to be similar throughout the world. A particularly high incidence among an Indian community in Britain has been interpreted as possibly being due to a higher mutation rate (Roddie and Bundey 1992), but this requires confirmation.

Changes in incidence in recent years

In recent years and perhaps more so in future, some reduction in the incidence of Duchenne muscular dystrophy might be expected as a result of several factors.

Beginning in the 1950s there was an increase in interest in genetic counselling, and the mid-1960s saw the advent of carrier detection tests. Later, prenatal fetal sexing became possible so that a mother who was at high risk

Table 8.2 *Results of various neonatal screening programmes for Duchenne muscular dystrophy reported at the 14th ENMC Sponsored Workshop 'Screening for Muscular Dystrophy', March 5–6, 1992, Baarn, The Netherlands (Chairman: Professor G-J. van Ommen)*

Centre	Start of programme	Age tested	Total screened (x 10³)	False positive (%)	Proven DMD	Author
Manitoba, Canada	1986	1–5 d	54	0.10	10	H. K. Jacobs
Lyons, France	1975	5 d / 3 d	328	0.19 / 0.40	60	C. Dorche
Philadelphia, USA	1986	1–4 d	49	0.30	10	E. W. Naylor
Antwerp, Belgium	1975	5–7 d	150	0.02	25	F. J. M. Eyskens
Cardiff, Wales	1990	6–7 d	24	0.02	9	D. M. Bradley
Germany*	1977	4 wks–6 months	358	0.02	78	G. Scheuerbrandt
TOTAL			963		192	$(I = 199 \pm 14 \times 10^{-6})$

*Voluntary screening.

of having an affected son could request selective abortion of any male fetus in any subsequent pregnancy. Finally, in the recent past prenatal diagnosis of affected male fetuses has become possible by the use of DNA probes (p. 243). Although this latter development is too recent to have had any significant effect itself on incidence, genetic counselling and carrier detection studies in affected families might be predicted to have resulted in some reduction in incidence. Hurse and Kakulas (1974) claim there had been a decrease in Perth, Australia, over the period 1950-69. However, latterly there was a decrease in isolated cases with no family history which can only mean that ascertainment may not have been complete. Some boys may have developed the disease subsequent to the completion of the study. Monckton and colleagues (1982) also noted an apparent decrease in incidence in the latter part of their study period (1970-74) and concluded that this might be due to some potential cases having been born during this period but which had not yet been diagnosed. In a well designed and careful study in Western Japan a decrease in incidence from 223×10^{-6} for the period 1956-60 to 145×10^{-6} for the period 1976-80 was noted and attributed to the effects of genetic counselling (Takeshita *et al.* 1987).

In these sorts of studies it is important that the period covered should be such that there is a reasonable chance that all potential cases are likely to have developed clinical manifestations and to have been diagnosed. As a test of the completeness of the study, and provided the population itself remains the same, the number of isolated cases should remain unchanged. In the South East of Scotland, a small and well defined region which is well endowed with medical and genetic services, no familial cases have been reported since 1969, presumably as a result of genetic counselling, whereas the number of isolated cases has remained more or less the same (Table 8.3). Somewhat similar findings have been reported in Wales (Harper 1982).

Table 8.3 *Incidence of Duchenne muscular dystrophy in the South East of Scotland*

Period	Number		Incidence ($\times 10^{-6} \pm$ SE)
	Affected	Total	
1953–56	12	41 254	291 ± 84
1957–60	9	44 347	203 ± 68
1961–64	13	46 300	281 ± 78
1965–68	13	45 512	286 ± 79
1969–72	10	41 118	243 ± 77
1973–76	9	40 358	223 ± 74

Mutation rate

The rate at which the gene causing Duchenne muscular dystrophy mutates may be estimated either indirectly or directly.

Indirect estimation of mutation rate

For any X-linked recessive disorder (Haldane 1935) if the reproductive fitness of affected individuals is f, and the incidence of the disease is I, then the mutation rate is:

$$= \frac{1}{3} I(1 - f)$$

However, in Duchenne muscular dystrophy biological fitness is zero because affected boys do not procreate. Therefore the mutation rate is given by $I/3$. If the incidence of the disorder is assumed to be around 200 to 300 $\times 10^{-6}$, then the mutation rate is around 70 to 100×10^{-6} genes per generation.

Direct estimation of mutation rate

In the direct method an attempt is made to estimate the actual number of new mutations among isolated cases. If a out of b known female carriers have an abnormal SCK level, then the detection rate of carriers is a/b. If n isolated cases are born in a given period among N males born in the same period, and if c is the number of mothers of these n males who have an *abnormal* SCK level, then among these isolated cases (subject to sampling error) the number of *new* mutations will be:

$$n - \frac{bc}{a}$$

and therefore the mutation rate is:

$$\frac{\left(n - \dfrac{bc}{a}\right)}{N}$$

In one study (Gardner-Medwin 1970), 22 out of 35 known carriers had raised SCK levels. Of 56 mothers of isolated cases, 15 had raised levels. Thus the proportion of new mutations (mothers are non-carriers) among isolated cases is:

$$\frac{[56 - (35/22)\,15]}{56}$$
$$= 0.574$$

Over a 9-year period (1952–60), 43 isolated cases were born and therefore the number of new mutations is:

$$(43)(0.574)$$
$$= 24.682$$

The total number of males born in this period who survived to age 5 (by which time almost all cases of Duchenne muscular dystrophy are diagnosed) was 236 200. Thus the mutation rate is:

$$\frac{24.682}{236\,200}$$
$$= 105 \times 10^{-6}$$

The estimates of the mutation rate by both these methods are considerably greater than values obtained for other X-linked disorders (Vogel 1990). For comparison some representative values for various genetic disorders are given in Table 8.4. The only disorder with a comparable mutation rate is neurofibromatosis but this is now known *not* to be a single genetic disease. The very high mutation rate in Duchenne muscular dystrophy is probably a reflection of the enormous size of the dystrophin gene which therefore provides a bigger target for mutagenic agents.

Parental age and mutation rate

In X-linked recessive disorders possible effects of maternal or paternal age on mutation rates can be assessed separately by considering respectively

Table 8.4 *Average estimates of mutation rates for various genetic disorders (data from various sources)*

Disorder	Mutation rate ($\times 10^{-6}$)
Autosomal dominants	
Achondroplasia	6–13
Retinoblastoma	5–12
Tuberous sclerosis	6–10.5
Polyposis coli	13
Neurofibromatosis	44–100
Huntington's chorea	5
Myotonic dystrophy	8–11
Autosomal recessives	
Albinism	28
Total colour blindness	28
Phenylketonuria	25
X-linked recessives	
Haemophilia A	32–57
Haemophilia B	2–3

maternal age in the case of mutant males, and *maternal grandfather's* age in the case of mutant heterozygous mothers. The latter are mothers with no affected relatives other than sons (or have only one affected son but a significantly elevated SCK level) where the new mutation can have occurred in the X-chromosome she inherited from her father (Penrose 1955).

None of the studies which have considered this problem have found any significant increase in the age of mothers of presumed new mutants (Hutton and Thompson 1970; Pellié *et al.* 1973; Emery 1977*b*; Becker 1980; Yasuda and Kondo 1982).

With regard to presumed mutant heterozygous mothers, the mean ages of both grandparents at the birth of these mothers can be compared with the mean ages of the mothers' spouses' parents at the birth of their spouse. In one study the mean maternal grandfather's age seemed ($P = 0.05$) greater than expected from appropriate demographic data (Emery 1977*b*). Furthermore, in this study and in two others (Becker 1980; Yasuda and Kondo 1982) the mean maternal grandfather's age was greater than the mean paternal grandfather's age (Table 8.5), but the differences were not statistically significant.

If there is any paternal age effect on the mutation rate in this disorder it would seem to be negligible. The results of these studies do not support the idea that the mutation rate in males is significantly different from that in females.

Sex difference in mutation rate

It can be shown that if a mother has an affected son but no one else in the family is affected, then the probability of her being a carrier is:

$$\frac{\mu + \nu}{2\mu + \nu}$$

where μ = mutation rate in female germ cells,
and ν = mutation rate in male germ cells.

The probability that she is *not* a carrier and that the son is therefore the result of a new mutation is:

$$1 - \frac{\mu + \nu}{2\mu + \nu}$$

$$= \frac{\mu}{2\mu + \nu}$$

which represents the proportion of new mutants, often designated as 'x' (Haldane 1956). If the mutation rates are the same in both males and females then x is a third; if mutations occurred more frequently in the male then x

Table 8.5 *Ages of grandparents of cases of Duchenne muscular dystrophy where the mother is presumed to be a mutant heterozygote*

MGF			PGF				MGM			PGM			Reference
No.	Mean	s.d.	No.	Mean	s.d.	Diference	No.	Mean	s.d.	No.	Mean	s.d.	Difference	
26	34.3	6.14	22	30.9	6.42	+3.4	26	30.5	4.87	24	27.8	5.47	+2.7	Emery (1977b)
15	35.1	7.03	15	31.4	6.43	+3.7	14	30.4	6.63	16	27.4	5.48	+3.0	Becker (1980)
82	34.4	7.33	81	33.9	7.56	+0.5	82	30.3	7.06	82	29.0	6.07	+1.3	Yasuda and Kondo (1982)

MGF, maternal grandfather; PGF, paternal grandfather; MGM, maternal grandmother; PGM, paternal grandmother.

approaches zero; and if mutations occurred more frequently in the female then x approaches a half.

This is not just of academic importance because if mutations were found to occur exclusively in the male then all mothers with an affected son would be carriers, and this would be important in genetic counselling.

Several different methods have been devised for estimating x. Essentially there are three approaches:

(1) analysis of sibships (method of Haldane (1956), a modification of this (C), and an independent method (B) by Cheeseman *et al.* (1958), methods of Morton (1959) involving complex segregation analysis (Morton 1969) as well as maximum likelihood methods);

(2) sex ratio of unaffected sibs (Davie and Emery 1978); and

(3) methods based on the results of carrier detection tests.

The statistical methods used in sibship analysis are somewhat complex and details are given in the relevant publications.

With regard to the sex ratio method, this is independent of ascertainment, and is based on the assumption that among offspring of a *carrier* affected boys, unaffected boys and girls will, on average, occur in the ratio 1:1:2. Therefore the sex ratio (M:F) among unaffected sibs will be 1:2 (or 1:1.89 if corrected for the deviation of the sex ratio from 1). However among the sibs of *new mutants* the sex ratio will be 1:1 (or 1:0.94 if corrected). The proportion of new mutants among isolated cases can be estimated by determining the sex ratio among the sibs of isolated cases.

Finally, with regard to carrier detection methods, this has usually been based on comparing the proportion of abnormal test results (the most reliable in the past being the SCK level) in known carriers with mothers of isolated cases. Thus if:

i = proportion of mothers of isolated cases with an elevated SCK level;

d = proportion of known carriers with an elevated SCK level; and

P_i = proportion of isolated cases among all cases assuming *complete ascertainment* in a given population; then

$x = (1 - i/d)P_i$ (Moser 1984).

There are also more sophisticated methods for tackling this problem (Winter 1980). Some representative values are given in Table 8.6, from which it will be seen that the 95 per cent confidence limits ($x \pm 1.96\,\mathrm{SE}$) of almost all these estimates would accommodate a value of 0.33 which assumes that mutation rates are equal in males and females. However, occasionally significantly lower values have been obtained, particularly with carrier detection methods other than SCK levels. But in these cases the value of the methods used for detecting carriers (serum LDH–5 (Roses *et al.* 1977), lymphocyte capping (Pickard *et al.* 1978), and polyribosomal protein synthesis (Bucher *et al.* 1980)) have been questioned, and it is possible that they could lead to

Table 8.6 *Estimation of the proportion (x) of new mutants in Duchenne muscular dystrophy. Values have been rounded off to two decimal places*

Method	$x \pm$ SE	Reference
Sibships analysis		
Haldane	0.51 ± 0.08*	Cheeseman *et al.* (1958)
	0.52 ± 0.10†	
Cheeseman (B)	0.39 ± 0.16*	
	0.37 ± 0.19†	
Cheeseman (C)	0.34 ± 0.14*	
	0.40 ± 0.18†	
Maximum likelihood	0.32 ± 0.14*	Smith and Kilpatrick (1958)
	0.39 ± 0.17†	
Morton	0.35 ± 0.05	Morton and Chung (1959)
Haldane	0.29 ± 0.07	Danieli *et al.* (1980)
Cheeseman (B)	0.22 ± 0.08	
Cheeseman (C)	0.19 ± 0.07	
Maximum likelihood	0.29 ± 0.05	Yasuda and Kondo (1980)
Morton (modified)	0.17 ± 0.08	Bucher *et al.* (1980)
Cheeseman (B)	0.13 ± 0.11	Lane *et al.* (1983)
Segregation analysis	0.27 ± 0.08	Williams *et al.* (1983)
Segregation analysis	0.23 ± 0.05	Danieli and Barbujani (1984)
Segregation analysis	0.31 ± 0.07	Kanamori *et al.* (1987)
Maximum likelihood	0.23 ± 0.05	Danieli and Barbujani (1984)
Sex ratio in sibs		
	0.44 ± 0.12††	Davie and Emery (1978)
	0.32 ± 0.12**	
	0.23 ± 0.20††	Bucher *et al.* (1980)
Carrier detection	0.32 ± 0.05	Gardner-Medwin (1970)
(based on SCK)	0.32 ± 0.06	Moser (1971, 1977)
	0.12 ± 0.04	Roses *et al.* (1977)
	0.28 ± 0.04	Davie and Emery (1978)
	0.30 ± 0.09§	
	0.34 ± 0.06 (est).	Caskey *et al.* (1980)
	0.12 ± 0.03	Danieli *et al.* (1980)
	0.35 ± 0.03***	Zatz (1986)

* Northern Ireland data (Stevenson 1958).
† Utah data (Stephens and Tyler 1951).
†† Uncorrected, or ** corrected.
§ Pedigree *and* SCK data.
*** Personal communication to the author.

an excess of false positive results and thereby overestimate the proportion of carriers among mothers of isolated cases. But the possibility of germ-line mosaicism (p. 246) must also be considered as a possible explanation for lower values of x (Fu and Barbujani 1990). In an extensive study of a pooled sample of 1885 sibships from 7 different countries, the proportion of sporadic cases was estimated to be 0.229 ± 0.026 (Barbujani *et al.* 1990). From this data it can be calculated that the upper 95 per cent confidence limit for x is 0.280 and therefore the proportion due to mosaicism in apparently non-carrier mothers would be expected to be at least 16 per cent. This figure is close to that obtained from molecular studies.

The increasing election by mothers, after the birth of an affected son, of family limitation and selective abortion in future pregnancies, may well invalidate the assumptions underlying these various approaches. These practices will lead to an increasing proportion of isolated cases and a decreasing sex ratio (M:F) in subsequent sibs.

Finally a recent collaborative international investigation of the problem using DNA haplotypes in order to identify the origin of mutations within families indicates that the mutation rates in males and females are roughly equal (Müller *et al.* 1992).

So far it has been assumed that all cases result from a mutation in the germ cells. But if the male twins discordant for Duchenne muscular dystrophy reported by de Grouchy *et al.* (1963) were in fact identical, as the authors stated, then this raises the possibility that mutations may also occur *after* conception. Post-zygotic mutation would also account for a reported pair of MZ twins being discordant for tuberous sclerosis (Northrup *et al.* 1990). There could be other examples.

Clinical heterogeneity

The consensus view is that Duchenne muscular dystrophy is a well defined and homogeneous disorder. However, we have seen already that there is a wide spectrum of clinical severity (see Chapter 3). Furthermore, the very high incidence of the disorder cannot be accounted for by heterozygous advantage (Skolnick *et al.* 1977), but is due to mutations at different points in the very large Xp21 locus.

Correlations between relatives regarding age at onset and of becoming confined to a wheelchair have been interpreted as indicating heterogeneity (Feingold *et al.* 1971). In addition, Samaha and Congedo (1977) have reported two different patterns of muscle sarcoplasmic reticulum membrane proteins in affected boys, and Cohen *et al.* (1982) have shown that decay rates in muscle strength in affected boys are not homogeneous but may be at least bimodally distributed. Finally, we found that in affected boys with *severe* mental handicap (IQ < 50), the age at onset and of becoming confined

Table 8.7 *Age at onset and of becoming confined to a wheelchair in patients with normal intelligence (N) or with severe mental handicap (MH)*

	Onset							Chairbound							Reference
	N			MH				N			MH				
	No.	Mean	s.d.	No.	Mean	s.d.	P	No.	Mean	s.d.	No.	Mean	s.d.	P	
	15	2.20	0.78	15	2.43	1.03	NS	12	8.77	1.12	13	9.65	1.60	NS	Emery *et al.* (1979*b*)
	29	3.64	1.72	10	3.61	2.01	NS	24	9.49	1.70	11	10.83	1.65	< 0.05	Bortolini and Zatz (1986)

to a wheelchair was somewhat later; the fall in SCK levels with age less marked; and the urinary excretion of certain amino acids somewhat greater than in a group of carefully *matched* affected boys with normal intelligence (Emery *et al.* 1979*b*). It was suggested that perhaps affected boys with *severe* mental handicap might possibly represent a small subgroup of patients genetically distinct from most other patients with the disease. It was not suggested that the presence or absence of lesser degrees of mental handicap could be a criterion for dividing patients into different genetic groups because this is obviously not valid. Bortolini and Zatz (1986) have also examined the possibility of genetic heterogeneity on the basis of various clinical criteria and SCK levels in affected boys with normal intelligence or severe mental handicap. They felt their data did not reveal any evidence of heterogeneity though boys with severe mental handicap did become confined to a wheelchair somewhat later than boys with normal intelligence. Comparable data from these two studies are summarized in Table 8.7.

Clinical evidence of allelic heterogeneity has therefore been rather unconvincing. The relationship between phenotype and molecular pathology has been more helpful in resolving this problem and will be discussed in Chapter 9.

Summary and conclusions

Evidence from various sources, including pedigree studies, affected girls with Xchromosome abnormalities, and statistical methods have shown that Duchenne muscular dystrophy is inherited as an X-linked recessive trait. The mutant gene is always fully penetrant and a subclinical, as opposed to a preclinical, form of the disease does not exist. There is a suggestion that the rates of spontaneous abortion and male stillbirths may be increased in affected families, but this requires further evaluation. Estimates of the incidence of the disorder, based on population surveys and neonatal screening, vary but are probably around 200 to 300 $\times 10^{-6}$. This puts the mutation rate at around 70 to 100 $\times 10^{-6}$ genes per generation which is considerably greater than any other X-linked disorder and reflects the enormous size of the dystrophin gene and therefore a greater target for mutagenic agents. A possible difference in mutation rates in male and female germ cells has been studied by considering maternal and grandpaternal age effects, as well as the proportion of isolated cases which could be due to new mutations. The results of these investigations indicate that the mutation rates in male and female germ cells do not differ significantly and around one-third of isolated cases of the disease are due to new mutations.

Finally, the wide spectrum of clinical severity, and correlations between relatives, suggest that there may be genetic (allelic) heterogeneity. This problem has not been resolved satisfactorily on the basis of clinical criteria, although it is clear that heterogeneity exists at the molecular level (see Chapter 9).

9 Molecular pathology

In order to unravel the molecular pathology of a disease where the basic biochemical defect is unknown, various approaches are possible. These have been well exemplified in the case of Duchenne muscular dystrophy. First, the gene has to be localized to a specific chromosome and then to a particular site on the chromosome. Secondly, armed with such information DNA markers can be selected which are located in this particular region of the chromosome and if they prove to be closely *linked* to the disease locus they can be used *indirectly* for carrier detection and prenatal diagnosis. Thirdly,

Table 9.1 *Summary of some salient features in girls with a Duchenne-like disorder and various X/autosome translocations*

| Autosome breakpoint | Parents' karyotype | Parental ages | | Probability mother is a carrier | Age | | |
		Maternal	Paternal		Onset	Chairbound	At reporting
11q13	N	NR	NR	SCK normal	NR	NR	16 yrs
21p12	N	21	25	SCK normal	2 yrs	—	20 yrs
3q13	N	28	40	Possibly a carried on SCK and EMG but no details	10 mths, generalized hypotonia	—	45 mths
1p34 (+inversion)	N	NR	NR	$P = 0.01$	Walked at 15 mths, but unsteady	8 yrs	8 yrs
5q35	N	39	39	SCK normal	4 yrs	—	9 yrs
6q21	N (mother)	29	26	$P = 0.06$	5 yrs	10 yrs	11½ yrs
11q23	N	NR	NR	SCK normal	?	—	13 yrs
9p22	N	18	22	SCK normal	<2 yrs	—	9 yrs
2q36	N	NR	NR	NR	19 mths generalized hypotonia and delayed milestones	Requires assistance in walking	14 yrs
6q16	N	NR	NR	SCK normal	<3 yrs	—	4½ yrs
9p21	N	NR	NR	SCK normal	<2 yrs	12 yrs	Died at 23
8q24	N	25	29	SCK normal	2–3 yrs	—	6 yrs
4q26	N	NR	NR	SCK normal	2 yrs	—	3 yrs
5q31	N	20	23	SCK normal	2½ yrs	—	6½ yrs
15q26	N	31	34	SCK normal	4–5 yrs	—	9⅔ yrs

N, normal; NR, not recorded; MH, mentally handicapped; ?, not clear.

it may be possible, using molecular techniques, to 'walk the genome' from the DNA markers toward the mutant gene so as to eventually include the gene itself. As will be seen, however, there have been several other strategies pursued to isolate the Duchenne locus. Fourthly, having isolated the gene, or at least part of it, this can then be used as a 'gene-specific' probe for *direct* prenatal diagnosis and carrier detection. Finally, having isolated the gene then it is possible by DNA sequencing and other techniques to define the nature of the molecular defect and its product. Each of these steps will be described in relation to Duchenne muscular dystrophy, although much of the detail is really outside the scope of this book and is furnished in the relevant bibliography.

Localization of the Duchenne gene

An early clue as to the specific location of the Duchenne locus came from the study of rare cases of a Duchenne-like disorder in girls. The first cases

Severity	IQ	Active der X (%)		Comment	Reference
		Fibroblasts	Lymphocytes		
?	NR	NR	NR	—	Greenstein *et al.* (1977, 1980)
Mild	N	95	93	—	Verellen *et al.* (1977, 1978)
					Verellen-Dumoulin *et al.* (1984)
? Severe	MH	—	93	Certain dysmorphic features (hypertelorism, facial assymetry, etc.)	Canki *et al.* (1979)
Severe	N	—	100	—	Lindenbaum *et al.* (1979)
Severe	N	100	98	—	Jacobs *et al.* (1981)
Severe	N	—	98	—	Zatz *et al.* (1981*a*)
? Mild	N	—	?	—	Bjerglund Nielsen *et al.* (1983)
? Severe	MH	—	99	—	Emanuel *et al.* (1983)
? Severe	MH	NR	NR	Course has fluctuated with SCK ranging from normal to 27 000 iu	MacLeod *et al.* (1983)
? Severe	NR	NR	NR	—	Perez Vidal *et al.* (1983)
Severe	MH	—	100	Idiopathic ketonic hypoglycaemia; epilepsy and features of Turner's syndrome	Bjerglund Nielsen and Nielsen (1984)
Mild	N	98	75	—	Narazaki *et al.* (1985)
?	?	—	100	—	Saito *et al.* (1985)
Severe	MH	—	100	—	Nevin *et al.* (1986)
? Severe	N	95	93	—	Ribeiro *et al.* (1986)

were described in the late 70s (Verellen *et al.* 1978; Lindenbaum *et al.* 1979), but there were soon many others. The salient features of some published cases are summarized in Table 9.1. Since the first edition of this book other cases have also been reported (Kimura *et al.* 1986; Bodrug *et al.* 1990; Lucci *et al.* 1991), and there are probably many others in the population. In each case the findings have been consistent with the diagnosis of a muscular dystrophy with grossly elevated SCK levels and myopathic changes on electromyography (EMG) and muscle pathology. Most have been clinically similar to Duchenne muscular dystrophy although in some cases the disorder seemed less severe and perhaps more like Becker muscular dystrophy. Some have been mentally retarded. All, however, have had a reciprocal translocation between an autosome and the X chromosome, and since these are balanced translocations with no apparent loss of chromosomal material these girls might have been expected to be normal. In such X/autosome translocations however it is the normal X which tends to be preferentially inactivated, with the result that genes on the derived (der) X are expressed. It could therefore be that the mothers of these girls were heterozygous carriers and the maternal X chromosome carrying the mutant gene was involved in the translocation. However, this is unlikely because in only two instances (Canki *et al.* 1979; Verellen-Dumoulin *et al.* 1984) has there been any suggestion that the mother *might* be a carrier, and at least in one of these this now seems very unlikely (C. Verellen-Dumoulin 1986, personal communication) and that the translocation chromosome was in fact of *paternal* origin (Kean *et al.* 1986). The paternal origin of a translocated chromosome has also been reported by Bodrug *et al.* (1990). Also the parents of these girls have had normal chromosomes and we are therefore left to conclude that both the translocation as well as the disease must have arisen *de novo* in the affected girls.

Since different autosomes were involved in the translocations but the breakpoint on the X chromosome was always *in the region of Xp21*, the most likely explanation is that the translocation in some way disrupted the normal gene at Xp21 which then resulted in the disease. The mutant gene is therefore presumed to be located at this point on the X chromosome (Fig. 9.1). X/autosome translocations involving this region of the X chromosome have occasionally been described in which muscular dystrophy was *apparently* not a feature (for example, Laurent *et al.* 1975). However, the region identified by studies of banded chromosomes covers a relatively large segment of DNA and is likely to involve loci other than Duchenne muscular dystrophy.

There is considerable variation in clinical severity in girls with X/autosome translocations and a Duchenne-like disorder. It seems possible that the phenotype may well depend on the proportion of cells in which the der X is presumably active. The milder the phenotype the lower the proportion of cells in which the active X chromosome is the der X, and therefore the greater

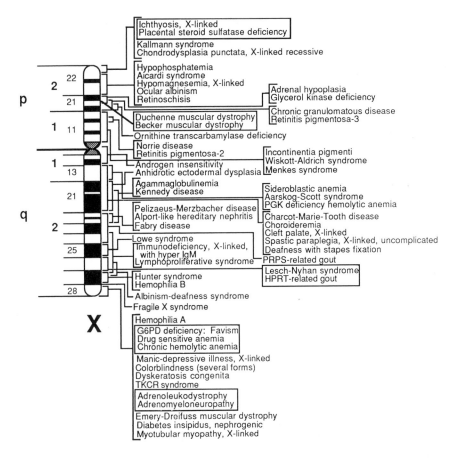

Fig. 9.1 Gene map of the X-chromosome and its banding pattern. (From McKusick, V.A. (1992). *Mendelian inheritance in man*, (10th edn). Johns Hopkins University Press, Baltimore, p. cci, reproduced with kind permission.)

the proportion of cells in which the active X chromosome is the normal X. For example, the proportion of cells in which the active X is the der X is somewhat lower in two cases considered to be mild (Verellen-Doumoulin *et al.* 1984; Narazaki *et al.* 1985). Alternatively in these milder cases the translocation has more likely interrupted the chromosomal Xp21 region concerned with Becker muscular dystrophy.

X/autosome translocations involving *other* breakpoints on the X chromosome have also been described. In these cases as well the expression of various X-linked disorders could be attributed to the disruption of the normal alleles at the respective loci (Table 9.2).

Table 9.2 *Expression of X-linked disorders in females with various X/autosome translocations*

Disorder	X breakpoint	Reference
Duchenne and Becker muscular dystrophy	Xp21	
Anhidrotic ectodermal dysplasia	Xq12	Gerald and Brown (1974)
Aicardi's syndrome	Xp22	Ropers *et al.* (1982)
Hunter's syndrome	Xq26 or Xq27	Mossman *et al.* (1983)
Aarskog syndrome	Xq13	Bawle *et al.* (1984)
Incontinentia pigmenti	Xp11	Gilgenkrantz *et al.* (1985)
Lowe's syndrome	Xq25	Hodgson *et al.* (1986*a*)
		Mueller *et al.* (1991)
Menkes syndrome	Xq13	Kapur *et al.* (1987)
		Verga *et al.* (1991)

While studies of X/autosome translocations in females with muscular dystrophy were in progress, a unique case was described which further confirmed the location of the Duchenne locus. This concerned a boy with Duchenne muscular dystrophy and some degree of mental retardation, but who also exhibited chronic granulomatous disease, McLeod syndrome (reduced antigenicity of the red cell Kell blood group), and a form of retinitis pigmentosa (Francke *et al.* 1985). High resolution chromosome banding studies revealed that the band Xp21 appeared to be slightly reduced in size, and molecular studies confirmed that the affected boy had a small interstitial deletion in this region. This deletion presumably removed DNA sequences at the Duchenne muscular dystrophy locus as well as at other adjacent loci so producing the clinical phenotypes. This case further supported the idea that the Duchenne locus is at Xp21. It also indicated that the loci for these different disorders are clustered together. In fact various associations of these different disorders have been reported in males: chronic granulomatous disease with McLeod syndrome (Marsh 1978); McLeod syndrome with raised SCK levels (Marsh *et al.* 1981) and a subclinical myopathy (Swash *et al.* 1983; Carter *et al.* 1990); chronic granulomatous disease with McLeod syndrome and raised SCK levels (Marsh *et al.* 1981); chronic granulomatous disease with Duchenne muscular dystrophy (but no mention of McLeod syndrome, Kousseff 1981); chronic granulomatous disease, McLeod syndrome, Duchenne muscular dystrophy, and a form of retinitis pigmentosa (Francke *et al.* 1985).

The gene for ornithine transcarbamylase (OTC) is also localized to Xp21

(Lindgren *et al.* 1984) and has been shown to be relatively closely linked to the Duchenne locus (Davies *et al.* 1985*a,b*). A small but visible deletion associated with OTC and glycerol kinase deficiencies and X-linked adrenal hypoplasia has been described (Hammond *et al.* 1985). Also, a deletion in the same region of the X chromosome has been found in boys with a myopathy, glycerol kinase deficiency, and adrenal insufficiency (Bartley *et al.* 1986; Saito *et al.* 1986). This triad has also been reported when there is no *visible* deletion (Renier *et al.* 1983), but a deletion may then be detected using an appropriate DNA probe (Dunger *et al.* 1986). The triad may also be associated with other abnormalities (Guggenheim *et al.* 1980). Glycerol kinase deficiency and adrenal hypoplasia have been recorded in different male members of a family but in the absence of a myopathy (Bartley *et al.* 1982), and the glycerol kinase locus is clearly distinct from the Duchenne locus (Seltzer *et al.* 1989).

Finally, Åland Island eye disease can also occur in association with Duchenne muscular dystrophy, glycerol kinase deficiency, and congenital adrenal hypoplasia (Pillers *et al.* 1990*a,b*).

Based on these reports of overlapping phenotypes it is possible to order the responsible gene loci (Fig. 9.2). Because of the involvement of contiguous genes, these have been referred to as *contiguous gene syndromes*. This arrangement of the disease gene loci around the Duchenne locus has

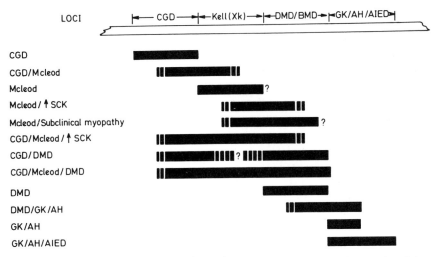

Fig. 9.2 Diagrammatic representation of *contiguous gene syndromes* involving chronic granulomatous disease (CGD), McLeod syndrome, Duchenne and Becker muscular dystrophies (DMD, BMD), glycerol kinase deficiency (GK), adrenal hypoplasia (AH), and Åland Island eye disease (AIED).

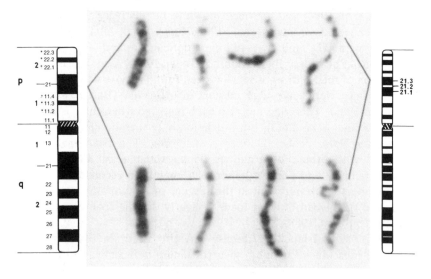

Fig. 9.3 High resolution banding patterns of X chromosomes from boys with Duchenne muscular dystrophy (*above*), and healthy boys (*below*). The possible appearance with techniques which identify a total of 400 bands (*left*), and 850 bands (*right*) are also illustrated. (From Spowart *et al.* (1982) with permission.)

now been confirmed by detailed gene mapping studies (*see*, for example, Ho *et al.* 1992).

It should be noted that deletions in the region of Xp21 result in various abnormal phenotypes only in males. In females such deletions have minimal clinical effects, presumably because the deleted X is preferentially inactivated (Herva *et al.* 1979).

Cases of Duchenne muscular dystrophy with *no* other associated abnormalities but with a microscopically evident interstitial deletion at Xp21 are very much the exception. Such cases have been described by Wilcox *et al.* (1986), Greenberg *et al.* (1987) and Werner and Spiegler (1988), where the deletion was large enough to be visible but was presumably not sufficiently extensive as to include any adjacent gene loci. In the vast majority of cases however no deletion or any other alteration is microscopically evident in the region of Xp21 (Fig. 9.3) even with high resolution banding (Spowart *et al.* 1982). Such techniques reveal that the band Xp21 can be subdivided into three regions (Fig. 9.4) and when applied to lymphoblastoid cell lines from females with a Duchenne-like disorder and an X/autosome translocation, the breakpoint has been found to be in sub-band Xp212 or in Xp211 (Boyd and Buckle 1986). It can be calculated that the DNA represented in the sub-

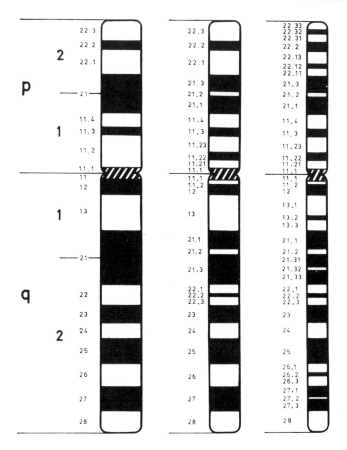

Fig. 9.4 Diagrammatic representation of the high resolution banding patterns which can be delineated on the X chromosome by various techniques.

bands Xp211, Xp212, and Xp213 is around 5000 kb, 2000 kb, and 4000 kb respectively (1 kb = 1000 base pairs of DNA). From these cytogenetic studies the chromosomal region involved in some way with Duchenne/Becker muscular dystrophy would therefore span more than a thousand kilobases of DNA.

Linked DNA markers

Between functioning genes there are large stretches of DNA, the functions of which are still largely unknown. Within this DNA are variations in nucleotide sequences which have no apparent phenotypic effects on the host organism and are inherited in a Mendelian fashion. These changes in base sequence, which occur about once in every 100 base pairs, can be identified because they can alter the DNA site normally cleaved by a particular restriction enzyme since these enzymes cleave DNA at sequence specific sites. Thus, a change in base sequence in a segment of DNA will, with a particular restriction enzyme, result in different sized fragments in different individuals. These genotypic changes can be recognized by the different mobilities of the restriction fragments on gel electrophoresis. The fragments are identified by using an appropriate 'probe' which is a labelled DNA fragment that will hybridize with, and thereby detect, complementary sequences among the DNA fragments produced by a restriction enzyme (Southern blot).

These variations in nucleotide sequences are referred to as *restriction fragment length polymorphisms (RFLPs)*. Their interest lies in the fact that the demonstration of linkage between an RFLP and the locus for a particular genetic disease can be useful for carrier detection and prenatal diagnosis. Also, if the chromosomal site of an RFLP were already known then it could furnish information on the site of a disease locus to which it proved to be

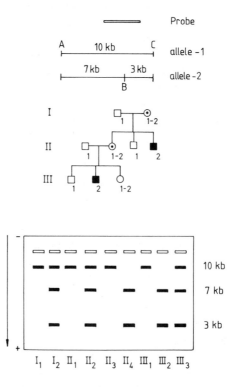

Fig. 9.5 Pedigree of an X-linked recessive disorder linked to an RFLP (the alleles of which are represented below the pedigree symbols) and the appearance of the corresponding Southern blot.

closely linked. A hypothetical example of the co-inheritance of an RFLP and an X-linked recessive disorder is given in Fig. 9.5. Here it is assumed there is a polymorphism at restriction site *B*, the absence of the site is called allele-1 and the presence of the site is allele-2. When the restriction enzyme cuts the DNA in one chromosome at sites *A* and *C* it generates a single fragment of size 10 kilobases (10 kb) which corresponds to allele-1. If the enzyme cuts the DNA not only at sites *A* and *C* but also at *B*, two fragments will now be generated of sizes 7 kb and 3 kb which correspond to allele-2. Polymorphic genotypes can therefore be deduced from the pattern of bands on an electrophoretic gel. In this example, grandmother (I_2) and mother (II_2) are both heterozygous for the RFLP and both carry the X-linked recessive disorder. Since both affected males have allele-2 it would appear that allele-2 and the disorder are co-inherited. That is, they are both on the same X chromosome. By studying individuals in a family in which an RFLP and an X-linked recessive disorder are inherited it is possible to estimate how frequently crossing-over occurs between them. Thus, in this example, if the unaffected son III_1 had also inherited allele-2 there would appear to have been at least one cross-over (or recombinant) out of four meioses. By studying a number of informative families in this way, the frequency of recombination can be determined. Recombination frequency, usually designated as θ, is related to the distance between the gene loci concerned — one per cent recombination being equivalent to a distance of one map unit, or one centiMorgan (cM), which is roughly equal to 1000 kb, or 10^6 base pairs. When loci are some distance apart then the error rate in diagnosis will be equal to θ at each meiosis. The details of the calculation of genetic distances from linkage data are simply explained in Emery (1986). A more detailed and authoritative up-to-date discussion is given in Lalouel and White (1990) which also provides an extensive bibliography on the subject.

With regard to linkage with Duchenne muscular dystrophy, the first step was to isolate a relevant DNA sequence. In 1981, Davies and her colleagues isolated the first DNA sequences from cloned fragments derived from the human X chromosome, the so-called X genomic library. The location of these cloned sequences was then determined by various methods. These included studying somatic cell hybrids with a full complement of Chinese hamster or mouse chromosomes and different extents of the human X chromosome. Another method of localizing a DNA sequence was by *in situ* hybridization whereby the sequence was labelled and hybridized directly to a metaphase chromosome preparation. One of the cloned sequences, designated RC8, turned out to be located on the short arm of X chromosome. Using this as a probe, it detected a polymorphism with the restriction enzyme *Taq* I, and by studying several families the polymorphism detected by RC8 (now called DXS9) proved to be linked to Duchenne muscular dystrophy (Murray *et al.* 1982). Shortly afterwards a different probe (L1.28) detected another polymorphism (DXS7) on the opposite side of Xp21, and it was found that the Duchenne locus lay between the two (Davies *et al.* 1983). Both markers eventually turned out to be about 15 cM on either side (referred to as 'flanking' or 'bridging') the Duchenne locus. Not only was this a landmark in the history of the disease but it was the first disorder shown to be linked to an RFLP.

At the same time Kingston and her colleagues (Kingston *et al.* 1983) showed that Becker muscular dystrophy was linked to DXS7 (L1.28). Subsequently it was also shown to be linked to DXS9 (RC8) and to other DNA markers at roughly similar genetic distances to Duchenne muscular dystrophy (Kingston *et al.* 1984; Fadda *et al.* 1985; Brown *et al.* 1985; Wilcox *et al.* 1985). These findings therefore indicated that Duchenne and Becker muscular dystrophies could either be allelic or the two loci be very close together in the same region of the X chromosome. We now know that they are in fact allelic. Interestingly, Emery–Dreifuss muscular dystrophy appears to be linked to colour blindness and to DNA markers located at Xq28 (p. 90), which indicates that the responsible gene mutation is *not* be allelic with Duchenne and Becker muscular dystrophies.

A number of polymorphic loci have now been detected around the

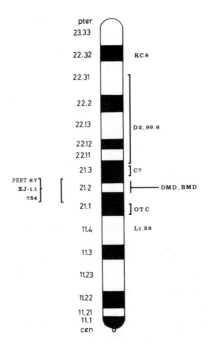

Fig. 9.6 Localization of various RFLPs around the Duchenne/Becker locus. (Reproduced by kind permission of Dr Kay Davies.)

Duchenne locus. Their ordering and exact distances apart are not yet entirely certain but the current situation is summarized in Fig. 9.6. The subject of DNA markers in X-linked dystrophies has been reviewed in a series of articles in the *Journal of Medical Genetics* (1986, Vol. 23, No. 6, p. 481 *et seq.*).

Isolation of the Duchenne gene

The most obvious approach to eventually isolating the Duchenne gene itself would be to 'walk the genome' from a closely linked probe toward the gene, so as to eventually include it. This could be done by studying overlapping clones of DNA sequences. There are several reasons, however, why this approach is difficult. Even a very closely linked marker only 1 cM from the disease locus is a million base pairs away, and it would be extremely difficult to know if one was moving closer or further away by this strategy. Other methods seemed more likely to succeed.

One approach pursued by Worton and his colleagues in Toronto, Canada, was to isolate the junctional region in an X/autosome translocation associated with a Duchenne-like disorder in a female. They chose a translocation involving chromosome 21 (described by Verellen-Dumoulin *et al.* 1984), which they showed split the block of genes encoding ribosomal RNA on the short arm of chromosome 21 (Worton *et al.* 1984). They then used ribosomal DNA probes to identify the junctional fragment in clones derived from the region of the translocation site. The region spanning the translocation breakpoint, and which presumably contained at least part of the Duchenne locus, was then cloned. A sequence derived from the clone was found to detect an RFLP which was very closely linked to Duchenne muscular dystrophy. This probe (referred to as XJ probe), failed to hybridize with DNA from the occasional patient with Duchenne muscular dystrophy indicating that in these boys there is a deletion of the region complementary to the probe (Ray *et al.* 1985).

Kunkel and colleagues in Boston approached the problem in a particularly ingenious way. They extracted DNA from a patient with the deletion described previously by Francke and her colleagues (p. 172). The DNA was then sheared by sonication which produces DNA fragments with irregular ends. DNA from a 49, XXXXY lymphoid cell line was cleaved with the restriction enzyme *Mbo* I. The two sets of fragments were then mixed and heated in order to disassociate the DNA strands. These were then allowed to reassociate in the presence of phenol (so-called phenol enhanced reassociation technique — PERT). Under appropriate conditions, and with the patient's DNA in excess, most of the reassociated molecules will have sheared ends and a few will be hybrid molecules with one sheared end and one *Mbo* I 'sticky end'. However, those sequences in the control *not* represented in the patient's DNA (where they are deleted) will not hybridize with the patient's DNA. By perforce they will only hybridize between themselves and therefore consist of perfectly reassociated molecules with two *Mbo* I ends. Only the last can be ligated into an appropriately cleaved plasmid and be cloned (Kunkel *et al.* 1985). In this way a library of cloned sequences (referred to as PERT probes), corresponding to the portion of DNA deleted in the affected boy, was produced. These have detected several RFLPs closely linked to the Duchenne locus and, like Worton's probes, they also detected small deletions in a proportion of affected boys (Monaco *et al.* 1985) which are of different lengths in different families (Kunkel *et al.* 1986).

It should be noted that the probes isolated by Worton (XJ) and Kunkel (PERT) have shown recombination with Duchenne muscular dystrophy ($\theta \simeq 0.05$) thus further indicating that the Duchenne locus is very large (Fischbeck *et al.* 1986). In fact recombination between markers at the two *extremes* of the locus is around 10 per cent (Abbs *et al.* 1990; Oudet *et al.* 1991). But recombination may not be uniform throughout the locus, a hotspot, for example, being centred around DXS 164 (PERT 87) (Grimm *et al.* 1989).

Deletions

The Xp21 locus has been cloned (see below) and using cDNA probes derived in this way approximately 70 per cent of cases of Duchenne muscular dystrophy (Forrest *et al.* 1987b) and over 80 per cent of cases of Becker muscular dystrophy (Bushby *et al.* 1992) have been found to have gene deletions. These findings have two important implications. First, if the deletion involves a significant part of the gene, then it might be expected that the affected individual could amount an immune response if exposed to the missing gene product and this could make replacement therapy difficult. Secondly, in cases associated with a deletion it is possible to identify new mutations. This is illustrated in Fig. 9.7 based on two families reported by Monaco *et al.* (1985). Using a particular probe (PERT 87-8) an RFLP was detected with the enzyme *Bst* XI reflected in two DNA fragments of sizes 4.4 kb and 2.2 kb (say allele-1 and allele-2).

In family A, grandmother (I_2) is either homozygous for allele-2 or hemizygous because one allele has been deleted. Her daughter (II_1) has no allele-2 which she should have inherited from her mother. She is therefore heterozygous for the deletion which is evident in her affected son (III_1) who is therefore *not* a new mutation.

In family B both grandmother and mother are heterozygous for the RFLP and neither allele is deleted. However, one of the alleles is deleted in the affected son who must therefore be a new mutation.

Though up to 70 per cent of cases of Duchenne muscular dystrophy have a deletion, about 5 to 10 per cent have a gene *duplication* (Hu *et al.* 1988,

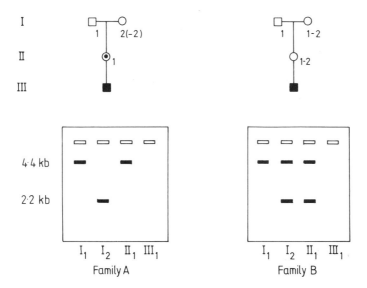

Fig. 9.7 Two families in which affected boys have a gene deletion. The alleles of an informative RFLP are represented below the pedigree symbols and the appearances of the corresponding Southern blots are shown.

1989) which probably results from unequal sister-chromatid exchange. The remaining cases are presumed to be caused by *point mutations*, about which little is known at present. However the construction of a yeast artificial chromosome (YAC) containing the complete Duchenne gene will no doubt make the investigation of such mutations easier (Monaco *et al.* 1992; Den Dunnen *et al.* 1992).

Origin of deletions

Deletions in dystrophy, whether in-frame or frame-shift, no doubt result from the effects of environmental mutagenic agents. This has been well documented in many animal species with similar mutations. But it is also possible that in some cases they may arise as a result of micro-inversions within the very large Xp21 locus itself. If the inversion occurred in a female then at meiosis mispairing between the two X chromosomes would result in a loop. If intra-chromosomal breakage–fusion occurred at the junction of the loop, then this would maintain the integrity of both chromosomes but generate a deletion of the inverted sequence at the site of breakage-fusion. If so, then the maternal grandmother, as well as the mother, might be expected to carry the inversion. Such 'micro-inversions' could generate 'micro-deletions' involving only a few kilobases. If such inversions were relatively frequent among females in the general population, then isolated affected males could occasionally be due to perturbations resulting from breakage-fusion (Fig. 9.8).

Interestingly there is a bimodal distribution of recombination hot spots within the dystrophin gene (Oudet *et al.* 1992) and these *coincide* with the distribution of deletions (p. 72), which also supports the idea that the former is related to, or even generates, the latter!

Molecular pathology and phenotype

There is no simple relationship between the *extent* of a mutation and the resultant clinical disease. For example, a comparatively minute deletion of 52 bp out of 88 bp in exon 19 has been reported in a boy with classical Duchenne muscular dystrophy (Matsuo *et al.* 1990). On the other hand, a massive duplication of more than 400 000 bp within the central region of the gene resulted in a dystrophin of approximately 600 kDa, yet the patient only had a mild Becker dystrophy (Angelini *et al.* 1990). The effects on the phenotype depend not so much on the extent of a deletion/duplication but on whether or not it disrupts the reading frame.

Frame-shift hypothesis

We have seen (p. 87) that the milder Becker muscular dystrophy results from mutations which maintain the reading frame (in-frame) resulting in an abnormal but partially functional dystrophin, but in Duchenne muscular dystrophy mutations disrupt the reading frame (frame-shift) so that virtually no dystrophin is produced. This reading frame hypothesis (Monaco *et al.* 1988) holds for over 90 per cent of cases. But exceptions do occur such a mild Becker muscular dystrophy with a frame-shift deletion. These cases could be explained if, for example, synthesis of dystrophin was reinitiated from an internal start codon further along the gene (Malhotra *et al.* 1988). This is shown in Figure 9.9. In an extensive study of patients with Duchenne dystrophy with frame-shift mutations, the size of muscle dystrophin, *detected at greatly reduced levels*, agreed closlely with that expected if the reading frame were restored and translation proceeded (Nicholson *et al.* 1992*a*). In fact there is a suggestion of a correlation between the amount of dystrophin in these cases and the severity of the disease as assessed by the age at becoming confined to a wheelchair (Nicholson *et al.* 1992*c*). Even the very low levels of muscle dystrophin in Duchenne muscular dystrophy may therefore have some functional significance. Exceptional cases of severe Duchenne dystrophy with an in-frame deletion may be due to the resultant truncated transcript not being translated or translated into an unstable protein (Chelly *et al.* 1990*a*, 1991).

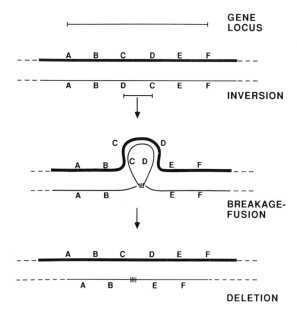

Fig. 9.8 Diagrammatic representation of how a micro-inversion *within* a large gene locus could generate microdeletions.

Mutation site

Although deletions (and occasional duplications) can occur almost anywhere in the dystrophin gene, most occur in two 'hot-spots'. These have been referred to as the *Central* High Frequency Deletion Region (HFDR) and the *Proximal* HFDR (Fig. 4.17, p. 72). The Central HFDR is located approximately 1200 kb from the 5′ end of the gene, clustered around exons 45–55 where most deletions can be detected with the P20 probe (cDNA probes 7–8). The Proximal HFDR is located approximately 500 kb from the 5′ end of the gene, clustered around the first 20 exons where most deletions can be detected with PERT and XJ probes (cDNA probes 1–3) (Lindlöf *et al.* 1989; Gilgenkrantz *et al.* 1989; Cooke *et al.* 1990; Covone *et al.* 1991). Roughly 85 per cent of deletions can in fact be detected using only two cDNA probes (1–2a and 8).

It seems that proximal (5′) deletions are commoner in familial cases and distal deletions in isolated cases. A 'proximal' new mutant has a greater risk of recurrence, of about 30 per cent, and a 'distal' new mutant has a lesser risk of recurrence of about 4 per cent (Passos-Bueno *et al.* 1992).

The majority of *out-of-frame* (frame-shift) deletions in these regions, as well as elsewhere, result in severe Duchenne muscular dystrophy. Most of these cases have virtually no dystrophin. In Becker muscular dystrophy

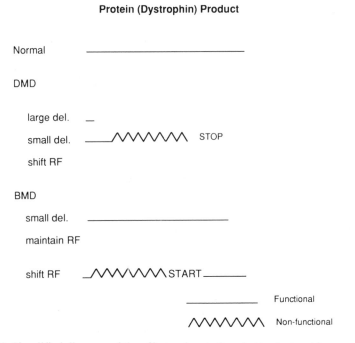

Fig. 9.9 Simplified diagram of the effects of mutations in the dystrophin gene on the gene product which maintain or disrupt (shift) the reading frame (RF).

there is no clear correlation between abundance of dystrophin and clinical course (Bushby *et al.* 1992) and there is no overlap in dystrophin levels in these two disorders. Furthermore, the C-terminal region is usually absent in Duchenne muscular dystrophy but present in the milder Becker dystrophy, though it has been argued that this distinction may, at least in part, be artefactual (Nicholson *et al.* 1992*b*).

With regard to mental retardation in Duchenne dystrophy, there is some grouping of deletions in the region of exons 50–52 in such cases. This may therefore represent a crucial region for mental development. It is unlikely however that the brain-specific promoter of dystrophin (which is located 5′ to the muscle dystrophin promoter) is itself involved in the aetiology of mental retardation in this disorder (p. 123).

With *in-frame* deletions the spectrum of phenotypes is much wider (Fig. 9.10). Though there are exceptions, deletions in certain regions tend to be associated with particular phenotypes (Koenig *et al.* 1989; Beggs *et al.* 1991; Love *et al.* 1991). Deletions of exons 45–57, for example, tend to be associated with typical fairly mild Becker muscular dystrophy with loss of ambulation after the age of 40 (Bushby *et al.* 1992).

A most interesting finding is that deletions of the central region of the gene

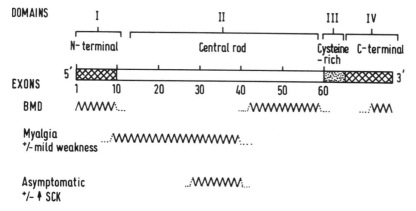

Fig. 9.10 Regions of the dystrophin gene and protein associated with particular phenotypes resulting from in-frame mutations.

which remove almost 50 per cent of the dystrophin can result in a very mild phenotype. The resultant significantly truncated dystrophin is therefore adequate for almost normal muscle function (England *et al.* 1990; Love *et al.* 1991). Furthermore, some deletions within this region may produce myalgia and muscle cramps but no weakness (Gospe *et al.* 1989), or even no symptoms at all or merely a raised SCK level (Beggs *et al.* 1991).

Mutations *outside* the Xp21 locus have also been described in patients with dystrophy. If a deletion involves adjacent genes as well as the dystrophin gene, then the resulting phenotype will reflect the involvement of these contiguous genes (p. 173). Thus a large deletion of the glycerol kinase and adrenal hypoplasia gene loci also involved the 3′ end of the dystrophin gene in three brothers who clinically exhibited features of glycerol kinase deficiency and adrenal hypoplasia as well as Becker muscular dystrophy (Love *et al.* 1990). At the other end of the Xp21 locus, a mutation of the muscle specific promoter resulted in a patient with mild Becker dystrophy with a full-sized dystrophin of reduced abundance (Bushby *et al.* 1991*b*). However, when specifically sought for, mutations in the muscle promoter region in Duchenne and Becker dystrophies are apparently rare (Vitiello *et al.* 1992).

There is a suggestion that a gene for X-linked cardiomyopathy (in which there is usually no skeletal muscle involvement) may be located at the 5′ end of the Xp21 locus (J. Towbin, personal communication, 1992) and conceivably could therefore also become involved in any extensive deletion of this latter locus.

Thus the idea discussed previously (p. 77), that there is a wide spectrum of abnormalities associated with mutations at the Xp21 locus, finds support from molecular studies. In fact there may be healthy males in the population who have small defects in the central rod region of the dystrophin protein which may only be expressed under stress, such as muscle cramps after exercise or excessive muscle fatigue in later life. We have no idea what effects different mutations within the Xp21 locus might have on cardiac function. For example, a mutation which does not cause weakness might conceivably affect cardiac muscle in some way in later life in an otherwise healthy individual.

The dystrophin gene

The dystrophin gene was isolated and characterized by first using PERT (Monaco *et al.* 1986) and XJ (Burghes *et al.* 1987) probes to identify relevant mRNA transcripts in human skeletal muscle. The corresponding cDNA was then cloned and sequenced (Koenig *et al.* 1987, 1988). The gene proved to be some 2400 kb in length, consisting of over 70 exons of mean size 0.2 kb and introns of mean size 35 kb. The gene is transcribed into a 14 kb mRNA. Thus the actual coding sequences represent less than 1 per cent of the nucleotide composition of the gene locus.

Muscle dystrophin is not the only product of the Duchenne gene locus. There is also a slightly different brain dystrophin, and another transcript for example consists only of the carboxy-terminal region (of 4.8 kb) and is particularly abundant in Schwann cells where the 14 kb dystrophin transcript is absent (Blake *et al.* 1992). Several other isoform of dystrophin also exist (p. 188). Furthermore, with a gene as large as the dystrophin gene, there is the remote possibility that it may contain a gene *within itself*. Support for this idea would be the identification of so-called 'CpG islands' within the gene. These are regions of CG dinucleotide pairs which contain *Hpa* II restriction sites and are known to be located near the 5′ ends of active genes.

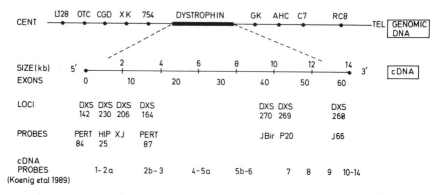

Fig. 9.11 Some flanking genes and intragenic markers of the Xp21 locus. The positions are relative and *not to scale* (data from various sources and Dr Donald R. Love (Oxford)).

At present there is no information on CpG islands within the dystrophin gene. But this has been found in the factor VIII gene which is very much smaller (187 kb with 26 introns) (Levinson *et al.* 1990).

The linkage relationships between the Xp21 locus and some flanking genes and intragenic markers are given in Figure 9.11 and Appendix G.

It should be noted that different notations for cDNA probes are often used. For example, cDNA probes 7 and 8 are the same as probes Cf 23a and Cf 56a respectively, and Cf 115 is contained within the cDNA probes 11–14 (for example, Passos-Bueno *et al.* 1990*a*).

Dystrophin

Using polyclonal antibodies directed against fusion proteins produced in bacteria from cDNA, the protein product of the Xp21 locus has been identified (Hoffman *et al.* 1987*a*). It has been named *dystrophin* and as would be predicted is a very large protein (Fig. 9.12).

It has a molecular weight of 427 kDa consisting of 3685 amino acids. It is a rod-shaped protein composed of four domains (Koenig *et al.* 1988):

- N-terminal domain with homology to α-actinin and composed of 240 amino acids;
- central rod domain formed by a succession of 25 triple helical repeats similar to spectrin, and composed of roughly 3000 amino acids;
- cysteine-rich domain composed of 280 amino acids;
- C-terminal domain composed of 420 amino acids.

That dystrophin shares many features with spectrin and α-actinin indicates that this too is a cytoskeletal protein. Early on it was shown to be localized to muscle cell membranes (Sugita *et al.* 1988; Zubrzycka-Gaarn *et al.* 1988). It is a costameric protein forming a lattice which encircles the muscle fibre and attaches the sarcomeres to the sarcolemma (Minetti *et al.* 1992). But it is not directly inserted into the membrane but via a glycoprotein with which it forms a dystrophin–glycoprotein complex (Campbell and Kahl 1989) with

427 kD with 4 domains of 3685 aa

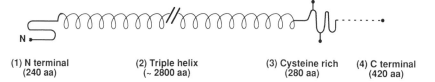

| (1) N terminal | (2) Triple helix | (3) Cysteine rich | (4) C terminal |
| (240 aa) | (~ 2800 aa) | (280 aa) | (420 aa) |

Fig. 9.12 The dystrophin molecule.

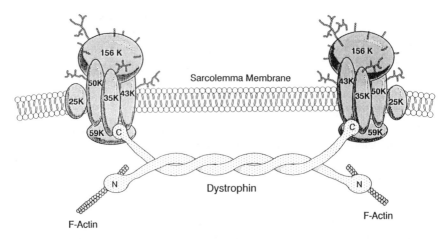

Fig. 9.13 The dystrophin–glycoprotein complex. (From Ervasti and Campbell (1991) and reproduced with kind permission of the authors and publishers.)

intermembrane and extramembrane components (Ibraghimov-Beskrovnaya *et al.* 1992) (Fig. 9.13). The role of this complex in the pathogenesis of muscular dystrophy will be discussed in Chapter 10.

But dystrophin is not a single protein but exists as a number of isoforms (or dystrophin-related proteins) of which at least six have been identified so far: adult skeletal muscle, embryonic muscle, cardiac muscle, diaphragmatic muscle, brain, and liver isoforms. Currently three of these have been characterized (14 kb muscle and brain transcripts, and a 6.5 kb liver transcript—Nudel *et al.* 1992). They have slightly different structures generated as a result of alternative splicing (Feener *et al.* 1989; Nudel *et al.* 1989; Klamut *et al.* 1990; Bies *et al.* 1992). There are probably many others. For example, there is probably more than one dystrophin isoform present in developing muscle alone (Clerk *et al.* 1992).

As Byers and colleagues (1991) have suggested, 'Isoform differences and the presence of dystrophin on different specialized membrane surfaces imply multiple functional roles for the dystrophin protein'. The nature of these roles is as yet unknown, but such a mechanism could well explain the distribution and extent of involvement of different tissues in Duchenne and Becker muscular dystrophies as a consequence of mutations at the Xp21 locus.

Summary and conclusion

Several females with Duchenne muscular dystrophy and X/autosome translocations have been described, the breakpoint on the X chromosome always being at Xp21. This, and the fact that a unique case of Duchenne muscular dystrophy has been found with a microscopically visible deletion in this same region of the X chromosomes, pointed to the disease locus being located at this point. Several restriction fragment length polymorphisms (RFLPs), which are polymorphisms due to the presence or absence of a particular restriction site, have been identified around Xp21 and linked to the Duchenne locus. Information on linked RFLPs can be used for prenatal diagnosis, and in conjunction with SCK levels can be used in carrier detection. Intragenic probes are now also available where the possibility of errors due to recombination are significantly reduced. Such probes have shown that 70 per cent of cases of Duchenne and Becker muscular dystrophy have submicroscopic gene deletions.

Finally, the Duchenne gene has been cloned and studied and has proved to be at least 2000 kb in length and to consist of at least 70 exons. The gene product has been identified and called *dystrophin*. This is a very large protein which is present in only very small amounts in normal muscle. It is virtually absent or nonfunctional in muscle in patients with Duchenne muscular dystrophy and truncated, presumably semifunctional, in Becker muscular dystrophy. It is associated with muscle cell membranes via glycoprotein forming a dystrophin–glycoprotein complex. Disruption of this complex, consequent on a deficiency of dystrophin, initiates the train of events which ultimately leads to muscle cell death. Dystrophin exists in a number of different isoforms (dystrophin-related proteins) with different tissue distributions. The effects of mutations at the Xp21 locus on these dystrophin isoforms might well explain the distribution and extent of involvement of different tissues in Duchenne muscular dystrophy.

10 Pathogenesis

When this book was first being written in 1985, much space was given to an examination of the evidence for what were referred to as the vascular, neurogenic, and membrane hypotheses of causation. But with the discovery that the *primary* cause was a deficiency of muscle dystrophin located at the cell membrane, there seemed no longer any reason to consider much previous research on the subject. However, I suspect that among these research findings may be important ideas necessary for a full and complete understanding of the disease process. Thus, although a vascular or neurogenic defect is definitely not the *primary* cause, nevertheless some minor changes in the microcirculation consequent on the replacement of muscle tissue by fat and connective tissue (Carry *et al*. 1986) could conceivably compromise the blood supply to any surviving muscle fibres and thereby aggravate the disease process. We have also seen how innervation is essential for complete maturation of the muscle fibre (p. 139). Possibly such innervation, as well as a deficiency of muscle dystrophin and other factors, is necessary for the full expression of an abnormal phenotype. As Hoffman and Kunkel, who first identified the primary defect in Duchenne muscular dystrophy have said, there may well be '. . . defects of the vasculature and nervous system in addition to the more obvious striated muscle involvement' (Hoffman and Kunkel 1989).

Vascular abnormalities

Evidence of possible abnormalities in the circulation came from early work by Démos (Démos 1961; Démos and Maroteaux 1961; Démos *et al*. 1962) and Engel (Engel 1975). Though these early findings have now been thrown into question, there is a need to study the matter with modern techniques of electron microscopy (Koehler 1977) and immunohistochemistry. It certainly seems possible that defects in the microcirculation of muscle might well occur as the tissue undergoes degeneration and is replaced by relatively avascular connective tissue. Furthermore, dystrophin has been found to be localized in the surface membrane of smooth muscle fibres in the tunica media of blood vessels (Miyatake *et al*. 1989). Could therefore its absence in Duchenne muscular dystrophy cause vascular dysfunction resulting in an increase in nerve growth factor receptor activity (Zhao *et al*. 1991)?

Neurogenic abnormalities

There is no doubt that the central nervous system is involved in the disease process (p. 115). But here we are concerned with possible involvement of muscle innervation in the disease process. Much of the earlier work, based largely on electromyographic studies reviewed in the first edition, has been refuted (Bradley *et al.* 1975*a*, *b*; Panayiotopoulos 1975). But it is difficult to avoid remembering that many characteristics of fast and slow muscles, their enzyme profiles and physiological properties, are dependent on appropriate innervation (Buller *et al.* 1960). It might be revealing to consider the relationship between the development of innervation in early fetal muscle and the expression of dystrophin in such tissues. Interestingly a dystrophin–like protein (utrophin, p. 75) is normally localized at the neuromuscular junction only, but in Duchenne muscular dystrophy it appears at the sarcolemma (Nguyen thi Man *et al.* 1991), whereas dystrophin itself is normally localized at the sarcolemma where it is absent in dystrophy (Bonilla *et al.* 1988*a*). Could the expression of this dystrophin–like protein in the sarcolemma in dystrophy be the result of a compensatory process, and if so how is this brought about, and does it have any physiological significance? There is some evidence that in regenerating fibres there is a compensatory increase in defective dystrophin transcription (Scott *et al.* 1988).

Membrane abnormalities

It is difficult to be sure when the idea was first considered that a significant defect in Duchenne muscular dystrophy might reside in the muscle cell membrane. Even in the 1950s this possibility was mooted when certain muscle enzymes were found to be increased in the serum of affected boys (p. 46). There is little doubt however that considerable impetus was given to the idea by the work of Roses and colleagues in the mid-1970s when they reported an apparent abnormality of the membrane-associated protein spectrin in *erythrocyte membranes* in Duchenne muscular dystrophy (Roses *et al.* 1975; Roses and Appel 1976; Roses *et al.* 1976*a*). This finding had instant appeal for many investigators working in the field. It not only satisfied the biochemists who needed a biochemical basis for any proposed membrane defect, but also those who expected that the basic genetic defect might possibly be expressed in tissues other than muscle.

Cell membranes in general consist of a lipid bilayer. On the extracellular surface are located various hormone receptor and ouabain binding sites as well as externally orientated enzymes, such as acetylcholinesterase. Within the membrane are located certain other enzymes, such as proteases, while on the intracellular surface are located other enzymes, such as glyceraldehyde-3-phosphate dehydrogenase, and cytoskeletal proteins, such as ankyrin,

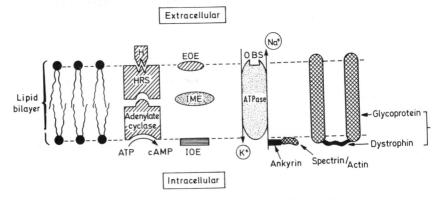

Fig. 10.1 Diagrammatic representation of a *generalized* cell membrane. HRS, hormone receptor site; EOE, externally oriented enzymes; IME, intramembrane enzymes; IOE, internally oriented enzymes; OBS, ouabain binding site.

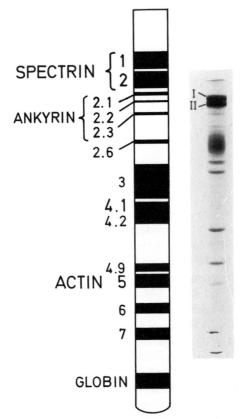

Fig. 10.2 SDS (sodium dodecyl sulphate) polyacrylamide gel electrophoresis pattern of the proteins in the erythrocyte membrane as visualized by staining with Coomassie blue.

spectrin, actin, and dystrophin (Fig. 10.1)

If erythrocyte ghost protein is subjected to polyacrylamide gel electrophoresis (PAGE) then with appropriate staining a number of bands are revealed (Fig. 10.2). Band 2 is a component of spectrin and Roses and colleagues reported an apparent increase in phosphorylation of this peptide in Duchenne muscular dystrophy.

Since this original work a variety of other membrane abnormalities have been reported, not only in erythrocytes but also in lymphocytes, fibroblasts, and muscle (Table 10.1).

Table 10.1 *Some reported membrane-associated abnormalities in Duchenne muscular dystrophy*

A. *Erythrocytes*
    1. Morphology
       echinocyte formation
       intramembranous particles ↓
    2. Biochemical
       K ′flux ↑
       Na, K-ATPase ouabain inhibition ↓
       Ca-ATPase ↑
       adenylate cyclase, epinephrine stimulation ↓
       phospholipids abnormal
       protein kinase (phosphorylation) ↑
       acetyl cholinesterase ↓
    3. Physical
       deformability ↓
       shear modulus ↑
       electron spin resonance abnormal
       osmotic fragility ↑
       electrophoretic mobility ↑
B. *Lymphocytes*
    capping ↓
C. *Fibroblasts*
    intercellular adhesiveness ↓
D. *Muscle*
    1. Morphology
       membrane discontinuities
       intramembranous particles ↓
    2. Biochemical
       adenylate cyclase, epinephrine stimulation ↓
       phospholipids abnormal
       Na, K-ATPase ouabain inhibition ↓
    3. Physical
       penetration by dyes, etc. ↑

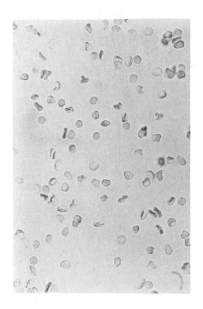 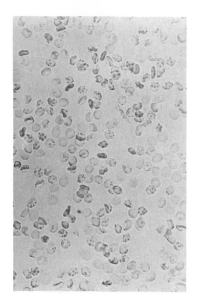

Fig. 10.3 (*Left*) normal appearance of erythrocytes. (*Right*) echinocytes.

The most obvious morphological abnormalities which have been reported include changes in erythrocyte shape, numbers of intramembranous particles, and lympocyte capping. Under certain *in vitro* conditions, erythrocytes may adopt a 'spiney' sea-urchin-like appearance which are therefore referred to as echinocytes, and such distortion has been reported to occur more frequently in Duchenne muscular dystrophy (Figs. 10.3 and 10.4). The membrane lipid bilayer may be freeze-fractured and on subsequent electron microscopy particles on both membrane fracture faces can be visualized and counted. In Duchenne muscular dystrophy it has been reported that the number of intramembranous particles, which represent membrane transport proteins, is reduced (Fig. 10.5).

Finally, protein receptors on the surface of peripheral blood lymphocytes can be visualized by using fluorescent-labelled polyvalent anti-human immunoglobulin producing so-called 'caps'. In Duchenne muscular dystrophy lymphocyte capping has been reported to be reduced compared with normal (Fig. 10.6).

Many of the reported physicochemical abnormalities could be explained on the basis of reduced membrane fluidity—that in some way *the membrane is more rigid than normal.*

These various findings have been critically reviewed by Rowland (1976,

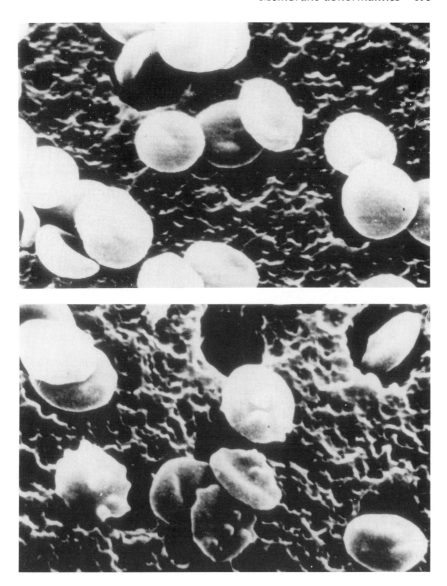

Fig. 10.4 Erythrocytes as seen with scanning electronmicroscopy. (*Above*), normal appearance, (*below*) echinocytes.

CONTROL   DUCHENNE

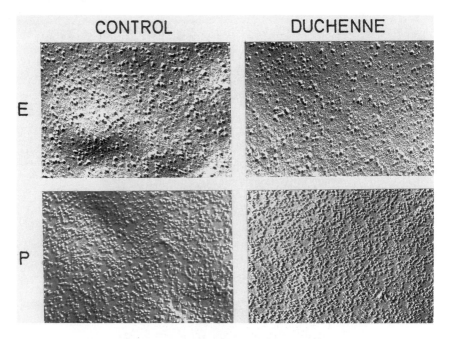

Fig. 10.5 Freeze-fracture electron micrograph of erythrocyte membranes showing the intramembranous particles on the P (protoplasmic) and E (external) faces. We have found no significant difference in the numbers of particles in controls and Duchenne muscular dystrophy (Lloyd *et al.* 1981).

1980) who provides an extensive bibliography. It appears that in many cases, even including the original report of abnormal band 2 phosphorylation, the findings are controversial. Either the abnormality in question has not been reproducible in different laboratories, or it has been found to occur in normal as well as affected boys. Of 27 erythrocyte abnormalities reported from 102 different laboratories, 9 are single reports, and of the remaining 18 there is controversy in all but one, namely increased Ca^{2+}-ATPase activity (Rowland 1980). However, even this latter finding is something of an enigma. Although it appears the activity of this enzyme, responsible for pumping calcium out of the cell, may be increased in erythrocytes (Hodson and Pleasure 1977; Luthra *et al.* 1979; Ruitenbeek 1979), there is apparently no abnormality of calcium efflux (Shoji 1981; Szibor *et al.* 1981), and calcium levels are normal (p. 205). There is also no apparent abnormality in calcium exchange in cultured skin fibroblasts (Statham and Dubowitz 1979).

It is not at all clear why there should be so much difficulty in reproducing observations in different laboratories, but it may be in part a reflection of

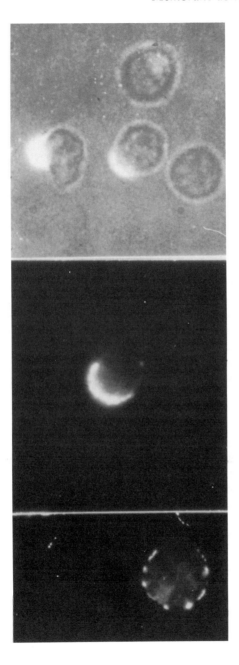

Fig. 10.6 Formation of 'caps' (from below to above) of fluorescent-labelled polyvalent anti-human immunoglobulin on peripheral blood lymphocytes.

the complexities of the various technologies involved as well as the need for their standardization.

It would be unwise, however, to dismiss all these findings since many have been reported by very reputable and established investigators. And they are all consistent with the notion that there *is* an abnormality in cell membranes in Duchenne muscular dystrophy—even though these studies themselves gave little idea as to the nature of the basic underlying defect. Time is now ripe to reconsider these reported abnormalities in the light of the proven deficiency of dystrophin as the primary cause. The problem is that the estimated amounts of dystrophin transcript (Chelly *et al.* 1988), at least in lymphocytes and fibroblasts, are so low (less than 0.05 per cent relative to 100 per cent in skeletal muscle) that it is difficult to imagine that they can be of any physiological significance. But in these tissues transcription may be under the control of different promotors and the products may not be strictly identical to muscle dystrophin (*see* for example Feener *et al.* 1989). This has been proposed as an explanation for impaired lymphocyte capping in dystrophy (Baricordi *et al.* 1989). Alternatively, the effects of a deficiency of dystrophin may not be the same in all tissues. For example, whereas enzyme efflux (at least LDH) is increased in muscle it is not significantly increased in erythrocytes and lymphocytes (Somer 1980), and whereas osmotic fragility is *increased* in erythrocytes, it is *decreased* in dystrophin-less muscle cells (Menke and Jockusch 1991). A defect in the interaction between various cytoskeletal components, including dystrophin(s), might explain the reported abnormalities in tissues other than muscle (Ferretti *et al.* 1990).

Table 10.2 *Proportion (%) of calcium-positive fibres in cryostat sections of gastrocnemius muscle biopsy samples in various neuromuscular disorders (unpublished data)*

Disorder	No.	Ca-positive fibres
Controls	7	<0.1
Muscular dystrophies		
Duchenne		
preclinical	2	5.3, 18.3
clinical	5	1.8–6.5
Becker	2	2.4, 5.5
limb girdle	2	–
facioscapulohumeral	2	–
Miscellaneous		
central core disease	2	–
nemaline myopathy	2	–
Werdnig–Hoffmann	2	0.0, 0.2

Calcium abnormalities

Around the time that the idea was being seriously considered that a membrane defect might be important in Duchenne muscular dystrophy, another idea was also gaining ground. This concerned the possibility that increased intracellular calcium might also be a significant factor in pathogenesis (Wrogemann and Pena 1976; Duncan 1978). There are a number of lines of evidence which now favour this idea.

There is histochemical and biochemical evidence of increased intracellular calcium in muscle in Duchenne muscular dystrophy, even from a very early age (p. 59), as well as in Becker muscular dystrophy, but to a much lesser degree in other neuromuscular disorders (Table 10.2) in which, incidentally, dystrophin is normal (Patel *et al.* 1988; Hoffman *et al.* 1988).

A significant increase in calcium-positive fibres has also been found in male fetuses at-risk for Duchenne muscular dystrophy (Emery and Burt 1980; Bertorini *et al.* 1984) when there is no evidence of muscle fibre necrosis (Fig. 10.7). We have examined 54 male fetuses at-risk for the disease with data on calcium-positive fibres in 37. Of these 37, 6 were considered to be affected, there being a good correlation between the presence of calcium-positive fibres and other variables (eosinophilic fibres and increased variance in muscle fibre size) which we have shown probably represent the earliest pathological manifestations of the disease (Toop and Emery 1974; Emery 1977*a*; Emery *et al.* 1979*a*) (Table 10.3).

Increased intracellular calcium has also been found in the *mdx* mouse (Fong *et al.* 1990) and in the dystrophic dog (Valentine *et al.* 1990) and, as in Duchenne muscular dystrophy, can be found in muscle fibres which appear normal. In female carriers of Duchenne dystrophy non-necrotic fibres devoid of dystrophin also contain increased amounts of calcium (Morandi *et al.* 1990). Thus the fact that increased intracellular calcium is found in normally appearing fibres deficient in dystrophin in affected individuals and carriers, as well as in at-risk fetuses, indicates that this must be an early and significant biochemical change in the dystrophic process. Furthermore increased levels of calcium are also found in *cultured* Duchenne muscle (Mongini *et al.* 1988; Fong *et al.* 1990). Increased intracellular calcium could also explain several of the membrane changes which have been reported (references in Emery and Burt 1980). Also the efflux of creatine kinase from skeletal muscle, one of the most consistent features of the disease, can be induced *in vitro* by increasing the concentration of calcium in the incubating medium. The efflux of lactate dehydrogenase and alanine and aspartate aminotransferases is also increased (Anand and Emery 1980). And CK efflux from Duchenne muscle *in vitro* is reduced in a calcium-free medium (Jackson *et al.* 1991).

Finally, increased intracellular calcium might also account for muscle

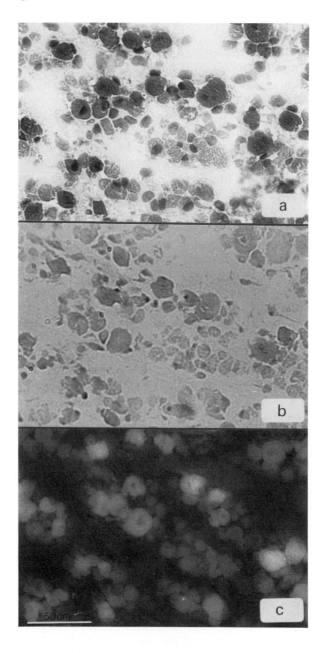

Fig. 10.7 Serial sections of muscle from an at-risk male fetus (B118) stained with (*a*) haematoxylin and eosin (note the dark-staining 'opaque' eosinophilic fibres), (*b*) alizarin red S, (*c*) fluorescent Morin.

Table 10.3 *Male fetuses at-risk for Duchenne muscular dystrophy and considered to be abnormal. Values outside the normal range are italicized (unpublished data)*

	P*	Gestation (weeks)	Fibre Diameter Mean (μm)	Variance	Eosinophilic fibres (%)	Ca-positive fibres (%) (1)	(2)
Controls (16)	—	14–21	6.9–10.7	0.8–3.6	0–5.0	0–3.9	0–7.0
At-risk							
B118	0.90	19	9.6	2.5	8.0	*12.0*	*10.5*
B132	0.20	16	10.0	4.3	6.9	8.4	*7.0*
B145	0.50	21	9.4	*5.4*	9.9	6.8	*7.5*
B150	0.18	12	9.5	3.2	7.5	6.5	*7.0*
B166	1.00	19	7.9	4.0	6.1	4.3	*7.5*
B188	1.00	20	9.1	*6.1*	5.3	5.4	*7.3*

* Probability of the mother being a carrier.
(1), alizarin red S; (2), fluorescent Morin.

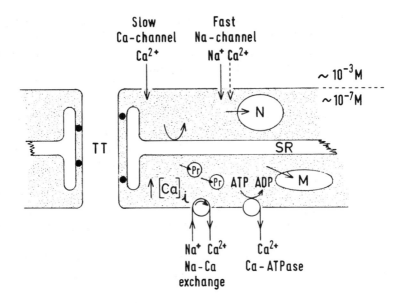

Fig. 10.8 Diagrammatic representation of a muscle cell and the factors which influence the intracellular concentration of calcium. (N, nucleus; M, mitochondria; SR, sarcoplasmic reticulum; TT, transverse tubule.)

necrosis through the enhancement of calcium-activated proteases (Sugita *et al.* 1984). It might also explain the development of muscle contractures since the binding of calcium to troponin C allows myosin to bind with actin which results in muscle contraction.

The regulation of intracellular calcium levels in normal and dystrophic muscle is complex (Martonosi 1989). Normally the concentration of calcium in extracellular fluid is considerably greater than in the cytosol (Fig. 10.8), and therefore any defect in the calcium pump or the cell membrane would automatically result in a massive influx of calcium. For example, increased intracellular calcium has been shown to occur if the Ca^{2+}-ATPase pump is inactivated by an inhibitor, such as phenylhydrazine (Shalev *et al.* 1981), or if ATP is depleted due to anoxia, as in myocardial ischaemia following coronary occlusion (Nayler 1980).

But what is the mechanism which causes the increase in intracellular calcium in Duchenne muscular dystrophy? Theoretically this could result from increased influx or decreased efflux of calcium but there is no evidence for the latter being a significant factor (Turner *et al.* 1991).

Dystrophin is associated with glycoprotein at the cell membrane forming a dystrophin–glycoprotein complex (Ervasti *et al.* 1990, 1991; Ohlendieck *et al.* 1991) and the absence of dystrophin in Duchenne muscular dystrophy leads to the loss of the dystrophin–glycoprotein complex (Ervasti *et al.* 1990). The complex consists of transmembrane and extracellular components. The former attaches dystrophin to the sarcolemma and the latter provides linkage between the sarcolemma and the extracellular matrix. In Duchenne muscular dystrophy the resultant absence of interaction between the sarcolemma and extracellular matrix could well render muscle fibres more prone to necrosis by perhaps altering calcium regulatory mechanisms (Ibraghimov-Beskrovnaya *et al.* 1992). This might occur by merely rendering the muscle fibres more susceptible to mechanical disruption or by increasing membrane permeability in general. But the situation may be more complex than this. Changes in stretch-activated cation channels may be involved (Duncan 1989). In both the *mdx* mouse and Duchenne muscular dystrophy there is in fact increased activitiy of leak channels which appears to be specific to calcium as it does not affect other ions such as sodium (Fong *et al.* 1990; Turner *et al.* 1991). Like similar channels in normal skeletal muscle, these calcium channels are rarely open at rest and only open when the muscle is stretched, but in dystrophy they behave differently (Franco and Lansman 1990).

Apart from increased activity of calcium-leak channels, calcium may enter the cell through the Na^+–Ca^{2+} exchange mechanism (Bkaily *et al.* 1990). Furthermore, in cultured dystrophic muscle, increased intracellular calcium is induced by acetylcholine which may indicate the role of neurogenic factors (Mongini *et al.* 1988). Finally, arguments have been advanced by J. P. Infante and V. A. Huszagh (personal communication, 1990) and Tay and colleagues (1990) that changes in dystrophin itself may be causally related to increased intracellular calcium.

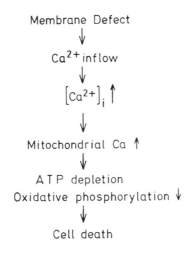

Fig. 10.9 Calcium influx and cell death.

On present evidence the most rational explanation for the increased intracellular calcium in Duchenne muscular dystrophy would appear to be a disturbance of the physiological relationship between the dystrophin-glycoprotein complex and calcium-leak channels.

But whatever the mechanism, there then follows enhancement of calcium-activated proteases as well as mitochondrial overload, resulting in a reduction in oxidative phosphorylation and eventually cell death (Fig. 10.9). The dependence of cell death on calcium influx is nicely demonstrated in the study of Schanne *et al.* (1979). These investigators showed that the exposure of rat hepatocytes in short-term culture to a variety of agents known to disrupt cell membranes in one way or another only resulted in cell death if the medium contained calcium (Table 10.4).

Taking into account all these various observations, it seems quite clear that increased muscle intracellular calcium is a very early manifestation of the disease, which eventually triggers off muscle fibre necrosis. It has been suggested that intracellular calcium levels might possibly be increased in skin fibroblasts (Fingerman *et al.* 1984) but using electron probe X-ray microanalysis we have been unable (Freeman and Emery, unpublished) to detect any consistent abnormality in calcium levels in *single* red cells in affected boys or carriers (Table 10.5), and levels in lymphocytes are normal (Klip *et al.* 1985). There is no evidence that cell death occurs in any tissue other than muscle in Duchenne muscular dystrophy.

Table 10.4 *Viability (trypan blue exclusion) of rat hepatocytes in short term culture in the presence or absence of calcium in the medium (from Schanne et al. 1979, with permission)*

	Viability (%)	
Treatment	Medium plus Ca^{2+}	Medium minus Ca^{2+}
None	100 ± 3	101 ± 3
A23187 (ionophore)	6 ± 1	98 ± 5
Lysolecithin	19 ± 1	97 ± 9
Amphotericin B	30 ± 3	98 ± 3
Melittin	46 ± 1	103 ± 6
Phalloidin	38 ± 3	103 ± 5
Methylmethanesulphonate	48 ± 8	99 ± 2
Ethylmethanesulphonate	36 ± 6	106 ± 2
N-Acetoxyacetylaminofluorene	58 ± 3	101 ± 3
Silica	26 ± 9	100 ± 6
Asbestos	45 ± 6	104 ± 11

Table 10.5 *Mean intracellular calcium concentrations ($\mu mol.ml.$ cell water^{-1}) in single erythrocytes in healthy controls and affected boys and carriers of Duchenne muscular dystrophy (unpublished data)*

Controls	
females (5)	0.20, 0.46, 0.98, 1.01, 1.38.
males (2)	0.42, 1.56
Duchenne muscular dystrophy	
carriers (3)	0.55, 0.96, 1.52.
affected (5)	0.35, 0.49, 1.30, 1.64, 1.90

It has been argued that the release of basic fibroblast growth factor (bFGF) from necrotic muscle fibres may be an important mechanism in initiating and maintaining fibrosis in Duchenne muscular dystrophy (Hoffman and Gorospe 1991). However the fact that fibrosis only occurs in the human disease and the dystrophic dog but not in the dystrophic cat or *mdx* mouse, raises some important questions regarding pathogenetic mechanisms in these different species (p. 146).

Immune factors

Although most emphasis in the past has been on the efflux of protein from dystrophic muscle fibres, there is also experimental evidence which indicates that substances may actually *enter* affected muscle fibres (p. 130). Also, histochemical studies have demonstrated that *in vivo* there is ingress not only of calcium but also IgG, complement (Engel and Biesecker 1982), and albumin (Cornelio and Dones 1984). Based on the findings of Cornelio and Dones (1984) as well as our own unpublished data, it would seem that there is first an ingress of calcium and albumin into eosinophilic 'opaque' fibres

Table 10.6 *Histochemical reactions of muscle fibres in Duchenne muscular dystrophy*

	Muscle fibres			
	'Normal'	Eosinophilic 'opaque'	Necrotic	Regenerating
Calcium	+	+ + +	+ / −	−
Albumin	−	+ +	+ +	−
Complement	−	−	+ + +	−
RNA (acridine orange)	−	−	−	+ +

(Table 10.6). The muscle fibre then begins to undergo necrosis and while still staining for calcium now also becomes positive for complement (Engel *et al.* 1984). This ingress of complement components with their subsequent activation would accentuate the process of muscle fibre lysis and destruction.

It has been recognized for many years that necrotic fibres are invaded by macrophages. However, it has now been shown by immunocytochemical methods using labelled monoclonal antibodies to surface antigens on various mononuclear cells, that many of these are in fact T cells (Arahata and Engel 1982; Engel and Arahata 1986), a view supported by ultrastructural studies (Fidziańska *et al.* 1984). This then raises the important possibility that cell necrosis may be accentuated by T-cell-mediated injury as occurs in poly myositis (Rowe *et al.* 1983; Olsson *et al.* 1984). May be '. . . abnormal muscle fibre components in Duchenne muscular dystrophy instigate a secondary autoimmune response' (Engel *et al.* 1984). That is, abnormal muscle fibre components could lead to a change in surface antigens which cytotoxic lymphocytes then recognize as foreign (non-self) and attack the muscle membrane which then results in the ingress of complement and calcium with subsequent fibre necrosis.

Kiepiela *et al.* (1988) have reported a significant increase in the number of T suppressor/cytotoxic cells in the peripheral blood in Duchenne muscular dystrophy. Furthermore, it has been found that HLA class I antigens (MHCI) are expressed in skeletal muscle in various muscular dystrophies but not in normal muscle (Rowe *et al.* 1983; Appleyard *et al.* 1985). Subsequent more detailed studies have confirmed these findings (Emslie-Smith *et al.* 1989). The expression of these surface antigens would render the dystrophic muscle susceptible to T-cell-mediated attack and cause membrane damage *in addition* to any mechanical damage consequent on a defective cytoskeleton. But as Andrew Engel (personal communication, 1991) has pointed out, the expression of MHC class I antigens '. . . is clearly not limited to X-linked dystrophies and the autoimmune phenomena occurring in Duchenne dystrophy as well as in other dystrophies are probably epiphenomena'. Nevertheless, it seems reasonable that though this is an epiphenomenon the expression of a surface antigen which then renders the cell susceptible to T-cell attack has a number of important implications. (1) Cell necrosis would be restricted to those tissues which not only express the antigen but are also exposed to possible T-cell attack, such as skeletal and cardiac muscle. It could be that though mononuclear cells may be associated with affected muscle fibres in a fetus (Fidziańska *et al.* 1984), cell destruction does not occur because of 'immaturity' of the immunological system. Also minimal muscle membrane damage at this stage in development is presumably adequate for the ingress of calcium but not for other factors (? complement) which are necessary to produce visible evidence of necrosis. (2) The expression of the genetic defect in an organ which is in an immunologically 'privileged' (protected) position, such as the brain, might interfere with its normal functioning but would not lead to T-cell attack with subsequent cellular necrosis. (3) Such a mechanism might explain why full expression of the genetic defect with muscle fibre necrosis does not occur in cultured myoblasts because of the absence in the system of immunologically competent cells, antibodies, and complement components. The addition of these factors to culture media might possibly result in muscle cell necrosis.

Finally, if T-cell attack is a factor in muscle cell necrosis in certain forms

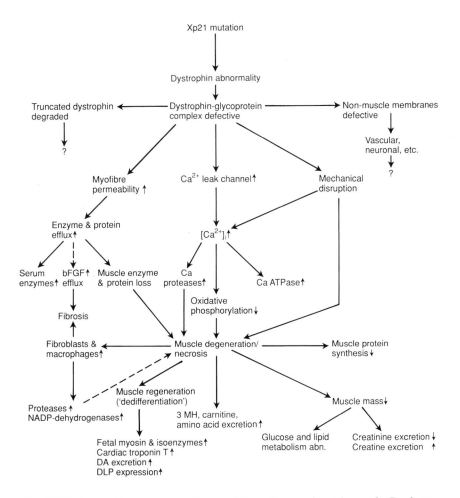

Fig. 10.10 A tentative scheme of the possible pathogenetic pathways in Duchenne muscular dystrophy. (DA, dimethyl arginine; DLP, dystrophin-like protein; MH, 3-methyl histidine; bFGF, basic fibroblast growth factor).

of muscular dystrophy, possibly some therapeutic value might be obtained with monoclonal antibodies to T lymphocytes, as has been discussed in general terms by Hohlfeld and Toyko (1985), or more likely by pharmacological suppression of the immune response. In the latter regard it is therefore of considerable interest that in Duchenne muscular dystrophy treatment with prednisone produces a marked reduction in T cells in muscle tissue (total, CD8 and cytotoxic/suppressor) and a reduction in the number of fibres focally invaded by lymphocytes (Kissel *et al.* 1991). Furthermore, such treatment improves muscle strength in these patients (Chapter 13). Perhaps a more vigorous immunosuppressive therapy might be even more effective.

Conclusions

The primary defect in Duchenne muscular dystrophy is a deficiency of dystrophin, the results of which may vary in different tissues in which this defect is expressed. Evidence from various sources suggests there is a widespread defect in cell membranes but it is in skeletal muscle where this defect has its most profound effects. Dystrophin is associated with glycoprotein to form a dystrophin–glycoprotein complex which when deficient (in some way that is not as yet entirely clear) results in calcium influx and eventually cell degeneration and cell death. Based on current information, a tentative scheme of the possible pathogenetic pathways in Duchenne dystrophy has been drawn up (Fig. 10.10).

But such a scheme, though it may concentrate the mind, gives no indication as to the *primary* cause of muscle weakness, why this is progressive, affects different muscles differently, and is milder in Xp21 myopathies other than Duchenne muscular dystrophy. There is also the possibility that immune factors may cause muscle membrane damage *in addition* to any other mechanism more directly related to the deficiency of dystrophin. The biggest challenge to future research in this disease is the detailed understanding of how the clinical phenotype can be related to a deficiency of dystrophin.

11 Prevention

Since Duchenne muscular dystrophy is a serious disorder for which at present there is no effective treatment, a great deal of emphasis has been given to prevention. This involves the ascertainment of women likely to have an affected son, and the provision of genetic counselling and prenatal diagnosis for such women.

Ascertainment of families at risk

The ascertainment of women at risk of having an affected child is the first prerequisite of prevention. Logically this would seem best achieved by screening all females to determine which ones are likely to be carriers. This is impractical, however, because there is as yet no single test which could be used to detect all carriers, and in any event the cost of such screening would be prohibitively expensive. Furthermore, as already observed, in one-third of cases the mother is not a carrier, the affected son being the result of a new mutation (p. 161).

Another approach might be to screen all pregnancies for affected males. However, quite apart from technical and economic considerations, this would raise a number of serious ethical problems. At present the only practical solution is to ensure that all affected boys in the community are ascertained, and that their mothers, and subsequently other female relatives, are then tested to determine their carrier status and the likelihood of the disorder recurring.

Population screening

Because SCK levels in affected boys are grossly elevated from birth, there is the potential for detection in the neonatal period (p. 46). This can be achieved by determining the SCK level in dried blood spots obtained from a heel prick. The blood spots are placed on a filter paper card and the air-dried specimen can then be assayed immediately or stored. Enzyme activity remains stable for several weeks at room temperature provided direct heat and sunlight are avoided. Specimens can therefore be conveniently sent by post. It should be emphasized, however, that it is not possible to screen for female carriers in this way because the probability of any female at random *not* being a carrier far outweighs the possibility of her being a carrier based on a slightly elevated SCK level.

A sensitive assay for creatine kinase activity in minute quantities of dried blood was first introduced by Antonik and further developed by Scheuer-brandt (Zellweger and Antonik 1975; Beckmann and Scheuerbrandt 1976). This is a bioluminescence assay and depends on the generation of ATP by creatine kinase (p. 45). The ATP then reacts with luciferin in the presence of the enzyme luciferase to produce light — a reaction employed by fireflies. A sensitive but less expensive fluorimetric/electrophoretic method has also been developed for measuring creatine kinase activity in dried blood spots (Adriaenssens and Vermeiren 1980; Lloyd *et al.* 1982). Essentially, this method consists of separating creatine kinase isoenzymes from the haemo-globin of the blood spot and from each other by electrophoresis, the enzyme substrate being in a gelatin or agarose matrix. The activities of creatine kinase isoenzymes (particularly the MM isoenzyme) are determined by com-paring the UV fluorescence of the samples with standards of known activities. Several other methods are also available for measuring creatine kinase levels in dried blood spots.

Extensive experience of the luciferin/luciferase method indicates that the false positive rate is between 0.2 and 0.06 per cent, and may even be less (Scheuerbrandt *et al.* 1984, 1986). With the fluorimetric/electrophoretic method we have found a false positive rate of at most 0.2 per cent, and this will no doubt be reduced further with more experience. Furthermore, none of the false positives in our series was found to have a grossly elevated creatine kinase level when a subsequent *serum* sample was tested. When a serum sample also yields a grossly elevated SCK level then the diagnosis has to be confirmed by appropriate investigations. There will always be some false positives with this test because it has to be sufficiently sensitive to detect *all* cases. It seems likely, therefore, that the false negative rate among those tested will be low, if not zero. The problem here is more likely to result from a laboratory or administrative error or failing to test an infant who subse-quently develops the disease.

The results of neonatal screening for Duchenne muscular dystrophy have already been discussed (p. 156).

However, the important question remains as to whether such screening is really justified. It can be argued that if an affected boy was detected suf-ficiently early and his mother proved to be a carrier and was counselled, second cases in the family might be prevented. It has been estimated that up to 15–20 per cent of cases might be prevented in this way. In the present series of patients in which precise information was available, there were 67 families in which an affected boy was born but at the time no one else was affected in the family and the mother subsequently became pregnant. The average time between the birth of this son and the birth of the next child was 2.71 years (s.d. 1.45; range 1.0–7.0 years). Thus the next pregnancy was con-ceived on average less than two years after the birth of a son who *sub-sequently proved to be affected*. Since at least 75 per cent of affected boys present suspicious signs *after* this age (p. 28) and the mean age at diagnosis is around 5 years of age with a range of 2 to 8 years (Crisp *et al.* 1982), most parents would have been completely unaware of the risks in the next pregnancy. In fact, 10 sons in the next or a following pregnancy subsequently proved to be affected.

Neonatal screening has also been justified on financial grounds, it being argued that the tests are relatively cheap to carry out and prevention compared with management would be cost effective (Zellweger *et al.* 1975; Grimm 1981). It can also be combined with neonatal screening for other genetic disorders such as cystic fibrosis (Prior *et al* 1990).

Finally, most parents of affected boys appear to favour such screening when questioned (Firth and Wilkinson 1983; Smith *et al.* 1990*b*) for a number of reasons: it would prevent the anxiety which results from the long delays and unfounded reassurances often experienced between the first symptoms and the establishment of the diagnosis; parents have a 'right' to know as soon as possible; it would help prevent further affected children; it has practical advantages in affording an early opportunity to obtain appropriate housing for example; and, finally, it has emotional advantages. However, those questioned in this study were all parents who had already had an affected son. The concern is of presenting a couple with the devastating news that their newborn son has a serious genetic disorder when they were completely unprepared for this. Furthermore, the parents have to cope with the problem some four or five years sooner than they would otherwise have had to. Some have therefore advocated a compromise, that screening might be restricted to those boys who are not walking by the age of 18 months (Gardner-Medwin *et al.* 1978; O'Brien *et al.* 1983), or when there is a delay in motor and mental development for no obvious reason (Crisp *et al.* 1982). The age of 18 months was selected because by this time almost all normal boys have learned to walk but only about 50 per cent of affected boys (p. 27). It has been reasoned that this more restricted screening would have the advantages of involving fewer tests (and therefore lower costs), and that the results would be easier to interpret and less likely to cause anxiety because the parents' concern is already aroused. Of course, since the screening would be carried out later, fewer secondary cases (less than 10 per cent) could be prevented. It would therefore be less effective. It would also be necessary to establish procedures for informing all family doctors of the requirement for testing and the referral of blood samples to an appropriate centre. This could present organizational difficulties. In the event, screening of boys at 18 months who are not walking has been shown *not* to be justified because the detection rates are unacceptably low (Smith *et al.* 1989).

However the subject is viewed, screening for Duchenne muscular dystrophy has so far failed to generate a great deal of enthusiasm either among paediatricians or geneticists. There is little doubt, however, that when an effective treatment eventually becomes available interest will be rekindled. For it seems probable that the sooner any treatment is begun the more likely it is to be effective and arrest the course of the disease. A number of issues will then have to be faced including the for very careful and sensitive counselling of parents of proven positive cases.

At present most paediatricians and geneticists confine their activities to the family of an affected boy. All his female relatives can be screened in order to assess their carrier status, and records of those found to be at risk can be maintained on a genetic register system for subsequent follow-up.

Genetic registers

Viewed at the population level, any approach to prevention must first involve ascertaining all cases in the community. There are essentially three ways in which this may be achieved. First, by population screening which has already been discussed. Secondly, studying families in which an affected individual is known to exist. Thirdly, screening of hospital, public health, and special school records for affected individuals. Having now ascertained cases of the disease, the next step is to determine if there are any female relatives who could be at risk of having an affected son and may require genetic counselling. The procedure we adopted is that unless a family is already known through an affected boy and his parents, individuals who could be at risk are not contacted directly but only through their family doctor. This provides an opportunity to check that the diagnosis has been well established in the affected family member. It also protects individuals from being contacted who have either already had genetic counselling or where it would be imprudent, for religious reasons for example, or unnecessary if they have already completed their family. In Britain the relative's family doctor can be identified when the relative's name and address is known because each local Executive Council holds a list of patients in its area which shows the family doctor with whom they are registered. However, in small nuclear families such measures are usually not necessary. On average there are about three females at high risk (greater than 1 in 10) of having an affected son in each family with a serious X-linked recessive disorder (Emery and Smith 1970).

For ease of follow-up and recall and to maintain strict confidentiality, personal and genetic data on such females are best held in a computerized register. A number (Table 11.1) of such registers of genetic disorders have been developed in several countries (Emery and Miller 1976; Emery 1991c). A register designed specifically for the prevention of genetic disease was developed in Edinburgh with the acronym RAPID (*R*egister for the *A*scertainment and *P*revention of *I*nherited *D*isease) in the early 1970s (Emery *et al.* 1974). The system is outlined in Fig. 11.1. To maintain strict confidentiality a number of security checks have been incorporated into the system. Access is only possible when a valid password 'A' is used. If data are to be

Table 11.1 *General genetic register systems*

System	Centre	Reference
MEGADATS	Indiana, USA	Merritt *et al.* 1976
RAPID	Edinburgh, UK	Emery *et al.* 1974
National Register	Leuven, Belgium	Vlietinck and van den Berghe 1976
GENFILES	San Francisco, USA	Loughman *et al.* 1980
GENTIC	Marseilles, France	Ayme *et al.* 1982
PRUFILE	London, UK	Mutton *et al.* 1988

retrieved, the request is first checked for its validity, i.e. correct family name and number and disease code, etc. A second password 'B' allows data to be retrieved at various levels depending on the particular operator's password. The clinician or geneticist dealing with the family has access to all the medical and genetic information, but someone concerned with tracing relatives may retrieve only names and pedigree data. Information in the register is released only to other physicians and geneticists directly involved in the management of the patient and his family. Finally, no families are included on the register without their fully informed consent. The British Clinical Genetics Society has published a Working Party Report on genetic registers in which various technical and ethical matters are discussed in detail (Emery *et al.* 1978).

Data which can be stored in such a register include information on DNA polymorphisms (Read *et al.* 1986), for example in an affected boy against the day when he might die and the information is required to counsel a female relative. The register can also be designed to facilitate the later recall of female relatives who, *a priori*, are at risk but who are currently too young for counselling. Information on any aborted fetus (e.g. DNA polymorphisms and that it might have been affected, see p. 245) can also be stored which in future might be of additional help in counselling. However, apart from the prevention of Duchenne muscular dystrophy and other genetic diseases, a computerized genetic register system can also be of value in several other ways. For example, it can facilitate the recall of family members should there be new developments in carrier detection, prenatal diagnosis, and, hopefully one day, treatment. It can also be useful in putting families in contact with various welfare agencies and for informing them of changes in medical and social benefits. The European Alliance of Muscular Dystrophy Associations has recommended the setting up of a register of patients with neuromuscular diseases largely for epidemiological purposes (EAMDA 1984). However, many see the main function of a local genetic register system as facilitating the prevention of genetic disease within the community it serves.

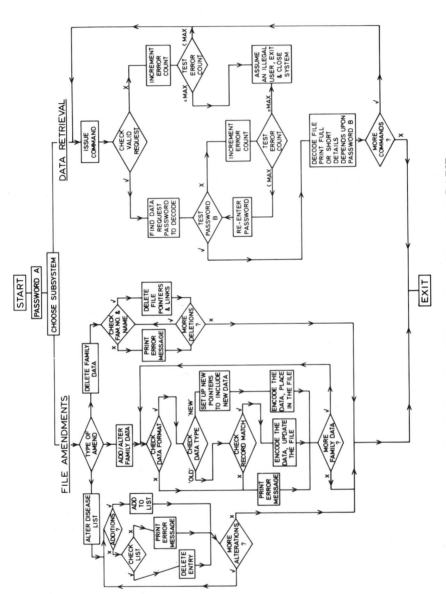

Fig. 11.1 Outline of the genetic register system RAPID.

Carrier detection

The whole problem of genetic counselling in Duchenne muscular dystrophy revolves around the detection of female carriers. If, as was suggested (Roses *et al.* 1976b), essentially all mothers of affected boys are carriers, the situation would be much simpler. This now, however, seems unlikely to be the case (p. 163; Nicholson *et al.* 1981), and in any event the carrier status of sisters and daughters of carrier mothers often has to be determined.

Definition of carrier status

First it is necessary to consider the definition of a carrier. In the past, confusion on this point has often lead to difficulties in interpreting the results of any proposed tests for detecting carriers. There are three accepted categories of carriers based on genetic considerations.

First, *definite (or obligate) carriers* who are mothers of an affected son but who also have an affected brother, affected nephew by their sister, or an affected maternal uncle or other maternal male relative. Included in this category are also mothers of affected sons by different non-consanguineous fathers.

Secondly, *probable carriers* who are mothers with two or more affected sons but with no other affected relatives. Such women could conceivably be heterozygous for the autosomal recessive limb girdle muscular dystrophy of childhood which clinically resembles Duchenne muscular dystrophy. However, since the latter is comparatively rare these women are usually included with the definite carriers.

Thirdly, *possible carriers* who are mothers of an isolated case as well as their sisters and other female relatives. This category also includes female relatives of definite and probable carriers. The probability of all such women being carriers has to be determined. The term *suspected carrier* is frequently used for any woman who is at risk of being a carrier.

Biological considerations

The evaluation of carrier detection tests has been bedevilled by several factors. Some of these are inherent in that Duchenne muscular dystrophy being an X-linked recessive disorder, there will inevitably be variability in expression in carrier females because of random inactivation of the X chromosome. This means that a proportion of carriers are unlikely to be detectable by any biochemical method except one employing cloned cells to identify two populations, or based on DNA studies. Furthermore, it may be difficult if not impossible to determine the rate of false positives with any test since a potential carrier informed of an abnormal result is unlikely to risk childbearing. However, if a subsequent pregnancy is terminated it may be possible in some cases to confirm the diagnosis by studying muscle dystrophin from the aborted fetus. Such information may also be used to confirm the carrier status of the mother.

Methodological considerations

Even though the cause of Duchenne muscular dystrophy is now known and abnormalities of muscle dystrophin and DNA are detectable in some carriers, as we shall see, this is not always so. If these molecular based tests prove uninformative in a particular case then information from other tests may have to be considered — though this is becoming less of a problem with improvements in molecular diagnosis. But with all tests on carriers there can be serious methodological problems.

Sometimes a test has been applied to carriers before its validity has been established in affected boys. Thus, a test which is positive in only a proportion of affected boys, or only in the later stages of the disease, is unlikely to be of much value in detecting healthy carriers. Only in occasional, and mainly early studies, has an attempt been made to compare the results of several different sorts of tests (SCK levels, EMG, muscle histology) on the same individuals (for example, Emery 1965a; Hausmanowa-Petrusewicz *et al.* 1968b; Radu *et al.* 1968; Dubowitz 1982). However, lack of correlation with SCK levels would not necessarily invalidate a new test. The two might be independent variables and the results of the two tests could then be combined to enhance carrier detection.

Another problem has been that definite carriers have sometimes not been clearly distinguished from possible carriers. For example, the results of a test on mothers of isolated cases have occasionally been reported when the actual carrier status of these mothers is not known. Furthermore, comparisons have often been made with poorly matched or an inadequate number of healthy controls.

Finally, as Harper has emphasized in a thought-provoking essay on the subject (Harper 1982), all too often the results of research investigations have been too hastily applied to service use.

Ideally, any proposed test should be subjected to the following evaluation. First, it should be positive in all affected boys, even from a very early stage in the disease process. There should be no false negatives and false positives should be acceptable only if they occur in conditions unlikely to be confused with Duchenne muscular dystrophy or can be readily distinguished from it. Secondly, its validity in carrier detection should be based on testing a significant number of definite carriers and an equal number of carefully matched healthy female controls. In both controls and carriers the material to be studied (say DNA) should be collected and processed in the same way and under identical laboratory conditions. Finally, the results of the test should be compared with an established test, such as the SCK level, carried out on the same individuals.

It could be argued that the advent of DNA markers for carrier detection has made other approaches to the problem redundant. But it is perhaps worth considering that a significant biochemical or related defect detectable not only in affected boys but also in healthy carriers would confirm its importance in relation to the pathogenesis of the disorder. Changes which take place in carriers with increasing age could be particularly informative in this regard (p. 242).

Carrier detection tests

Over the years there have been reports of various abnormalities in carriers of Duchenne muscular dystrophy. Some, such as total body potassium and rubidium, have been shown to be valueless in carrier detection. Others of more recent interest are listed in Table 11.2. The references have been

Table 11.2 *Some reported abnormalities in female carriers of Duchenne muscular dystrophy*

Abnormality	Reference
Clinical	
Muscle weakness	Reddy *et al.* (1984)
Cardiomyopathy	Wiegand *et al.* (1984)
Muscle pathology	
Histology	Schiffer *et al.* (1984)
Histochemistry	Maunder-Sewry and Dubowitz (1981)
Ultrastructure	Fisher *et al.* (1972); Afifi *et al.* (1973)
Ultrasound	Rott and Rödl (1985)
Computerized tomography	Stern *et al.* (1985)
Muscle biochemistry	
Nuclear calcium	Maunder-Sewry and Dubowitz (1979)
Ribosomal protein synthesis	Ionasescu *et al.* (1980)
Electromyography	Hausmanowa-Petrusewicz *et al.* (1982)
Electrocardiography	Lane *et al.* (1980)
Cell surface membranes	
Erythrocytes	
morphology/physicochemistry/biochemistry	Lucy (1980); Rowland (1980)
Lymphocyte capping	Ho *et al.* (1980)
Fibroblasts	Hillier *et al.* (1985)
Serum enzymes and proteins	
Creatine kinase (+ isoenzymes)	—
Pyruvate kinase	Falcão-Conceição *et al.* (1983*a*)
LDH-5	Somer *et al.* (1980)
Myoglobin	Nicholson (1981); Percy *et al.* (1984)
Haemopexin	Lössner *et al.* (1982)

selected in order to guide the reader to the related earlier literature.

It should perhaps be emphasized that some of these abnormalities are contentious whereas others have been more convincingly established. The value of ultrasound has been questioned (Heckmatt and Dubowitz 1983) and there are doubts as to whether serum levels of LDH–5, myoglobin, or haemopexin have any additional value over and above information provided by creatine kinase and pyruvate kinase. With regard to electromyography, some years ago we were unable to find any significant differences between 12 controls and 22 carriers regarding action potential duration and amplitude and the frequency of polyphasic potentials when measurements were made blind (Emery *et al.* 1966), although admittedly some others had a little better success (e.g. Moosa *et al.* 1972). Recently, sophisticated electromyographic techniques involving computer analysis appear to have been more successful but they require considerable expertise in their interpretation and are time consuming.

There is, however, general agreement that a proportion of carriers exhibit some degree of weakness, have abnormalities of muscle pathology, and have significantly raised serum levels of creatine kinase and pyruvate kinase.

Clinically manifesting carriers

It has been long recognized that females may have a Duchenne-like disorder. Two of Duchenne's original 13 cases were in fact girls and Gowers (1879*b*)

Table 11.3 *Possible explanations for a female having a 'limb girdle' type myopathy*

1. *Congenital myopathy*
2. *Spinal muscular atrophy*
3. *Duchenne-related disorder*
   - (*a*) Hemizygous
     XO, etc.
   - (*b*) Homozygous
     extremely rare
   - (*c*) Heterozygous
     'manifesting carrier'
   - (*d*) X/autosome translocation
4. *Limb girdle muscular dystrophy*
   - (*a*) Childhood
   - (*b*) Adult
5. *Polymyositis*
6. *Acquired myopathy*
   Sarcoidosis, thyrotoxic, metabolic bone disease,
   acromegaly, etc.
7. *Drug induced*

reported a Duchenne-like disorder in a girl with a clearly X-linked pedigree (case 8), in the sister of an affected boy (case 15), and in an isolated case (case 30). There are several reasons for females having a Duchenne-like or Duchenne-related disorder and these have been discussed in Chapter 5, and are summarized in Table 11.3. Some of the conditions listed however are unlikely to cause confusion but are included for the sake of completeness. Manifesting carriers of Becker muscular dystrophy have also been described but are rare. An adult female with muscle weakness may therefore present a difficult diagnostic problem in the absence of a family history of dystrophy (Barkaus and Gilchrist 1989).

It has been estimated that between 5 per cent and 10 per cent of carriers have some degree of weakness (Moser and Emery 1974). But this may be slight and only elicited on careful clinical examination. Calf enlargement has often been emphasized but is in fact an unreliable sign. Actual measurements of calf size reveal no significant difference between controls and definite carriers (Table 11.4 and see Cavanagh and Preece 1981).

Manifesting carriers of Duchenne muscular dystrophy have occasionally been described in the same family (Moser and Emery 1974; Frouhar *et al.* 1975; Falcão-Conceição *et al.* 1983*b*; Reddy *et al.* 1984), and this has also been observed in other X-linked disorders such as Fabry's disease (Ropers *et al.* 1977)(Fig. 11.2). A very large family with Duchenne muscular dystrophy extending over seven generations has been described, in which there were 14 affected males and four manifesting carriers (Spector *et al.* 1990).

Since such manifestations are a consequence of random X-inactivation (p. 100), their familial occurrence suggests that this process may be under genetic control and might be explained if there were an X-linked gene(s) which controls X chromosome inactivation. In the mouse there is certainly an X-linked locus which controls X-inactivation (X-chromosome controlling element or *Xce*) and can lead to non-random X-inactivation (Cattanach and Williams 1972; Cattanach 1975; Johnston and Cattanach 1981). The idea of

Table 11.4 *Calf sizes (mean ± s.d.) in female controls and carriers of Duchenne and Becker muscular dystrophies*

	No.	Calf size (cm)	CS/SA × 1000
Controls	100	34.7 ± 2.4	2.2 ± 0.1
Carriers — Duchenne	21	34.9 ± 2.4	2.1 ± 0.2
Carriers — Becker	30	35.5 ± 3.5	2.2 ± 0.2

Surface area = $(Wt)^{0.425} \times (ht)^{0.725} \times (71.84)$ (Du Bois and Du Bois 1916)

CS, calf size; SA, surface area.

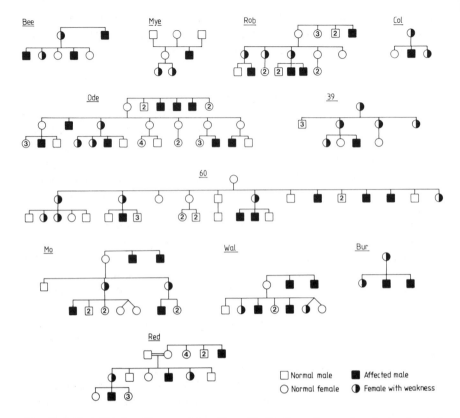

Fig. 11.2 Simplified pedigrees of families with Duchenne muscular dystrophy and several female relatives with weakness. *Bee* (Murphy and Thompson 1969); *Mye, Rob, Col,* and *Ode* (Moser and Emery 1974); *39* and *60* (Falcão-Conceição *et al.* 1983*b*); *Mo, Wal,* and *Bur* (unpublished); *Red* (Reddy *et al.* 1984).

an 'X chromosome controlling element' segregating in families with more than one manifesting carrier is attractive.

Besides muscle weakness, there is evidence in a proportion of carriers of cardiac involvement. In 4 of 50 carriers the algebraic sum of the R and S waves in the right praecordial lead of the electrocardiogram was found to be outside the normal range, an abnormality similar to that found in affected boys (Emery 1969*a*). Similar findings have also been reported in a detailed study by Lane *et al.* (1980).

From a practical point of view it may well be that a proportion of carriers have a latent dystrophic cardiomyopathy. This could have important implications since they often have to lift and carry their affected sons. In fact mitral valve prolapse (Biddison *et al.* 1979), and even congestive cardiomyopathy have been described in the occasional carrier (Wiegand *et al.* 1984). Involvement of the myocardium leading to cardiac failure may be more common in manifesting carriers (Kamakura *et al.* 1990).

Muscle pathology

Abnormalities in muscle pathology in carriers have been known for some time (Dubowitz 1963*b*; Emery 1963, 1965*b*). These abnormalities include increased variation in fibre size, eosinophilic 'hypercontracted fibres', and even fibre necrosis and phagocytosis, although the latter are found only when there is florid muscle weakness. In only about 10 per cent of symptomless carriers is there usually any obvious abnormality on routine histology. However, careful quantitation of muscle fibre size, internal nuclei, and histochemical fibre type proportions has been claimed to demonstrate abnormalities in around 70 per cent of carriers by Maunder-Sewry and Dubowitz (1981). These investigators believe that significant abnormalities can occasionally be detected even when the SCK level is within the normal range. This has yet to be corroborated. What does seem clear however is that two populations of muscle fibres, one normal and the other abnormal, are not found in carriers as was originally suggested by Pearson *et al.* (1963). Instead a wide spectrum of abnormalities can be seen from muscle fibres which appear to be normal through to those which are clearly undergoing necrosis. The explanation lies in the way multinucleate muscle fibres originate and develop. If the myotomes were mosaics of nuclei in some of which the active X chromosome is the one bearing the normal gene and in others the active X chromosome is the one bearing the Duchenne gene, then fusion between mononucleate myoblasts derived from the myotomes would result in muscle fibres possessing different proportions of the two types of nuclei. The proportion in any one fibre would be determined to some extent by the proportion in the original myotome. The proportion of nuclei in any muscle fibre in which the active X chromosome is the one bearing the Duchenne gene presumably determines the degree of abnormality in that fibre (Fig. 11.3).

Thompson *et al.* (1974) noted a small (but not significant) decline in SCK levels with increasing age in carriers and interpreted this as perhaps being a reflection of a gradual reduction in the number of affected muscle fibres and their replacement (from proliferating satellite nuclei) by more normal fibres. However, so far there have been no reported studies of repeated muscle biopsies on carriers which is now feasible with needle biopsy. If anything, muscle weakness in manifesting carriers tends to get worse, not improve, over the years. Presumably, if there is any replacement of dystrophic fibres with age, mosaicism in satellite nuclei would tend to perpetuate the production of variably affected muscle fibres, unless they too participate in the selection process.

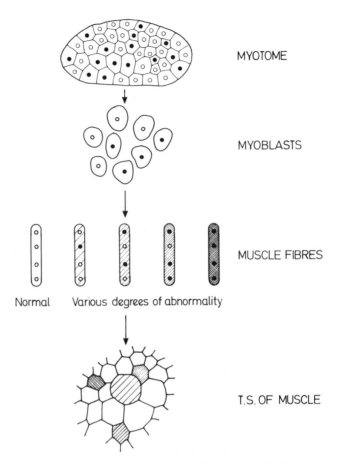

MYOTOME

MYOBLASTS

MUSCLE FIBRES

Normal   Various degrees of abnormality

T.S. OF MUSCLE

Fig. 11.3 Possible explanation for the muscle histological findings in carriers of Duchenne muscular dystrophy. (Nuclei in which the active X chromosome bears the normal gene, (○), or the Duchenne gene, (●).)

The distribution of muscle dystrophin shows variation between and within muscle fibres in manifesting carriers but not in non-manifesting carriers (p. 100).

Serum creatine kinase

For many years the the most widely used single test for detecting carriers was the SCK level. From the very early successful studies of Schapira and colleagues in 1960, the detection rate obtained by a number of investigators in the following 5 years was around 60–70 per cent (Emery 1967*b*), and has not changed significantly since. Its great advantage is its simplicity and further-more the results can be combined with data from linked DNA markers to provide valuable additional information for carrier detection. However, in applying the test, possible causes of variation both in female controls and carriers must be considered. This variability is partly technical and partly biological in origin. Considerable variability has been reported in values obtained when the same blood sample has been posted to different labora-tories for analysis (Bullock *et al.* 1979). Part of this variability may be due to lack of standardization of the assays used and for this reason recom-mended methods have been advocated (e.g. Moss *et al.* 1981). However, when different assay methods are carried out in a single laboratory on the same series of controls and carriers, the resulting probability estimates vary very little (Tippett *et al.* 1982). Thus, a laboratory may be able to produce risk estimates of *acceptable precision for genetic counselling purposes* with-out having to study a series of known carriers provided that the method used has first been standardized on an adequate number of controls and the values obtained are comparable to those in a centre where many carriers have been studied with the same method.

If specimens are stored at 4 °C for no longer than a few days there is little loss of activity. Exposure, however, to extremes of temperature and sunlight can have significant effects. A slight rise in activity over the course of the day (Thompson 1968), and slightly higher levels in summer compared with winter (Smith *et al.* 1979; Percy *et al.* 1982) have been reported. However, both diurnal and seasonal variations are small and from a practical point of view are relatively unimportant.

In our laboratory the coefficient of variation on replicate samples taken at the same time from any one individual was less than 2 per cent. However, in samples obtained from the same individual but at different times, the coef-ficient of variation ranged from 5–10 per cent. This added variation results from various biological factors. The stage of the menstrual cycle and the use of oral contraception have little effect, but vigorous exercise may cause significant increases though normal daily activity is without any material effect (Hudgson *et al.* 1967*b*). Age also has to be considered. After the menarche some reports have indicated a slight increase with increasing age (especially after the menopause) whereas others have found no significant effect (reviewed by Gale and Murphy 1979). It would seem that if there is any effect of age in adult women this is small and can be ignored in esti-mating the probability of a woman being a carrier. However, since most females are likely to be tested in their teens or in early adult life, it is impor-tant to consider the effects of age at these times. Several studies have indicated that levels are significantly *higher* in teenage (especially pre-menarchal) girls compared with adult women (Bundey *et al.* 1979*a*; Smith *et al.* 1979; Lane and Roses 1981; Livingstone *et al.* 1982; Passos *et al.* 1985).

Pregnancy is also an important factor, levels being significantly lower in the early stages (King *et al*. 1972), and significantly higher *immediately* post-partum (Emery and Pascasio 1965), when the latter is presumably due to the release of enzymes from the involuting myometrium.

Genetic factors also seem to influence SCK levels. Meltzer *et al*. (1978) have presented data on levels in 14 monozygotic and 14 dizygotic twins. Although their method of statistical analysis was not quite appropriate, intrapair variances calculated from their data for monozygotic (1312) and dizygotic (3877) twins differ significantly $(F = 2.96, P < 0.05)$, which indicates that variation in identical twins is significantly less than in non-identical twins. Racial factors may also be involved since the mean level in Negro females has been found to be significantly greater than in Caucasian females in the United States (Meltzer 1971; Meltzer and Holy 1974; Passos-Bueno *et al*. 1989*a*).

All these various factors also have an effect on SCK levels in carriers. *Standardized* exercise (on a walking machine or a bicycle ergometer) has been claimed by some to accentuate SCK levels in carriers more than controls provided that it is strenuous and the effects are followed for several hours afterwards (Emery 1967*b*; Gaines *et al*. 1982; Herrmann *et al*. 1982; Cordone

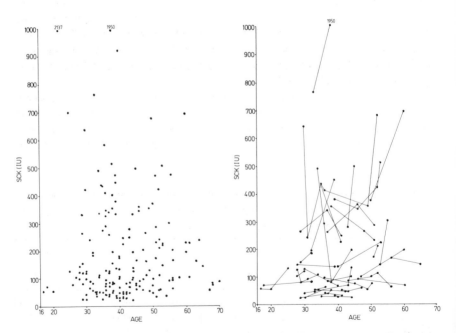

Fig. 11.4 SCK levels and age in definite carriers of Duchenne muscular dystrophy. (*Left*) all values (N = 180) (*Right*) values for individual carriers tested at different ages (N = 39). (Unpublished data.)

et al. 1984). It has therefore been recommended as a provocative test in suspected carriers with a borderline SCK level. Driessen-Kletter *et al.* (1990) have shown a significant increase in serum myoglobin as well as SCK levels in carriers after exercise.

We have determined SCK levels by the method of Rosalki (1967), assays being performed at 30 °C and the results expressed in International Units (iu) per litre. After the late teens there is no clear relationship between age and SCK levels in carriers (Fig. 11.4). In 180 measurements on definite carriers tested at different ages, neither the correlation with age ($r = -0.10$), nor the regression on age ($Y = 296 - 2.29X$) were statistically significant. There was also no consistent change in individual adult carriers tested at different ages.

However, a follow-up study by Moser and Vogt (1974) suggested that carrier detection might be better in childhood. Furthermore, Nicholson *et al.* (1979) found that the proportion of 52 daughters (mean age 16) of definite carriers who had raised SCK levels (above the normal 95 per cent confidence limits of 73 iu for girls under 16, and 60 iu for older women) was 45 per cent. Since half the daughters would be expected to be carriers, the detection rate would seem to be around 90 per cent compared with 53 per cent for their adult carriers. However, SCK levels are also higher in normal premenarchal girls, and it has been suggested that these results might be explained if this factor had not been very carefully controlled (Bundey *et al.* 1979*b*; Carter 1979). SCK levels in early adolescent carriers also decrease with age and conditional probabilities of heterozygosity have been determined for this group (Passos-Bueno *et al.* 1989*b*).

We refrained from testing very young girls who are at risk. However, among daughters of definite carriers who are age *15 and over* and who have not yet had any children, the proportion with SCK levels exceeding the normal 95 percentile (86 iu) for adult women was not significantly different

Table 11.5 *The proportion of daughters of definite carriers who have SCK levels which exceed the normal 95 percentile (86 iu) for adult women (unpublished data)*

| | No. | Age | | | | Proportion | |
		Range	Mean	s.d.		No.	%
Controls	200	18–52	27.06	9.10		11	5.50
Carriers	125	17–70	41.69	11.67		78	62.40
Controls	65	15–20	18.72	0.67		3	4.62
Daughters of carriers	49	15–20	17.33	1.84		16	32.65
	72	15–39	19.78	4.64		21	29.17

Table 11.6 *Correlations between SCK levels in females within families of definite carriers. The correlations between sisters (daughters of definite carriers) refer to all sisters (1), or where at least two sisters in a family had SCK levels in excess of 170 iu (2) and therefore likely to be carriers, or less than 86 iu (3) and therefore unlikely to be carriers (unpublished data)*

	Carrier mothers and daughters	Daughters of carriers		
		Sisters (1)	Sisters (2)	Sisters (3)
Number	101	111	20	41
Correlation	0.016	0.138	0.182	0.112
Students 't'	0.158	1.455	0.785	0.704

from the expected proportion (31.20 per cent) based on the findings in definite carriers (Table 11.5).

SCK levels in carriers may also be affected by genetic factors. Thus Sibert *et al.* (1979) found that the interfamilial variance of SCK levels in carriers was significantly ($P < 0.05$) greater than the intrafamilial variance, suggesting that there might be 'familial clustering' of SCK levels. In the present study this problem has been examined by considering correlations between SCK levels in various female relatives within families of definite carriers (Table 11.6). All the correlations were positive but none was significantly different from zero. If there are any familial similarities in SCK levels these would therefore seem to be relatively unimportant.

In view of the various technical and biological variations which may

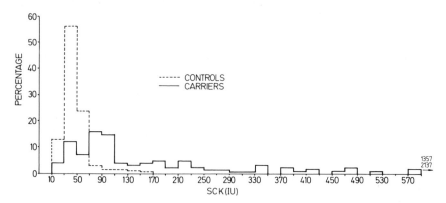

Fig. 11.5 Distribution of SCK levels determined under standardized conditions in 200 normal adult control females and 125 definite carriers.

Table 11.7 *Distribution of SCK levels in controls and carriers (unpublished data)*

SCK	Controls No.	Controls % (Y_1)	Carriers No.	Carriers % (Y_2)	h (Y_1/Y_2)
11–30	26	13.0	5	4.0	3.25
31–50	112	56.0	15	12.0	4.67
51–70	47	23.5	9	7.2	3.26
71–90	6	3.0	20	16.0	0.19
91–110	3	1.5	18	14.4	0.10
111–170	6	3.0	14	11.2	–
> 170	0	0.0	44	35.2	–
Total	*200*	*100.0*	*125*	*100.0*	*–*

influence SCK levels, it is therefore not surprising that there is a considerable spread of values in controls, the distribution being positively skewed. In carriers the spread is even greater and the distribution even more skewed, but there is no suggestion of any bimodality (Fig. 11.5). Since the distributions in the two groups are so different results have been expressed as the ratio (*h*) of normal homozygosity (Y_1) to heterozygosity (Y_2) as in Table 11.7. The normal 95 percentile (based on the cumulative distribution curve) is 86 iu; 78 (62 per cent) of definite carriers had levels which exceeded this, and 44 (35 per cent) had levels outside the upper limit of the normal range of 170 iu.

Because of the variability in SCK levels in carriers our practice, and that of others, has been where possible to take the mean of samples obtained on three separate occasions in the belief that this might provide a better guide to carrier status. However, compared with the values obtained with single determinations in controls, no matter how the upper limit of normal is

Table 11.8 *Proportion (%) of carriers (N = 94) with SCK levels which exceed the normal upper limit depending on whether the first, mean or highest of three determinations is used (Emery 1982)*

	95 percentile (86 iu)	Median × 2.5 (110 iu)	Median × 3 (132 iu)
First	58	49	40
Mean	64	46	40
Highest	65	52	41
Controls	*5*	*3*	*1*

defined, repeat testing seems to have little overall effect on the discriminatory value of the test (Table 11.8).

Linked DNA markers

There have been many attempts to improve the discriminatory value of the SCK test by combining the results with those of other tests, such as muscle pathology, electromyography, and particularly other serum enzymes and proteins such as haemopexin, myoglobin, and pyruvate kinase. But it is now clear, however, that the most useful information is obtained by combining SCK data with information from linked DNA markers. It should be emphasized however that it is entirely incorrect to consider the value of the SCK test purely in terms of 'detection rate'. It is much preferable to consider the probability (odds) of a woman being a carrier based not only on her SCK level but also on pedigree and DNA data. It usually then makes little difference to the final probability estimate in practical terms whether the test result is actually outside the normal range or lies in the upper part of the range.

Finally, the diagnosis of the affected male and the identification of a carrier female in a family has to be seen as an overall problem, data on the former helping to establish the status of the latter (Fig. 11.6).

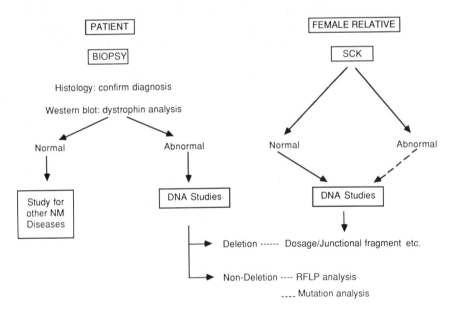

Fig. 11.6 The diagnosis of the affected male and identification of the carrier female in a family with an Xp21 disorder.

Calculation of risks

The estimation of genetic risks is usually, although not always (see Bundey 1978), based on Bayes' theorem (Emery and Morton 1968; Murphy and Mutalik 1969). In these calculations four probabilities are considered: *prior*, *conditional*, *joint*, and *posterior*. The prior probability is based on knowledge of the individual's antecedents and sibs. The conditional probability is the probability of being a carrier or not depending on the individual's SCK level, data from DNA markers, and the number of normal sons she may have had. The product of the prior and conditional probabilities is the joint probability. The final posterior probability of a woman being a carrier is the joint probability of getting the observed information given she is a carrier, divided by the sum of this probability plus the joint probability of getting the observed information if she is not a carrier. The method of calculation is illustrated in the following examples.

Consider the family in Fig. 11.7 where a daughter III$_3$ with a normal son seeks genetic counselling. It would appear that the Duchenne gene and RFLP allele-2 are co-inherited in the family (see p. 176). First, we consider the prior probability of III$_3$ being a carrier or not being a carrier which is 0.5. Let us assume that she has an SCK of 40 iu, that she has inherited RFLP allele-2 from her mother, and the frequency of recombination (θ) between the RFLP and the disease locus is 5 per cent (0.05). Then, if she *is* a carrier the (conditional) probability of her having allele-2 is 0.95 i.e. 1 minus θ, because crossing-over would *not* have to occur. Since 56 per cent of controls and 12 per cent of definite carriers have an SCK of 31–50 iu (Table 11.7, p. 227), the conditional probability of having an SCK of 40 iu if she is a carrier is 0.12. Finally, the conditional probability of having a normal son if she is a carrier is 0.50. On the other hand if she is *not* a carrier then these

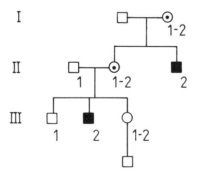

Fig. 11.7 Pedigree of Duchenne muscular dystrophy linked to an RFLP, the alleles of which are represented below the pedigree symbols.

conditional pro-conditional probabilities are respectively 0.05 (since crossing-over would now have to occur), 0.56, and 1.00. The calculations are set out as follows:

Probability	Carrier	Not a carrier
Prior	0.50	0.50
Conditional		
allele-2	0.95	0.05
SCK 40 iu	0.12	0.56
normal son	0.50	1.00
Joint	0.029	0.014

Posterior
  (of being a carrier)

$$= \frac{0.029}{0.029 + 0.014}$$
$$= 0.674$$

i.e. there is a very high probability (67 per cent) that she is a carrier and therefore any son she has would have a 1 in 3 chance of being affected.

However, suppose she had inherited allele-1, and therefore seemed unlikely to be a carrier (unless crossing-over occurred) yet her SCK level was 100 iu (i.e. in the upper part of the normal range), the calculations are then as follows:

Probability	Carrier	Not a carrier
Prior	0.50	0.50
Conditional		
allele-1	0.05	0.95
SCK 100 iu	0.144	0.015
normal son	0.50	1.00
Joint	0.002	0.007

Posterior
  (of being a carrier)

$$= \frac{0.002}{0.002 + 0.007}$$
$$= 0.222$$

Thus, the chance of being a carrier remains high and in this case the probability of a son being affected is roughly 1 in 9.

It should be noted that in these calculations for the sake of simplicity the linkage phase in the mother (whether allele-2 is co-inherited with the Duchenne gene) is assumed and with a closely linked probe ($\theta < 0.10$) this makes no practical difference to the results (Emery 1986). Other worked examples are given in Harper *et al.* (1983) and Pembrey *et al.* (1984).

However, nowadays in many families there is only one affected boy. The affected boy in such a family may represent a new mutation and there is also no certainty as to the linkage phase in the family. Let us first consider for the sake of simplicity that in such a family only data on SCK levels are available. Let us assume that a woman who seeks genetic counselling has an SCK of 80 iu, one normal brother, and a sister with an SCK of 60 iu who has an affected son, there being no one else affected in the family. We first have to go back one generation and consider the *mother* of these two sisters. Like any woman in the population she has a prior probability of being a carrier of 4μ, where μ is the mutation rate in both males and females. The reason, put simply, is that the chance of a mutation occurring in either of her maternally or paternally derived X chromosomes is 2μ and the probability that she might have inherited the mutant gene through her mother is also 2μ. We then consider the conditional probabilities, firstly of her having had a normal son and secondly of having had a daughter with an SCK of 60 iu and an affected son. In the case of the daughter we first determine the prior probabilities of her being a carrier or not a carrier given her mother is or is not a carrier. Secondly, we determine the conditional probabilities of the daughter having an affected son and a serum creatine kinase level of 60 iu assuming she is or is not a carrier, and finally we determine her joint probabilities. The final overall joint probabilities are arrived at by multiplying the daughter's joint probabilities by her mother's prior probabilities and her mother's conditional probabilities of having a normal son.

The calculations are set out as follows:

Probability	Carrier			Not a carrier	
Prior	4μ			$1 - 4\mu \simeq 1$	
Conditional					
a normal son	$1/2$			1	
daughter					
	Carrier	Not a carrier		Carrier	Not a carrier
Prior	$1/2$	$1/2$		2μ	1
Conditional					
⌠ affected son	$1/2$	μ		$1/2$	μ
⌡ SCK 60 iu	0.07	0.24		0.07	0.24
Joint	0.02	0.12μ		0.07μ	0.24μ
Joint	0.04μ	$0.24\mu^2$ (negligible)		0.07μ	0.24μ

The final posterior probability of the *mother* being a carrier, taking into account information on her daughter with an affected son, is the sum of the joint probabilities if she is a carrier (columns 1 and 2) divided by the sum of these probabilities plus the sum of the joint probabilities if she is not a carrier (columns 3 and 4) i.e.

$$\frac{0.04\,\mu}{0.04\,\mu + 0.07\,\mu + 0.24\,\mu}$$
$$= 0.11$$

We now consider the sister who came for counselling who now has a prior probability of being a carrier of 0.055, say 0.06:

Probability	Carrier	Not a carrier
Prior	0.06	0.94
Conditional		
SCK 80 iu	0.16	0.03
Joint	0.010	0.028

Her (posterior) probability of being a carrier is therefore:

$$\frac{0.010}{0.010 + 0.028}$$
$$= 0.26$$

Thus, despite the fact that both she and her sister have SCK levels within the normal range, the sister who requested counselling still has a high chance (i.e. about 1 in 4) of being a carrier.

A general formula for calculating the probability of a woman being a carrier of a *lethal* X-linked disorder, which affects either a brother or a son (*there being no one else affected in the family*) has been derived (Emery and Morton 1968). If h_c and h_m refer respectively to the relative probabilities of normal homozygosity to heterozygosity (Y_1/Y_2 in Table 11.7) in the suspected carrier and her mother, so that if there is no such information $h = 1$,

and if q = number of normal brothers
and r = number of normal sons
and if $s = 1$ where a son is affected and 0 if a brother is affected
and $t = 0$ where a son is affected and 1 if a brother is affected,

then the probability (P) of her being a carrier of a *lethal* X-linked disorder is:

$$P = \frac{1 + sa}{1 + sa + ab + tb}$$

where $a = h_m 2^q$
and $b = h_c 2^r$

It is also helpful to include in these calculations information on SCK levels in all the first degree postpubertal female relatives of a suspected carrier (Emery and Holloway 1977).

Over the years we tested some 1400 potential carriers in over 400 families, in many of which there was only one affected boy. By using Bayesian statistics and combining both pedigree and SCK data, rather than using pedigree data alone, this reduced considerably the proportion of women who fell into the intermediate risk range (Fig. 11.8). Even further separation is possible if DNA data are also included in the calculations.

Finally, even in families with an isolated case of Duchenne muscular dystrophy, carrier detection can be improved by using data from a linked

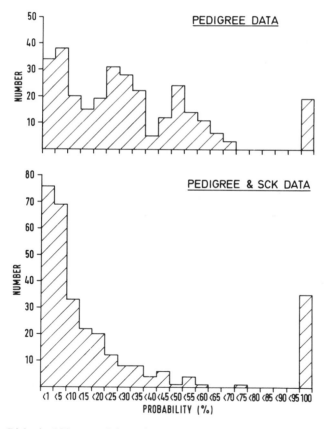

Fig. 11.8 Risks in 300 potential carriers based on: (*above*) pedigree data alone, (*below*) pedigree and SCK data combined.

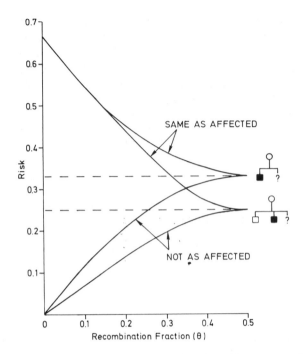

Fig. 11.9   Risks of the sister of an isolated case of Duchenne muscular dystrophy being a carrier (or a subsequent male fetus being affected) depending on whether the individual has the same or a different maternal RFLP allele from the affected boy.

RFLP. The probability of the sister of an affected boy being a carrier (or a subsequent male fetus being affected) depends on whether the individual has the same or a different maternal RFLP from the affected boy. If the sister has a different allele then, barring crossing-over, she is unlikely to be a carrier. The position is improved the closer the DNA marker is to the disease locus. If θ is, say, 0.05 and she has a different allele from her affected brother, her risk becomes about 1 in 16, or less than 1 in 30 if she also has an unaffected brother (Fig. 11.9). The risks could be reduced even further depending on her actual SCK level.

Information on DNA markers lying on either side of the locus (flanking or bridging markers) and from the maternal grandfather's haplotype are also important, and increase the precision (Clayton and Emery 1984; Clark 1985). The likelihood that information from a linked RFLP will be helpful (the mother will be heterozygous and the segregation pattern in the family will be informative) increases as the number of alleles at the RFLP locus increases (Asmussen and Clegg 1985).

Table 11.9 *Risks of the sister of an isolated case of Duchenne muscular dystrophy being a carrier (or of a subsequent male fetus being affected) for different values of* h *and recombination fraction* (θ), *and whether the sister* (*or male fetus*) *has the same* or a different† RFLP allele from the affected boy. (When* θ = 0.50 *there are no data on a DNA marker; when* h = 1.0 *there are no data on SCK)*

	Recombination fraction (θ)							
	0.01	0.05	0.10	0.15	0.20	0.30	0.40	0.50
h = 0.1								
Same:	0.950	0.938	0.923	0.908	0.892	0.863	0.841	0.833
Diff:	0.118	0.403	0.577	0.672	0.731	0.795	0.825	0.833
h = 0.2								
Same:	0.904	0.884	0.858	0.831	0.806	0.759	0.726	0.714
Diff:	0.063	0.253	0.405	0.506	0.576	0.660	0.702	0.714
h = 0.5								
Same:	0.790	0.753	0.707	0.664	0.624	0.558	0.515	0.500
Diff:	0.026	0.119	0.214	0.291	0.352	0.437	0.485	0.500
h = 1.0								
Same:	0.653	0.603	0.547	0.497	0.453	0.387	0.347	0.333
Diff:	0.013	0.063	0.120	0.170	0.213	0.280	0.320	0.333
h = 2.0								
Same:	0.485	0.432	0.376	0.330	0.293	0.240	0.210	0.200
Diff:	0.007	0.033	0.064	0.093	0.119	0.163	0.190	0.200
h = 3.0								
Same:	0.386	0.336	0.287	0.248	0.217	0.174	0.150	0.143
Diff:	0.004	0.022	0.043	0.064	0.083	0.115	0.136	0.143
h = 4.0								
Same:	0.320	0.275	0.232	0.198	0.172	0.136	0.117	0.111
Diff:	0.003	0.017	0.033	0.049	0.063	0.089	0.105	0.111
h = 5.0								
Same:	0.274	0.233	0.194	0.165	0.142	0.112	0.096	0.091
Diff:	0.003	0.013	0.027	0.039	0.051	0.072	0.086	0.091

$$\text{* Risk} = \left(1 + \frac{h(1 + 4\theta - 4\theta^2)}{2 - 4\theta + 4\theta^2}\right)^{-1} \qquad \text{† Risk} = \left(1 + \frac{h(3 - 4\theta + 4\theta^2)}{4\theta - 4\theta^2}\right)^{-1}$$

The calculations involved in determining the probability of the mother or sister of an isolated case being a carrier, which takes into account both SCK and RFLP data, are detailed in Emery (1986) and Young (1991). However, they can be somewhat tedious, especially when more than one DNA marker is involved and there are a number of relatives to be considered. Fortunately there are now computer programs available specifically for these calculations (for example, Clayton 1986; Sarfarazi and Williams 1986). Too much reliance on such programs, however, may lead to problems because serious errors can occur if mistakes are inadvertently made in inserting relevant data. When dealing with straightforward familial cases, and in isolated cases where one is only dealing with a single closely linked probe, the calculations can often be performed with a hand calculator.

A guide to the risks of a daughter being a carrier, whose brother is an isolated case, are given in Table 11.9. The risks depend on her SCK level (the relative probability of normal homozygosity to heterozygosity '*h*'), whether she has the same or a different RFLP allele as her affected brother, and the frequency of recombination (crossing-over) between the RFLP and the disease locus (0.01–0.50). The risks of the mother having another affected son correspond to the entries in the table where $h = 1$ (i.e. where in a potential carrier it is assumed there is no information on SCK levels). These risks, however, ignore additional information which might also be available including the number of normal sons and brothers the mother may have, the mother's SCK level, information from more than one probe, and the haplotype of the maternal grandfather. Nevertheless, the tabulated risks provide at least a first approximation. Note that until there is more information about subsequent sons and her daughter's status, the risks of the mother

Table 11.10 *Some DNA probes useful for carrier detection and prenatal diagnosis. The heterozygote frequencies and genetic distances are approximate (data from various sources)*

Probe	Restriction enzyme	Heterozygote frequency	Genetic distance (cM)
Distal (terminal)			
RC8	Taq I	0.25	15
99–6	Pst I	0.50	15
B24	Msp I	0.15	10
C7	Eco RV	0.25	10
PERT 87-8	Bst XI	0.50	
	Taq I	0.40	
PERT 87-1	Xmn I	0.40	~ 10
	Bst NI	0.50	
XJ-1.1	Taq I	0.30	
754	Pst I	0.45	10
OTC	Msp I	0.30	10
L1.28	Taq I	0.45	15
Proximal (centromere)			

See also Appendix G.

being a carrier are *a priori* 2 in 3 and obviously uninfluenced by DNA marker data on her affected son.

In order to determine the risks from Table 11.9 in a particular case using a particular probe, values of θ for various markers are given in Table 11.10. For example, consider the sister of an isolated case of Duchenne muscular dystrophy who has an SCK of 60 iu ($h = 3.26$, Table 11.7) and who has inherited a *different* C7 allele ($\theta = 0.10$, Table 11.10) from her affected brother, then her probability of being a carrier is roughly 0.04 or 1 in 25. Such an estimate of heterozygosity however, does not take into account any recombination which may occur within the Xp21 locus itself but is adequate for most practical purposes.

One further point is as follows. The carrier status of a female in an affected family with a deletion may be deduced from information obtained at prenatal diagnosis. If a male fetus is found to have a demonstrable gene deletion then clearly the mother must be a carrier (or a germ-line mosaic, p. 246). If the fetus has no demonstrable DNA abnormality then this of course tells us nothing of the mother's genotype.

Linkage with RFLPs can be very useful in deciding if a woman is a carrier (*see*, for example, Darras and Francke 1988; Liechti-Gallati *et al.* 1990). But RFLPs are not the only markers which can be used for this purpose, a particularly valuable polymorphism being so-called CA repeats (Clemens *et al.* 1991; Feener *et al.* 1991; Richards *et al.* 1992) (Fig. 11.10).

The particular value of linked markers is that they may provide helpful information even in a family where an isolated affected boy is now deceased. Here it may be possible to show, for example, that the male fetus of a sister of the affected boy has inherited the grandpaternal X chromosome haplotype and therefore is unlikely to be affected. Linkage studies may be

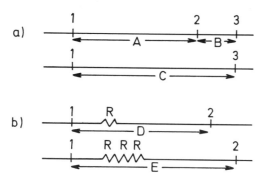

Fig. 11.10 DNA length polymorphisms due to: (*a*) variations in restriction sites, for example, with loss of a restriction site resulting in a larger DNA fragment (C); (*b*) variations in the number of repeats (R) between restriction sites (e.g. CA repeats). Restriction sites are indicated by numbers and the resultant restriction fragments by letters.

the only approach to carrier detection when there is not a deletion. But this situation will change with methods capable of identifying all mutations at the Xp21 locus (Roberts *et al*. 1992).

But the establishment of carrier status, or the diagnosis of an affected fetus, which depends on linkage, will always be subject to error due to recombination, though with intragenic and close flanking markers this error will be very small.

To reduce problems of recombination, a method has been devised (Orita *et al*. 1989) for identifying polymorphisms *within* a deleted PCR multiplex band; so-called single stranded conformation polymorphisms (SSCP). These sequence polymorphisms resulting from nucleotide substitutions are more common than RFLPs. For these reasons SSCP analysis has been recommended for carrier detection (Richards and Friend 1991; Zietkiewicz *et al*. 1992). But a conformational change induced by a *point mutation* (as well as a deletion) results in a mobility shift on an electrophoretic gel using appropriate primers and this method is therefore now being used to detect such mutations (Nigro *et al*. 1992).

Direct carrier detection

Methods of diagnosis which depend on linkage are referred to as *indirect* since they do not identify the mutation itself but only its location with respect to DNA markers. Methods which aim to identify the mutation are referred to as *direct*. These latter methods should, at least in theory, make a precise diagnosis possible.

Dosage

Theoreically using an appropriate cDNA probe, Southern blot analysis should reveal a dosage difference between controls and carriers in the ratio 2:1 for deletions and 2:3 for duplications (Laing *et al*. 1989; Prior 1991). Unfortunately in most carriers such differences are not convincing. The methodology (as in other carrier tests, p. 216) requires meticulous care and very good Southern blots, and each sample should be analysed in duplicate and compared with bands obtained under comparable conditions from healthy control females.

Approaches depending on PCR amplification with densitometric quantification of radioactivity, fluorescence, or ethidium bromide stained gels may prove more valuable (Abbs and Bobrow 1992).

Junction fragments

A deletion or duplication may generate a so-called 'junction fragment' of altered size if the breakpoint occurs close to a non-deleted exon so that it lies within the restriction fragment detected by a cDNA probe. This is recognized as an additional band on a Southern blot (Den Dunnen *et al*. 1989). If a

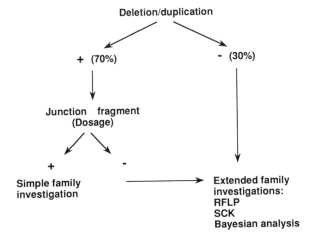

Fig. 11.11 Investigation of families with or without a gene deletion or duplication (unless a point mutation can be detected directly, e.g. by SSCP).

deletion-associated junction fragment occurs in a family then all affected males and all carrier females in the family will have this additional band. The presence or absence of an additional band is clearly less subjective than methods which depend on dosage. Unfortunately, with Southern blot analysis and cDNA probes, at most only 20 per cent of deletions are associated with an identifiable junction fragment. However, by using other techniques (Chen *et al.* 1988), such as field inversion or pulsed-field gel electrophoresis (FIGE, PFGE), the proportion of cases in which a junction fragment is seen can be increased to over 90 per cent. Unfortunately these techniques are technically demanding, time consuming, and require expensive equipment and at present would be impractical in a routine diagnostic service. Nevertheless, in a family with a deletion or duplication, search for a junction fragment can play a crucial role in the way the family is investigated (Fig. 11.11).

In situ *hybridization*

At first glance this would seem to provide the most obvious way of detecting a woman who carries a deletion on one of her two X chromosomes. By using a labelled probe (for example, a dystrophin cosmid), only one of her two X chromosomes should show a site-specific hybridization signal on a metaphase chromosome preparation (Ried *et al.* 1990). Unfortunately because of repetitive sequencs throughout the genome, such a probe is also likely to hybridize to other sites and to other chromosomes as well. The answer has therefore been to suppress these other sites by adding appropriate competitor DNAs to the probe mix (Lichter *et al* 1990). This method has therefore been referred to as chromosomal *in situ* suppression (CISS) hybridization. In cases where only one X chromosome shows a hybridization signal, this approach provides unequivocal evidence of carrier status (Ried *et al.* 1990). But the method is technically demanding though with refinement it offers an excellent direct means of detecting carriers.

Lymphocyte RNA

A particularly novel approach to carrier detection has been developed by Roberts and colleagues (1990, 1991). Essentially it consists of amplifying (by 'nested' PCR) reversely transcribed mRNA from peripheral blood lymphocytes in which dystrophin mRNA is 'illegitimately' transcribed. The products are visualized on a gel by ethidium bromide staining. Analysis of band sizes of the PCR products indicates whether a deletion or duplication is present. With modifications it can also detect point mutations. The main disadvantage of this method is its dependence on very high amplification of a very rare mRNA. However, since this approach is also applicable to other genetic disorders it may well attract technological refinements in future. It has the advantage of being rapid, non-radioactive, and qualitative. The preservation of material by lyophilization makes it possible to store and ship material to specialized centres for RNA-based diagnostic tests without deterimental effects (Anderson *et al.* 1992).

Automated DNA analysis

Automated methods of analysis are being developed. As Caskey has pointed out: 'The use of sequencing techniques for routine mutation detection is a relatively new concept but one which is gaining rapid use' (Caskey 1991). This has already been achieved in the case of Lesch–Nyhan syndrome. Even without material from a deceased male with Duchenne muscular dystrophy, theoretically DNA sequencing could identify female carriers in the family. A PCR-based linkage and carrier detection protocol with or without detectable deletions analysed on an automated sequencer has already been developed (Schwartz *et al.* 1992). Unfortunately an automated sequencer for the analysis of fluorescently labelled PCR products currently costs $120 000! No doubt the price will decrease as developments occur and usage increases.

The future

These novel and ingenious methods certainly demonstrate the resourcefulness of molecular biologists. As Bertolt Brecht has expressed, 'Beauty in nature is a quality which gives the human senses a chance to be skilful'. But at present it is difficult to see which method or methods will ultimately prevail. Personally I can imagine a situation one day where computerization will combine pedigree and SCK data with the results of automated DNA analysis to provide a solution to the problems of carrier detection and prenatal diagnosis. Who, for example, would ever have imagined 30 years ago that an average-sized hospital clinical chemistry department would be capable of analysing several thousand blood samples a day by automated methodology?

Muscle dystrophin

Muscle dystrophin investigations are very important in establishing the diagnosis of Duchenne and Becker dystrophies (Arahata *et al.* 1988; Hoffman *et al.* 1988). The distribution of dystrophin in muscle biopsy specimens is determined using immunohistochemical methods, and the abundance and size of dystrophin by Western blotting (p. 74). There is general agreement (Bonilla *et al.* 1988*b*; Arahata *et al.* 1989*a*; Morandi *et al.* 1990) that in *manifesting* carriers of Duchenne muscular dystrophy there is significant variation in dystrophin immunostaining both between and within fibres. Many fibres do not stain at all (Fig. 11.12). But in non-manifesting carriers variability in immunostaining is infrequent and negative fibres are rare, especially if the SCK level is normal (Morandi *et al.* 1990; Vainzof *et al.* 1991*b*). Also in symptomless carriers dystrophin abundance on Western blots is generally normal (Arahata *et al.* 1989*b*) and again especially if the

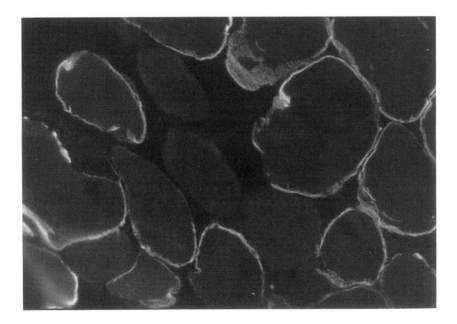

Fig. 11.12 Immunofluorescence staining of a muscle biopsy from a manifesting carrier of Duchenne muscular dystrophy. (Reproduced by kind permission of Dr Louise Nicholson.)

SCK level is normal (Morandi *et al.* 1990). On the other hand, Clerk *et al.* (1991) have reported variability in immunostaining and dystrophin of reduced abundance in at least a proportion of *younger* carriers. In the younger carrier of Becker muscular dystrophy *two* bands may be seen: normal and a reduced size dystrophin of reduced abundance (Chevron *et al.* 1992; Vainzof *et al.* 1992). It is therefore possible that these techniques *may* be more informative in younger women. A greater proportion of dystrophin-negative fibres are found in younger heterozygotes in the *mdx* mouse (Karpati *et al.* 1990; Weller *et al.* 1991) and the dystrophic dog (Cooper *et al.* 1990). But in Duchenne carriers no such relationship with age has been found by Vainzof *et al.* (1991*b*). In any event the weakness in manifesting carriers does not improve with age but invariably gets worse.

The consensus would seem to be that convincing and clear-cut muscle dystrophin abnormalities are infrequent in healthy carriers with a normal SCK level. Therefore such studies, which are both invasive and expensive, would seem at least at present to offer little additional information for carrier detection and genetic counselling (Fig. 11.13).

In conclusion, in *familial* cases where DNA samples from affected

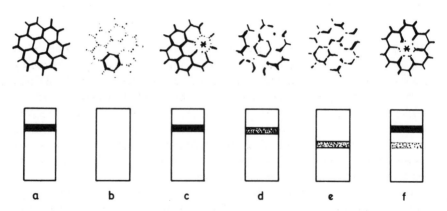

Fig. 11.13 Diagrammatic representation of possible findings on immunohistochemistry and Western blot analysis.

a) Control: normal size (427 kDa) and abundance.

b) DMD: occasional positive fibre, virtually no dystrophin.

c) Non-manifesting carrier of DMD: occasional negative fibre (*) and *possible* reduction in abundance of normal size dystrophin.

d) Manifesting carrier of DMD: variation in staining between and within fibres and reduction in abundance of normal size dystrophin.

e) BMD: variation in staining between and within fibres, and reduction in abundance and size of dystrophin.

f) BMD carrier: occasional negative fibre (*) and bands of normal and possibly reduced size dystrophin of reduced abundance.

Table 11.11 *Summary of approaches to carrier detection in families with Duchenne muscular dystrophy*: + *useful*; (+) *possible*; − *not indicated*

Affected male	Available		Unavailable
Deletion/duplication	+ (70%)	− (30%)	
Possible carrier			
(*i*) SCK	+	+	+
(*ii*) Linkage studies	+	+	(+)
(*iii*) DNA studies			
Dosage	+	−	(+)
Junction fragment	+	−	(+)
In situ hybridization	+	−	(+)
Lymphocyte RNA	+	−	(+)
DNA analysis	+	+	+
(*iv*) Muscle dystrophin	(+)	(+)	(+)

individuals are available and if a gene deletion or duplication is present, then carrier identification (and prenatal diagnosis) is usually straightforward by a combination of SCK, linkage, and gene studies (Table 11.11). Even when there is only one affected male in the family but DNA is available, then carrier identification is often possible using these methods. The main problem is when the only affected member of the family is now deceased. Reliance then has to be made on the SCK level and possibly, for example, a search for a junction fragment. Ultimately this problem will only be satisfactorily resolved by direct methods of DNA analysis.

It is salutary that in a detailed analysis of these problems in Finnish families (Kääriäinen *et al.* 1990) DNA analysis with flanking and intragenic markers gave confusing results in nearly 10 per cent of cases. Reasons included an increased SCK level when DNA studies indicated a low risk, the most likely explanation for which was intragenic recombination. But the possibility of a spurious SCK level has also to be considered. There is at present no simple answer and it remains necessary to combine all available data from the particular pedigree, SCK levels, and DNA studies. There is also the additional problem of germ-line mosaicism to be considered (p. 246).

Prenatal diagnosis

A woman at high risk of having an affected son may choose fetal sexing with selective abortion of any male fetus and in this way be guaranteed a daughter who will not be affected. However, this is unsatisfactory for two reasons. First, at least half of the aborted fetuses will in fact be normal. Secondly, sons who would not reproduce are replaced by daughters, a proportion of whom will be carriers and may in due course transmit the gene to their offspring. The effect is therefore dysgenic and would be expected to lead eventually to an increase in the incidence of heterozygous carriers. What is therefore required is a reliable test for the *affected* male fetus. At first it seemed that SCK levels in fetal blood obtained at fetoscopy might be valuable, but several false negatives soon invalidated this approach (Ionasescu *et al.* 1978; Emery *et al.* 1979*a*; Golbus *et al.* 1979). However, the advent of recombinant DNA technology has opened up an entirely different approach to prenatal diagnosis. Fetal DNA can be extracted from amniotic fluid cells obtained by transabdominal amniocentesis at about 16–18 weeks of gesta-

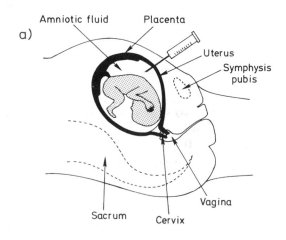

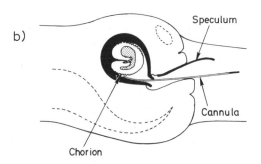

Fig. 11.14 Technique of: (*a*) transabdominal amniocentesis, (*b*) chorion biopsy. (From Emery (1985) reprinted with permission of John Wiley and Sons Ltd.)

tion. Then either using a gene-specific probe or a closely linked DNA marker the probability of the fetus being affected can be determined. The use of bridging markers reduces the probability of error due to crossing-over and prenatal diagnosis has been made on the basis of such markers (Bakker *et al.* 1985). In the case of the markers listed in Table 11.10, the probability that a woman would be heterozygous for at least one is 99.7 per cent. However, should she be homozygous for a possibly informative RFLP allele then it will not be clear which of her X chromosomes is carrying the Duchenne gene. Though errors due to recombination have been reported (Darras *et al.* 1987), the use of linked DNA markers as well as intragenic probes is informative and helpful in the vast majority of families (Cole *et al.* 1988). See Appendix G.

A more recent development has been the introduction of chorion biopsy for prenatal diagnosis (Rodeck and Morsman 1983; Hogge *et al.* 1985; Pescia and The 1986). Essentially the technique consists of inserting a flexible cannula/catheter either through the cervix or transabdominally into the uterine cavity. Chorionic villi (which are of fetal origin) are carefully removed for DNA, cytogenetic, and other studies (Fig. 11.14). Since this procedure can be performed as early as 10 weeks gestation and the material need not be cultured for DNA or chromosome studies, a prenatal diagnosis can be made much earlier than with amniocentesis and if an abortion has to be carried out it is therefore likely to cause less psychological trauma.

DNA studies on cultured amniotic fluid cells or chorionic biopsy material can establish fetal diagnosis on the basis of linkage studies when there is no deletion, or by demonstrating a deletion at Xp21 in other cases.

Fetal muscle biopsy

Fetal muscle biopsy has also been employed in the diagnosis of an affected fetus (Gustavii *et al.* 1983; Evans *et al.* 1991). The technique involves inserting a trocar and cannula through the myometrium into the amniotic cavity under ultrasonographic guidance in the second trimester of pregnancy. Diagnosis is then based on histological and dystrophin immunohistochemical studies on the biopsied material, and remarkably at birth there is little more than a small scar in the biopsy region. The technique however is difficult and the possibility of fetal loss is likely to be high.

Fetal muscle dystrophin

In the normal *embryo* dystrophin first appears in the sarcolemma at the peripheral ends of the myotubes immediately adjacent to the tendons. In the *fetus* it appears throughout the entire myofibre, becoming restricted to the sarcolemma only later (Prelle *et al.* 1991; Wessels *et al.* 1991).

Examination of muscle tissue from fetuses affected with Duchenne muscular dystrophy aborted in the second trimester of pregnancy has revealed a complete absence of dystrophin (Patel *et al.* 1988) as well as an increased variation in fibre size and an increased number of hypercontracted fibres (Boelter *et al.* 1990), which confirms that these histological changes are in fact an early manifestation of the dystrophic process (p. 199). Earlier in the first trimester of pregnancy however, truncated dystrophin is detectable. Using antisera specifically directed against various regions of the dystrophin molecule, positive reaction to the N-terminal region, different reactions to the central rod region, and negative reaction to the C-terminal region have been reported in affected fetuses (Ginjaar *et al.* 1991*a*). Since the C-terminal region is believed to be important in attaching dystrophin to the cell membrane, though this has been questioned (Helliwell *et al.* 1992, Récan *et al.* 1992), the presence of abnormal truncated unintegrated dystrophin early in development indicates that degradation occurs later. Most importantly this use of a series of antibodies covering the entire dystrophin molecule could be used to map mutations, so-called 'immunological mapping' of dystrophin mutations (Ginjaar *et al.* 1991*a*). This could be diagnostically important where no mutation is detectable at the DNA level.

Furthermore, such studies can be very important in helping to establish the carrier status of a mother when DNA is either unavailable from other affected relatives or is uninformative. The demonstration of a significant defect in fetal muscle dystrophin would confirm that the mother is a carrier. In other cases where haplotype information is available in an affected relative, fetal muscle studies may, in conjunction with these haplotype data, prove that a mother is *not* a carrier (Ginjaar *et al.* 1991*b*). This is clearly shown in the evolution over several years in the management of a family in which the only affected male was deceased (Fig. 11.15). The use of dystrophin genomic and cDNA probes for solving difficulties in carrier detection and prenatal diagnosis when there are no living affected members in a family has been critically and helpfully reviewed by Shomrat *et al.* (1992).

Germ-line mosaicism

In 1987 Bakker and colleagues reported two families with partial deletions of the Xp21 locus which were transmitted to more than one offspring by women who showed no evidence of the mutation in their own somatic (leucocyte) cells. Similarly, Darras and Francke (1987) reported a family in which a deletion had been transmitted twice by an unaffected male as proved by RFLP analysis (Fig. 11.16). Many other similar cases have since been reported (for example, Wood and McGillivray 1988, Bakker *et al.* 1989). These findings have been attributed to germ-line, germinal, or gonadal mosaicism. That is, individuals who are phenotypically normal and not genetic carriers nevertheless transmit a mutation to more than one offspring

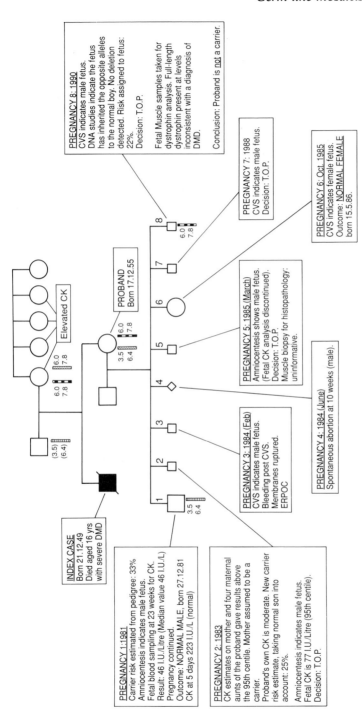

PREGNANCY 8: 1990
CVS indicates male fetus.
DNA studies indicate the fetus
has inherited the opposite alleles
to the normal boy. No deletion
detected. Risk assigned to fetus:
22%.
Decision: T.O.P.

Fetal Muscle samples taken for
dystrophin analysis. Full-length
dystrophin present at levels
inconsistent with a diagnosis of
DMD.

Conclusion: Proband is <u>not</u> a carrier.

PROBAND
Born 17.12.55

PREGNANCY 7: 1988
CVS indicates male fetus.
Decision: T.O.P.

PREGNANCY 6: Oct. 1985
CVS indicates female fetus.
Outcome: <u>NORMAL FEMALE</u>
born 15.5.86.

PREGNANCY 5: 1985 (March)
Amniocentesis shows male fetus.
(Fetal CK analysis discontinued).
Decision: T.O.P.
Muscle biopsy for histopathology:
uninformative.

PREGNANCY 4: 1984 (June)
Spontaneous abortion at 10 weeks (male).

PREGNANCY 3: 1984 (Feb)
CVS indicates male fetus.
Bleeding post CVS.
Membranes ruptured.
ERPOC

Elevated CK

INDEX CASE
Born 21.12.49
Died aged 16 yrs
with severe DMD

PREGNANCY 1: 1981
Carrier risk estimated from pedigree: 33%
Amniocentesis indicates male fetus.
Fetal blood sampling at 23 weeks for CK.
Result: 46 I.U./Litre (Median value 46 I.U./L)
Pregnancy continued
Outcome: NORMAL MALE, born 27.12.81
CK at 5 days 223 I.U/L (normal)

PREGNANCY 2: 1983
CK estimates on mother and four maternal
aunts of the proband gave results above
the 95th centile. Mother assumed to be a
carrier.
Proband's own CK is moderate. New carrier
risk estimate, taking normal son into
account: 25%.

Amniocentesis indicates male fetus.
Fetal CK is 77 I.U./Litre (95th centile).
Decision: T.O.P.

Fig. 11.15 The evolution over several years in the management of a family in which the only affected male was deceased. (Reproduced by kind permission of Dr David E. Barton and Dr Clare Davison.)

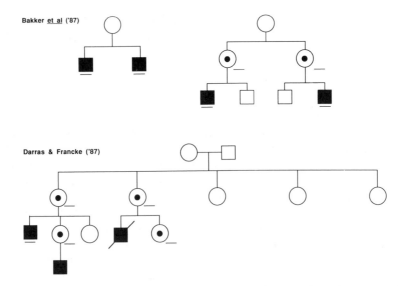

Fig. 11.16 Simplified pedigrees demonstrating germ-line mosaicism in transmitting parents. (−) indicates a demonstrable Xp21 gene deletion.

because they harbour a somatic mutation within a fraction of their germ-line cells.

The phenomenon is not restricted to Duchenne muscular dystrophy but has also been reported in a variety of other genetic disorders and has been extensively reviewed (Hall 1988, Edwards 1989). Though there is as yet no *direct* evidence of germ-line mosaicism in the case of Duchenne muscular dystrophy, in dominant lethal osteogenesis imperfecta the causative mutation was detected in 1 in 8 sperm of a normal father who had had two affected infants. In this case the transmitting father's germ-line mosaicism was a reflection of generalized somatic mosaicism (Cohn *et al*. 1990) which has also been described in a rare family with Duchenne muscular dystrophy in which a transmitting male appears to have been both a somatic and germ-line mosaic (Lebo *et al*. 1990).

Estimates of the frequency of germ-line mosaicism among families with Duchenne muscular dystrophy have been variously calculated to be between 12 and 20 per cent (Bakker *et al*. 1989, Passos-Bueno *et al*. 1990*b*, van Essen *et al*. 1992*b*). Formulae for incorporating germ-line mosaicism into calculations of genetic risk have been proposed (Grimm *et al*. 1990; Jeanpierre 1992). However from a practical point of view, it means that it can never be assumed that a male fetus born of a mother with a normal genotype will in fact be unaffected. It is therefore advisable to consider prenatal diagnosis in *all* pregnancies in at least the mother and sisters of an isolated affected boy.

In the case of a mother without a deletion who has an affected son, it is important to test with cDNA probes all her daughters to determine if she may be a germ-line mosaic (Prior *et al.* 1992).

Ova transfer and blastocyst biopsy

These procedures might be indicated in the case of a woman who is at high risk of having an affected son but who for various reasons may not be able to face prenatal diagnosis and abortion. Ova from an unrelated (non-carrier) female may be fertilized *in vitro* by the carrier's husband's sperm. A fertilized ovum is then implanted in the carrier's uterus where it develops normally.

Another possibility is to remove ova by laparoscopy from a carrier female and having fertilized them with her husband's sperm allow them to develop *in vitro* until, say, the early blastocyst stage. Or alternatively a few days after normal intercourse, a developing blastocyst is removed from the uterine cavity. Either way it is then feasible to remove a single cell without damaging the conceptus and by using appropriate DNA markers determine if it will be affected or a heterozygous carrier. Only unaffected male or non-carrier female conceptuses would be reimplanted in the uterus to undergo further development.

Yet an even more intriguing possibility is to remove an ovum and its associated polar body prior to fertilization, and by PCR amplify the relevant Xp21 sequence in DNA from the polar body. Any X-chromosomal defect detectable in the polar body cannot be present in the ovum which could then be fertilized *in vitro* and returned to the uterus to undergo further development.

All these techniques have been shown to be feasible in animal models and have already been applied in certain X-linked recessive disorders in humans (Van Voorhis *et al.* 1992). The author is not aware however, that any have yet been carried out on a carrier of Duchenne muscular dystrophy.

Summary and conclusions

Since Duchenne muscular dystrophy is a serious disorder for which at present there is no effective treatment, much emphasis has been given to prevention. This involves the ascertainment of women likely to have an affected son, and the provision of genetic counselling and prenatal diagnosis for such women. The ascertainment of women at risk could be achieved by screening the entire population for affected boys or by screening women within known affected families. Screening for affected boys in the newborn period has the advantage that such early detection might lead to the prevention of second cases in a family. A number of neonatal screening programmes have been developed with some success.

There are merits in recording affected families on a computerized register system with inbuilt safeguards for confidentiality and maintained on a local rather than a national basis. It can ensure that those in need of counselling, welfare services, and therapy can be readily contacted as developments in these various fields occur.

The major problem in prevention is the detection of female carriers. About 5-10 per cent have some degree of muscle involvement but this is rarely serious. The single most reliable test for detecting healthy carriers remains the SCK level, provided due attention is given to the various technical and biological factors which can affect it, including age (before 20) and pregnancy. Particularly valuable information is provided from linked DNA markers (Restriction Fragment Length Polymorphisms, RFLPs). The probability of a woman being a carrier is then based on combined pedigree, SCK, and DNA data using Bayesian statistics.

These indirect methods of carrier detection are being replaced by *direct* methods which depend upon identifying the mutation itself and include DNA dosage, detection of junction fragments, *in situ* hybridization, lymphocyte RNA analysis, DNA sequencing, and muscle dystrophin studies. The extension of DNA studies to the fetus has made prenatal diagnosis possible either through amniocentesis in the second trimester of pregnancy or chorion biopsy in the first trimester of pregnancy. This has also made possible the study of affected fetal muscle which is providing novel insights into the early stages of the dystrophic process.

Finally, because of the possibility of germ-line mosaicism, it is probably advisable to consider prenatal diagnosis in all pregnancies in at least the mother and sisters of an isolated affected boy.

12   Genetic counselling

Much emphasis has so far been placed on the probability of a woman being a carrier and the risks of her having an affected son. In genetic counselling these are important issues, but other matters also have to be considered and discussed.

Nature of genetic counselling

Genetic counselling is essentially a process of communication between the counsellor and those who seek counselling. Information to be communicated falls roughly into two main areas. First, information about the nature of the disorder: its severity and prognosis and whether or not there is any effective therapy, what the genetic mechanism is that caused the disease, and what are the risks of its occurring in relatives. Secondly, information on the available options open to a couple who are found to be at risk of transmitting the disease. This latter may include discussions of contraception, sterilization, prenatal diagnosis, and abortion.

When discussing the disease, the genetic counsellor has to present an accurate picture, even if depressing and disturbing if the parents are to make a reasoned decision about future children. Such discussions require considerable sensitivity and tact when the parents already have a young affected child. It is not uncommon for those involved in both the management of the disease as well as counselling to find themselves in the dilemma of having to maintain an optimistic outlook for the affected child and yet emphasizing the seriousness of the disorder when discussing its possible recurrence in any future children.

Having discussed at length the more medical aspects of the disease, the counsellor then proceeds to explain the genetic mechanism which caused it and the risks of recurrence in terms which are understandable to the individual couple. A preoccupation with risk figures can often be confusing and is best avoided. Often couples merely want to know if there is any chance at all that it could occur again. In many cases genetic mechanisms and recurrence risks need be discussed only in broad terms. In any event the actual interpretation of risks is very subjective: what might be an acceptable risk to one couple may be quite unacceptable to another. Nevertheless, risks form a useful basis for further discussions and can be a significant factor in influencing decision making. One important fact which may have to be explained is that being genetic the parents cannot hold themselves in any way responsible and every effort should be made to dispel feelings of guilt and recrimination which they may be harbouring.

If the risks are considered to be unacceptably high, then the options available include family limitation, contraception, prenatal diagnosis, and abortion, and perhaps one day blastocyst biopsy and other techniques. Contraception in this context requires expert advice because the results of failure will be far more devastating than when it is practised for purely social and economic reasons. A deep fear of having an affected child may well generate serious psychosexual problems and for this reason some definitive form of contraception may well have to be considered, such as tubal ligation or vasectomy. The effects of sterilization when performed on healthy women whose families are complete are likely to be entirely beneficial (Anon. 1984). But in a young woman in a family with Duchenne muscular dystrophy who either has no children or perhaps only the one affected child, it may have significant psychological sequelae. Counselling is especially important in these cases. To some couples sexual abstinence may be the only acceptable alternative.

Prenatal diagnosis has added a whole new dimension to genetic counselling, and when the result is negative the reassurance it gives is entirely beneficial. However, a proportion of mothers may decide to continue with the pregnancy after fetal sexing and learning that the fetus is male and therefore likely to be affected (Bundey and Ebdy 1982; Thompson 1984), presumably prepared to some extent to cope with the resultant problems (Golbus *et al.* 1974). Certainly therapeutic abortion can cause considerable psychological trauma in many women (Blumberg 1984), and in those genetic disorders where prental diagnosis is possible, after pregnancy termination following the diagnosis of an affected fetus, a significant proportion of mothers decline to undergo the procedure again. Sensitive counselling is therefore essential both at the time of prental diagnosis and during the period following a therapeutic abortion (Beeson and Golbus 1985). However, as Blumberg has stated, although 'Significant psychological trauma may be an unavoidable consequence of selective abortion, the alternative birth of a defective child is usually accompanied by even more intense feelings of guilt and depression' (Blumberg 1984).

As a prelude to genetic counselling it is important to divine a couple's educational and social background, their religious attitudes, and, if possible, something of their marital relationship if information is to be presented most effectively and sensitively. The counsellor may sense that for various ethical and other reasons contraception, sterilization, or prenatal diagnosis are unacceptable to a couple. These matters should then not be discussed further. The genetic counsellor's role is to inform and guide but not to coerce or impose his own views.

The various factors which influence the reproductive decision after genetic counselling are complex, variable, and personal and have been the subject of detailed studies by Frets and her colleagues (Frets *et al.* 1990*a*, 1990*b*, 1991).

Non-directive counselling

The genetic counsellor's role, until relatively recently, was often seen purely in medical and scientific terms: to establish a precise genetic diagnosis and to communicate factual information about the disease and its genetics. However, more emphasis is now being given to an appreciation of the psychological aspects of counselling. A change from what Kessler (1979) has referred to as *content-oriented* to *person-oriented* counselling. This change has been brought about by several factors. First, a disabling genetic disorder such as Duchenne muscular dystrophy often has profound psychological effects on the immediate family (Buchanan *et al.* 1979; Pullen 1984). Secondly, these effects may have long-term consequences and frequently extend to other relatives. Thirdly, it has been found that couples sometimes opt for a course of action which may well be at variance with what the counsellor might have regarded as 'reasonable'. For example, in a prospective follow-up study of 200 consecutive couples seen in a genetic counselling clinic with various genetic disorders, a proportion of those told that they were at risk of having an affected child were undeterred and actually planned further pregnancies (Emery *et al.* 1979*c*). At first sight such behaviour might seem irresponsible but on careful questioning in almost all cases the reasons for planning further children were often very understandable when considered from the parents' point of view. In some cases further pregnancies were planned because, after seeing the effects of a disorder in a previous child or in one of the parents, it was not considered sufficiently serious (congenital cataract, congenital deafness, peroneal muscular atrophy), or prenatal diagnosis was available (Sandhoff's disease, X-linked mental retardation),and yet in other cases the parents planned further pregnancies because if a subsequent child were affected it would not survive (renal agenesis), or if it survived it would succumb within a year or so (Werdnig–Hoffmann disease). There was a small but lamentable group of couples who had no living children and dearly wanted a family at whatever cost (Emery *et al.* 1979*c*).

Thus a course of action which might seem irresponsible to one person may seem eminently reasonable to another. The choice should be the individual's prerogative, always provided that it is made in the full knowledge of all the facts and possible consequences. Since the genetic counsellor's role is to help couples arrive at decisions which are *the best ones for themselves*, genetic counselling should never be directive. Nevertheless, because Duchenne muscular dystrophy is such a serious and distressing condition, most counsellors may hope that couples at risk will exercise caution.

Timing of counselling – the coping process

For really successful counselling it is essential to recognize the problems of attempting to communicate information of a personal and delicate nature in a situation when the parents may not yet have recovered from the shock of the diagnosis (Buchanan *et al.* 1979). They may well be harbouring feelings of guilt, recrimination, and lowered self-esteem. They may be angry and tense or just numbed by the situation. But all will be under considerable stress. The psychological sequence of events which follow the initial diagnosis is referred to as the *coping process* and is similar in other stressful situations such as bereavement. Thus parents with a child with Duchenne muscular dystrophy have to face two major stressful events – at the time the diagnosis is first made, and later when the affected boy dies. On both these occasions the family will require considerable support from all those concerned – paediatricians, physicians, geneticists, genetic associates, social workers, and nurses. It should also be remembered that the father may be just as affected as the mother, but since most men do not express their emotions readily, this may be underestimated or even go unrecognized.

Five sequential stages have been recognized in the coping process (Falek 1977, 1984):

- Shock and denial
- Anxiety
- Anger and guilt
- Depression
- Psychological homeostasis.

The duration of each stage varies from individual to individual. Very rarely, a parent may never progress beyond the stage of denial, while a few may reach the stage of depression and remain at this stage. The genetic counsellor has to recognize the existence of these stages and to tailor his counselling accordingly. He has to appreciate that the assimilation of information and the process of decision making will be very much influenced by the stage in the coping process that a parent has reached.

At the very beginning, the parent may be unable to accept that the child is affected, and at this stage sympathy and compassion are required until acceptance occurs. Anxiety impairs judgement and reason, and at this stage the counsellor should provide support and encourage the sharing of emotions. Information may have to be repeated on a number of occasions if it is to be fully understood and appreciated. The most difficult stage for the counsellor is when the parent is angry and resentful. Hostility may well be directed towards the counsellor himself. This has to be accepted as being part of the coping process and not taken personally. Gentle persuasion is indicated, although sometimes it may be necessary to withdraw temporarily and make arrangements for a later appointment when the parent's hostility and resentment may have been tempered. At the stage of depression the effects may be such as to necessitate some form of antidepressant therapy but it is probably at this stage that genetic counselling can begin more earnestly. Counselling should not be postponed until homeostasis has been reached, although obviously information will be better received and understood and decisions will be more rational at this last stage.

Genetic counselling is part of the general counselling which parents with an affected child are given, and which calls for special knowledge and skills on the part of the counsellor. These matters are discussed by Freeman and Pearson (1978), Parry (1984), Maguire (1984), and Charash *et al.* (1991) who provide references to the relevant bibliography.

Who should be offered genetic counselling?

Geneticists tend to consider risks greater than one in 10 as being 'high' and less than one in 20 as being 'low'. This is based on early studies which tended to show that, in general, couples are more likely to be deterred from planning a pregnancy when the risk is greater than one in 10, but less so if it is less than one in 20 (e.g. Carter *et al.* 1971; Emery *et al.* 1973b). However, it is difficult to extrapolate from responses to genetic disorders in general to one disease in particular, such as Duchenne muscular dystrophy, because into the equation has to be included the so-called 'burden' of a disorder. By this is meant the psychological, and to a lesser extent the social and economic problems attendant on having a child with a serious genetic disorder. The concept has been discussed in detail by Murphy (1973). In some disorders, such as congenital muscular dystrophy, although the burden is great it is of limited duration and therefore possibly more acceptable than in Duchenne muscular dystrophy where the affected child survives for many years, becoming progressively incapacitated. There is good evidence that couples are often more influenced by the burden of a disease than by the actual risks of recurrence (Carter *et al.* 1971; Leonard *et al.* 1972; Emery *et al.* 1973b; Hsia 1974; Stern and Eldridge 1975). Thus, concern among relatives about the disorder occurring in their children is only partly a reflection of their risk. It is also tempered by their individual views of the 'burden' of the disease.

In part for logistical reasons, it has sometimes been suggested that genetic counselling in Duchenne muscular dystrophy might be restricted to those women whose *a priori* risk is greater than 1 in 10. But this does not seem entirely justified because affected boys have sometimes been born to mothers whose risk had been estimated to be less than 1 in 20 (Hutton and Thompson

1976). There would seem every reason to offer counselling where appropriate to all first and second degree female relatives of affected boys as well as to any other relative who may be anxious. Some centres with considerable experience in the field offer their services to any woman who is concerned about the problem (Thompson 1984) and this would seem entirely commendable.

Effects of genetic counselling

The effects of genetic counselling and prenatal diagnosis in Duchenne muscular dystrophy can be assessed in various ways: in relation to changes in the incidence of the disorder in a community; the reproductive behaviour of those counselled; and the social and psychological effects on the family.

The effects on population incidence have already been discussed (p. 156) where it was concluded that at best this could be reduced to the occurrence of new mutations which in the past represented about a third of cases.

The effects on the reproductive behaviour of individual women who have been counselled have been assessed in several early studies, the results of which are summarized in Table 12.1. The definition of high, moderate, and low risks in each of the studies was similar, and only data on those women who were married and of reproductive age are included. Those who were deterred after counselling either avoided pregnancy altogether, or opted for prenatal diagnosis in any future pregnancy. Precise comparisons are difficult because of differences in the religious, cultural, economic, and educational levels of those counselled as well as presumably differences in the counsellors themselves. Nevertheless, it seems clear that those given a high risk are usually deterred from further pregnancies, unless coupled with prenatal diagnosis. In the study of Zatz (1983) from Brazil, the high proportion of those at low risk who were deterred may reflect the use of the information by women to gain priority help from family planning centres.

Follow-up studies have confirmed that the proportion of affected boys among births to mothers considered to be at high risk is significantly greater than among mothers considered to be at low risk (Hutton and Thompson 1976; Dennis *et al.* 1976).

But all these various studies were carried out before accurate carrier detection and prenatal diagnosis became possible using DNA markers. Now the element of uncertainty has been removed it would be interesting to compare these early findings with further studies to assess the effects of counselling and changes in population incidence of the disorder.

The social and psychological effects of genetic counselling in Duchenne muscular dystrophy are much more difficult to assess. A common complaint from parents is that at the time of diagnosis they were experiencing considerable stress, making it difficult to accept information at all (Buchanan *et al.*

Table 12.1 *The effects of genetic counselling in Duchenne muscular dystrophy on the reproductive behaviour of married women of reproductive age*

Period	High risk		Moderate risk		Low risk		Reference
	Total No.	% deterred	Total No.	% deterred	Total No.	% deterred	
1965–69	40	95	5	80	6	17	Emery *et al.* (1972)
1965–76	25	88	2	–	46	4	Dennis *et al.* (1976)
1965–74	45	82	33	51	29	24	Hutton and Thompson (1976)
1969–82	126	90	19	84	41	61	Zatz (1983)

1979). In one extensive study in the United Kingdom, Firth (1983) reported the results of interviews with 53 families. In only 18 were both parents told of the diagnosis together. Many of the parents who had been alone when told, described how their distress was heightened by having to break the news to their spouse. A third of the parents were not satisfied with the way the information had been conveyed which was often inadequate and with no follow-up. Although conveying information about a diagnosis is only part of counselling, it is an important part. It is difficult to see that if at this stage a good rapport has not been established with a couple, any meaningful dialogue can follow later. On the basis of her findings Firth made several recommendations: parents should be told of the diagnosis as soon as possible, together and in private, and a series of contacts should be planned not only with the paediatrician but with other health care professionals involved with the disease and who can provide long-term support for the family.

Since her report appeared in 1983 there have been changes. More help and guidance is now being given to families, but there is always room, for improvement. Some years ago a Working Party of the National Association for Mental Health concluded:

> . . . telling the parents is only a first step in the continuing management of the handicapped child. It is not an end in itself and unless it leads correctly on to the appropriate involvement of other professional workers it would largely have failed in its primary object of securing for the handicapped child the fullest possible developmental goals and an accepted place in the family.   (Carr and Oppé 1971)

Although these sentiments were expressed in regard to handicap in general, they are also relevant to Duchenne muscular dystrophy. Establishing the diagnosis and proffering genetic counselling should only be the beginning of the health professionals' involvement with the parents and the affected child. Their continuing support may well be required for several years to come.

A very readable series of reviews of the great variety of psychosocial problems associated with Duchenne and other neuromuscular disorders is provided by Charash *et al.* (1991). This and Firth's (1983) report should be carefully considered by anyone becoming involved in counselling families with Duchenne muscular distrophy.

Summary and conclusions

Genetic counselling is essentially a process of communication between the counsellor and those who seek counselling. The information to be communicated concerns firstly, the disease itself, the genetic mechanism which caused it, and the risks of recurrence; and secondly, the options available if the risks are considered unacceptably high. These include contraception, sterilization, prenatal diagnosis, and abortion, each of which may in itself have important psychological sequelae and require counselling. Some couples, for various ethical and other reasons, may be unable to accept these options. This is their prerogative for genetic counselling should not be directive but help couples reach a decision which is the best one for themselves.

It is particularly important to recognize the psychological aspects of genetic counselling and the sequence of events which follow the initial diagnosis and which are referred to as the *coping process*. This involves five sequential stages: shock and denial, anxiety, anger and guilt, depression, and finally, psychological homeostasis. Each stage requires counselling to be tailored accordingly for only in this way will it be at all effective and rational decisions made.

Concern about the disorder occurring in various relatives is tempered by considerations of the 'burden' of the disease as well as the individual's risks, and counselling should be offered to all those female relatives who are anxious about the problem.

The effects of genetic counselling can be assessed in several ways. There are indications that the population incidence is being reduced to the occurrence of new mutations which in the past represented about a third of cases. Studies of the reproductive behaviour of individual women who have been counselled indicate that those at high risk are very largely deterred from pregnancy unless coupled with prenatal diagnosis. Finally, the social and psychological effects of genetic counselling can be assessed, but so far this has received little attention in the case of Duchenne muscular dystrophy. Indications are that at least in the United Kingdom, there is often some dissatisfaction with the way in which the diagnosis is first made and lack of subsequent follow-up. There is a real need to ensure that parents are told accurately and compassionately as soon as possible. Thereafter a series of contacts can be offered and planned with various health care professionals involved with the disease. The latter can then provide, if need be, long-term support for the family as a whole.

13 Management

With the identification and charaterization of the defective protein in Duchenne and Becker muscular dystrophies, prospects for a rational therapy at last became a reality. But quite apart from such considerations, a great deal can also be done to improve the quality of life of affected boys. This involves maintaining their general well-being, preserving respiratory function, and preventing the development of deformities. Because of its unrelenting course, in the past there was a tendency among health care professionals to take a rather indifferent attitude to management. This view is no longer justified, however, as a great deal can be achieved by taking a positive approach, largely pioneered by Vignos in Cleveland, and Siegel in Chicago, which has now been adopted by most centres throughout the world. Much has been written on the subject and there are several helpful and detailed reviews (Walton 1969; Siegel 1977a, 1978; Bossingham et al. 1977; Rideau 1979; Vignos 1979; Dubowitz and Heckmatt 1980), as well as in the recent French publication *Cahiers de kinesitherapie* (part 155, No 3, 1992). Gardner-Medwin (1992) has written a particularly valuable lay guide to management for parents.

General management

Whatever stage the disease has reached there are certain general principles to be considered. It would seem hardly necessary to emphasize the need to maintain good health in general. There is no evidence that 'megavitamin therapy' is of any value in the disease, and in any event it may have serious side-effects (Evans and Lacey 1986), and could actually be harmful. Adequate intake of dietary fibre is important because of frequent problems with constipation. Excess weight gain should be avoided since it will overburden the already compromised musculature, and also add to the problems of lifting and carrying the patient when he is no longer able to walk. Griffiths and Edwards (1988) have published a chart which allows the ideal weight for a boy with Duchenne dystrophy to be determined. These authors have also produced a helpful leaflet on weight control in dystrophy for the Muscular Dystrophy Group of Great Britain. Oral hygiene is also essential.

In the early stages of the disease, and up to the time walking becomes difficult, parents should be encouraged to let their son lead as normal a life as possible. Prolonged bed rest for any intercurrent infection should be avoided, particularly after early childhood when it can precipitate loss of

Table 13.1 *Physical management in Duchenne muscular dystrophy*

---

1. *Promotion of ambulation*
   Weight control
   Exercise: active/passive
   Tenotomies
   Orthoses
2. *Prevention of deformities*
   Posture/support/orthoses
   Passive exercise/stretching
   Surgery
3. *Preservation of respiratory function*

---

ambulation. Some of the more important aspects of physical management are summarized in Table 13.1.

Active exercise

A question often asked is whether the parents should encourage active exercise in the belief that this might improve muscle strength or perhaps help preserve what strength remains. Muscle exercise has complex physiological and structural effects which vary from person to person, and in different forms of physical handicap.

Early studies of the possible beneficial effects of exercise in Duchenne muscular dystrophy are difficult to interpret for various methodological reason. However, in a study of the effects of a one year programme of active exercise against weight resistance in 14 affected boys (Vignos and Watkins 1966) some improvement in muscle strength at the beginning was noted, but this eventually levelled off. Any apparent beneficial effect was more marked in the less severely affected boys. An important general point emerges from this study. An apparent improvement is often detected at the beginning of such studies as the patients learn and become familiar with the methods involved. This we observed (Emery *et al.* 1982) in a double-blind study of a calcium blocker in Duchenne muscular dystrophy (Fig. 13.1), which incidentally was not recommended for treatment.

In another more recent study of 18 affected boys who were all still ambulant, there appeared to be no significant effect of resisted exercise on muscle strength (Dubowitz *et al.* 1984). However, the study period was only 6 months, and it would be valuable to know if a prolonged programme of resisted exercise would eventually have a beneficial effect on muscle strength.

Quite apart from any possible improvement in strength, such a regime has a beneficial psychological effect. Certainly these studies showed that active forms of exercise are not deleterious. However, such a regime requires a

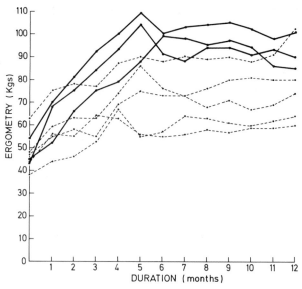

Fig. 13.1 Results of ergometry in patients taking a placebo (---), and those taking the active drug (−). Note the apparent increase in strength in all boys at the beginning as a result of 'training'.

considerable commitment in time since patients and their families may have to attend a special centre where such exercises can be performed, although, Scott *et al.* (1981) have shown that parents rapidly become competent to give such treatment at home.

Although it is not yet clear whether moderate exercise can actually increase muscle strength, an overly aggressive approach to physical activity could well be counterproductive and possibly aggravate the cardiomyopathy which is a concomitant of the disease (p. 109). In any event as Vignos (1979) has stated '. . . Activities involving recreational sports are generally more likely to win long-term adherence'. Swimming is particularly valuable as the buoyancy of the water makes exercises easier to perform. Cycling can also be beneficial although quite early on boys with Duchenne muscular dystrophy often find this difficult. The best advice would be to encourage normal physical activities as far as they are possible.

Passive exercise and physiotherapy

There seems little doubt that passive, stretching exercises can be valuable in preventing or at least delaying the development of muscle contractures, which are especially likely to develop once the child becomes chairbound. Such exercises include stretching of the Achilles tendon and the knee, hip, shoulder, elbow, and wrist joints. Sylvia Hyde (1984) has produced a helpful guide to such exercises for parents to use in the home, though it is advisable to have a professional physiotherapist explain and demonstrate the procedures at the beginning (Fig. 13.2). The emphasis is on firmness and kindness and the aim is to prevent contractures developing. Once they have developed then such passive stretching exercises are ineffective and the use of force can cause serious trauma. There is no doubt that a routine of passive exercises each day say after a nightly bath, will help prevent contractures. However, it is difficult and time consuming, but on the other hand it offers one of the few opportunities where parents can feel involved in doing something for their son.

Coupled with such exercises, the parents can also encourage deep breathing exercises and later postural drainage and assisted coughing. This will be discussed in more detail later (p. 275).

There are those who propose the use of night splints in order to help prevent the development of contractures of the ankle and knee joints. But while a boy is still ambulant it is doubtful if such measures have any real value, and in any event many children find them uncomfortable and, in our experience, compliance is not high.

Because of the growing awareness of the importance of physiotherapy in muscular dystrophy, an International Congress on the subject was held in

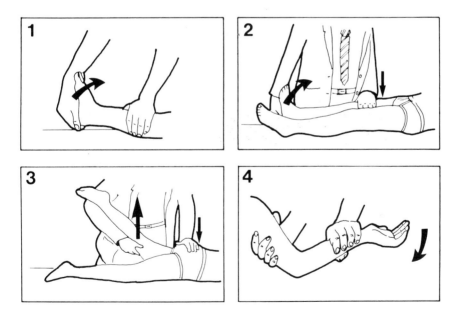

Fig. 13.2 Some of the passive stretching exercises to prevent contractures of the (1) tendo Achilles, and (2) knee, (3) hip, and (4) elbow joints. (After Hyde (1984) with permission.)

Italy in 1984, the Proceedings of which have now been published in detail (*Cardiomyology* Vol 3, nos 2–3, 1984) where the reader will find helpful information including some useful guidelines proposed by the European Alliance of Muscular Dystrophy Associations.

Finally, it should be mentioned that in the early stages of the disease there is no place for Achilles tenotomy. Later, when the boy is chairbound, tenotomy and the wearing of light-weight below knee orthoses and normal shoes helps maintain the feet in a satisfactory position, makes dressing easier, and although purely cosmetic, many find it worthwhile (Gardner-Medwin, 1992).

Chronic low frequency electrical stimulation

The possibility that chronic low frequency electrical stimulation might improve muscle strength has been studied (Scott *et al.* 1990; Zupan 1992) but the results have not been very encouraging. On present evidence the value of this technique in Duchenne muscular dystrophy is still not proven.

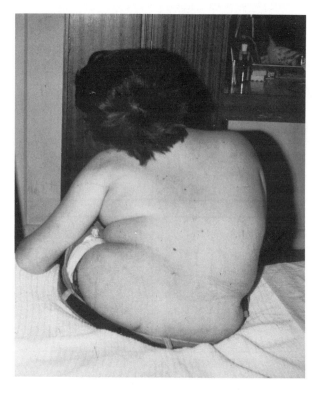

Fig. 13.3 Untreated scoliosis.

Scoliosis

Once an affected boy has lost the ability to walk, joint scoliosis soon follow. Although contractures are not a seri development does limit whatever limb movement remains and can ... dressing difficult. Scoliosis on the other hand is a serious complication (James *et al.* 1976). Sitting becomes difficult and uncomfortable but more importantly, the progressive thoracic deformity restricts adequate pulmonary ventilation and aggravates respiratory problems resulting from weakness of the intercostal muscles. Respiratory impairment becomes a major threat to life (p. 276) and increases once the child is chairbound (Fig. 13.3). It should be noted however that not all boys develop scoliosis. A small proportion develop hyperlordosis and a very few retain more or less normal spinal curvatures. On the other hand around 25 per cent of boys with scoliosis develop their spinal curvature *before* cessation of ambulation (Lord *et al.* 1990).

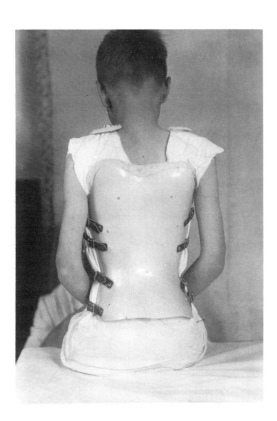

Fig. 13.4 Moulded and fitted back support.

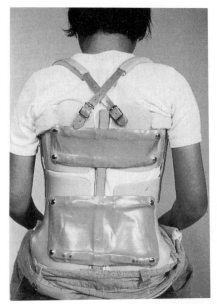
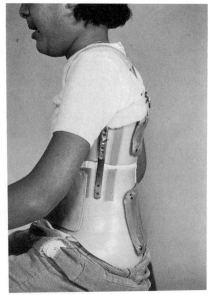
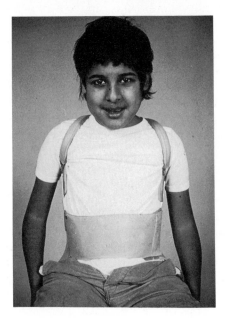

Fig. 13.5 Fitted spinal brace. (Reproduced by kind permission of Dr G. M. Cochrane and the Mary Marlborough Lodge.)

There are several ways in which the development of scoliosis can be limited: the adoption of a correct sitting posture; the fitting of an orthosis; prolongation of ambulation; and surgical intervention. From early on, even before ambulation is lost, it is important to emphasize a habit of adopting a correct sitting position. Once confined to a wheelchair this becomes especially important. A firm back support and special seating (for example, the Toronto seat) will help (Moseley 1984), but such measures on their own are likely to have only a limited effect. Individually designed body jackets or braces (Figs 13.4 and 13.5) fitted when a boy first becomes confined to a wheelchair and before the onset of scoliosis may be more helpful (Miller and Dunn 1982; Shapira and Bresnan 1982; Falewski de Leon 1984; Seeger *et al*.1984; Young *et al*. 1984). Such measures, however, although they may possibly impede the development of scoliosis, cannot prevent it (Robin 1976; Moseley 1984; Rideau *et al*. 1984; Rideau 1986; Seeger *et al*. 1984), and are not practical once it has progressed beyond about 40 degrees from the vertical.

The only real solution is to prolong ambulation or resort to surgery.

Prolongation of ambulation

There is no doubt that the development of contractures and spinal deformities is impeded by prolonging ambulation beyond the stage when this is normally lost (Swinyard grade 5: Vignos grade 7 — see Appendices C and D). This can be achieved by the application of light plastic or polypropylene long-leg fitted orthoses with an ischial supporting lip. This approach to management was first introduced by Vignos and Siegel in the 1960s (Spencer and Vignos 1962; Vignos *et al*. 1963; Siegel *et al*. 1968). If an equino varus deformity is already present, an Achilles tenotomy may be necessary in order to fit the orthoses. This can be performed percutaneously (Granata *et al*. 1984; Heckmatt *et al*. 1985), although others prefer open operation (Williams *et al*. 1984). Boys not requiring tenotomy at first and walking regularly in their orthoses may subsequently have problems with Achilles tendon tightening and require a tenotomy later. It may also be necessary for tenotomy of the hip flexors and tensor fascia lata (Siegel 1980; Rideau *et al*. 1983*a*). This can be combined with Achilles tenotomy in the one operation, which is relatively quick, requires brief anaesthesia, and entails minimal blood loss. If operation is necessary, long-leg plasters are fitted while the patient is under anaesthesia. A few days later these are replaced by fitted orthoses which are then regularly adjusted as the boy grows. The orthoses should have a knee-flexion device which permits sitting and also gives stability to the knee joint (Allard *et al*. 1981). Such orthoses can be worn with everyday shoes and beneath trousers (Fig. 13.6).

In a study of 57 affected boys (Heckmatt *et al*. 1985), all but 10 achieved useful independent walking by these measures. Among these 10, seven had

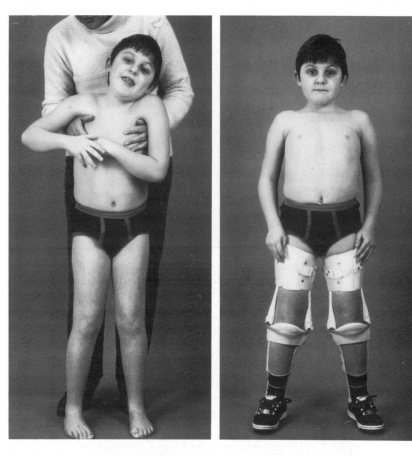

Fig. 13.6 Before (*left*), and after (*right*) fitting of long-leg orthoses to prolong ambulation. (Reproduced by kind permission of Professor V. Dubowitz.)

problems because of delays in providing their orthoses and as a result had to spend several months in plaster, one had severe asymmetrical hip and knee contractures, another lost confidence following a fall at home, and one regained the ability to walk independently without orthoses following tenotomy. It would therefore seem that provided orthoses are available at the time of operation, most boys will do well and retain the ability to walk. These measures prolong walking by about two years on average, but in some cases as long as five years (Heckmatt *et al.* 1985). However, success depends on several factors, and is most likely in those boys who are not obese or mentally handicapped, have good motivation, and where there is parental compliance. Timing is also particularly important. It should be commenced at the time ambulation is just beginning to be a serious problem. Once a child has been confined to a wheelchair for only a few months, rehabilitation becomes difficult, partly because of the severe loss of power, but also because marked contractures soon develop.

The application of orthoses does *not* accelerate the deterioration in muscle power, and in fact there may be a slight increase for a time (Hyde *et al.* 1982). The advantages include continued independence, easier management by the parents, slowing the development of contractures and spinal deformity, and psychological benefits. However, although there appear to be many benefits in such a regime, there is no evidence as yet that it prolongs life but some data from Western Australia indicate that this might be so (Miller and Dunn 1982).

Standing frames

In the last few years there has been much discussion of the value of standing frames/tilt tables. These are devices which allow a boy, who can no longer

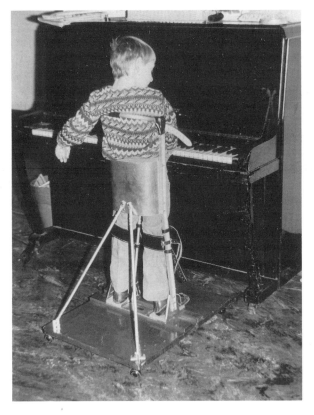

Fig. 13.7 A simple standing frame. (Reproduced by kind permission of Dr G. M. Cochrane and the Mary Marlborough Lodge.)

stand unaided, to achieve and maintain an upright position (Fig. 13.7). Modified wheelchairs have also been designed for the same purpose. The place of such equipment would be after a year or two in walking orthoses and the maintenance of an upright position after this stage could be both physiologically and psychologically beneficial. However, these aids in general have limited manoeuverability and are expensive. They seem likely to find use in adults with more slowly progressive forms of muscular dystrophy.

Swivel walkers

An extension of the standing frame is the swivel walker whereby the patient, while being maintained in an upright position, can progress forward by swinging forward the hips. But the main problem is stability which requires some careful engineering. Nevertheless, swivel walkers offer a dynamic alternative to standing frames.

Aids for the disabled

There are many commercially available aids for the disabled. In the United Kingdom much useful information has been compiled by the Mary Marlborough Lodge in Oxford. For example, *Walking aids* (Cochrane and Wilson 1991), *Hoists and lifts* (Cochrane and Wilson 1990), *Personal care* [Cochrane 1990*a*) and *Communication* (Cochrane 1990*b*).

Wheelchair-mounted robots manipulators are now also becoming available for boys with Duchenne muscular dystrophy. Control panels are suitably modified for the needs of a boy who is severely handicapped, with perhaps little more than residual finger movements, and in this way allow many activities of everyday living which would otherwise be impossible (Bach *et al.* 1990). They are, of course, expensive but the modification of commercially available equipment may well make them more freely available in future.

Surgery

Surgical correction of scoliosis using Harrington rods (Aprin *et al.* 1982) has the disadvantages of frequent post-operative pulmonary and other complications, and necessitates immobilization in a cast or brace for some time post-operatively. This approach has now been superseded by the Luque operation in which internal fixation is achieved by each vertebra being individually wired to two stainless steel rods (Luque 1982; Drennan 1984). The rigid stabilization obtained with this technique eliminates the need for postoperative immobilization and therefore reduces the loss of strength and

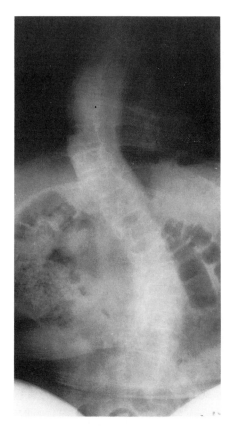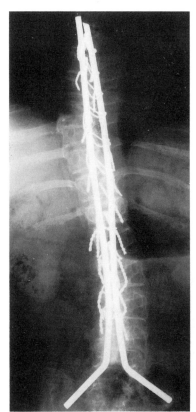

Fig. 13.8 Chest X-rays before (*left*), and (*right*) after surgical correction of scoliosis by the Luque operation. (Reproduced by kind permission of Mr G. R. Houghton.)

function which follows such immobilization. Postoperative complications are also less (Fig. 13.8).

Some have recommended the operation as a prophylactic measure before the development of scoliosis (Rideau *et al.* 1984), whereas others offer the operation only when scoliosis is approaching 30 degrees (Moseley 1984; Sussman 1984, 1985). The most important points when considering surgery are that spinal deformity is limited and that respiratory function is good. Surgery is indicated when the curve is less than 50 degrees and the forced vital capacity (FVC) is greater than 50 per cent of the expected value, and according to Sussman (1985):

... There is a 'window' of time between the point when the curve develops, but prior to a decrease in FVC below 50 per cent, during which the spinal surgery should be performed. If a patient is treated with an orthosis the 'window' will be narrowed, since the progression of the scoliosis will be temporarily slowed while pulmonary function continues to deteriorate.

Because of the resultant spinal rigidity and limited spinal movement, boys treated in this way often have to acquire new trick movements for everyday living, and may need more frequent turning in bed at night. However, boys with stable spines as a result of surgery can be confident that spinal deformity will not increase and often have an enhanced quality of life during the teenage period (Sussman 1984).

A careful follow-up study of the effects of spinal stabilization in Duchenne muscular dystrophy has recently been published (Galasko *et al.* 1992). Of 55 patients selected for surgery, 32 accepted and 23 refused. Both groups were then followed-up over a period of several years. In the non-operated group vital capacity deteriorated by a mean of 8 per cent per annum, whereas in the operated group it remained static for 3 years and thereafter diminished slightly. After 5 years there was a highly significant difference in survival in the two groups (over 70 per cent in the treated com-

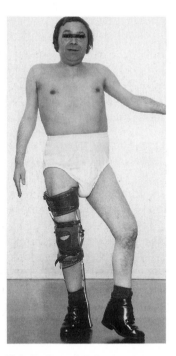
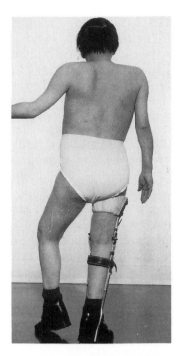

Fig. 13.9 Patient with Becker muscular dystrophy who, despite marked weakness of proximal lower limb girdle musculature, is sufficiently ambulant as a result of surgery and orthoses as to be gainfully employed.

pared with under 20 per cent in the untreated). Unfortunately not all have reported such success after spinal surgery (Shapiro *et al.* 1992).

In the more benign forms of muccular dystrophy there is no doubt that many years of useful and productive life are possible after various surgical procedures (tendon lengthening, arthrodeses, etc.) and with appropriate orthoses (Fig. 13.9).

An informative report, *Surgical treatment of spinal deformaties in neuromuscular diseases*, has been published by the European Alliance of Muscular Dystrophy Associations (EAMDA) in 1990, copies of which are available (*see* Appendix H, EAMDA, The Netherlands).

Surgical–anaesthetic risks

Many children with Duchenne muscular dystrophy tolerate surgery and general anaesthesia well, but there are recognized dangers. During anaesthesia sinus tachycardia, atrial and ventricular fibrillation, and cardiac arrest may occur, even in very young boys aged 3–5 in whom there is no evidence pre-operatively of cardiomyopathy (Seay *et al.* 1978; Boltshauser *et al.* 1980) or even before the diagnosis of Duchenne dystrophy has actually been made (Larsen *et al.* 1989).

Postoperatively other complications may occur, including gastric dilatation and myoglobinuria (rhabdomyolysis). Myoglobinuria does not normally occur in Duchenne muscular dystrophy (p. 142). However, it is frequently found postoperatively (Table 13.2), and reflects enhanced muscle breakdown. Some patients with myoglobinuria postoperatively have been noted subsequently to be somewhat weaker. In one case (Boltshauser *et al.* 1980) SCK levels were repeatedly normal for 8–12 days after operation, and the authors suggested that this might have been due to a temporary depletion of muscle enzyme as a result of excessive 'leakage' during the acute stage of rhabdomyolysis. An important danger with acute rhabdomyolysis and myoglobinuria is the possible development of renal impairment and even acute renal failure postoperatively (McKishnie *et al.* 1983).

The myoglobinuria (and myoglobinaemia) is probably a direct effect of the anaesthetic agents. In most, but not all reported cases (Table 13.2), succinylcholine has been used. Succinylcholine is known to occasionally cause myoglobinuria in normal children (Ellis and Heffron 1985), and the apparent increased incidence of myoglobinuria in patients with Duchenne muscular dystrophy is probably related to the pathophysiology of the disease. Unfortunately there do not appear to be any factors which pre-operatively identify patients likely to develop anaesthesia-related problems (Sethna *et al.* 1988). Certainly succinylcholine should be avoided and some other non-depolarizing neuromuscular blocking agent used instead (Buzello and Huttarsch 1988).

Table 13.2 *Occurrence of myoglobinuria (rhabdomyolysis) postoperatively in patients with Duchenne muscular dystrophy*

Age	Surgical procedure	Anaesthetic agents	Reference
NR	Adenoidectomy	Succinylcholine, halothane	Watters *et al.* (1977)
NR	Adenoidectomy	Succinylcholine, halothane	Watters *et al.* (1977)
NR	Strabismus correction	Succinylcholine, halothane	Watters *et al.* (1977)
4 yrs	Calcaneal osteotomy	Succinylcholine, N_2O, halothane	Miller *et al.* (1978)
3 yrs	Tonsillectomy	Succinylcholine, nembutal, cyclopropane	Seay *et al.* (1978)
4 yrs	Tonsillectomy	Succinylcholine, nembutal, N_2O, halothane	Seay *et al.* (1978)
5 yrs	Adenoidectomy	Succinylcholine, N_2O, halothane	Boltshauser *et al.* (1980)
21 mths	Ankyloglossia	Succinylcholine, N_2O, halothane	Oka *et al.* (1982)
5 yrs	Dental extraction	Succinylcholine, N_2O, halothane	Brownell *et al.* (1983)
3 yrs	Orchidopexy	Succinylcholine, N_2O, halothane	McKishnie *et al.* (1983)
4 yrs	Muscle biopsy	Protoxide/halothane	Fiacchino *et al.* (1984)
8 yrs	Orchidopexy	N_2O/isoflurane	Chalkiadis and Branch (1990)
7 yrs	Dental	N_2O/halothane	Bush and Dubowitz (1991)

NR, not recorded.

Much has been made of the possible dangers of malignant hyperpyrexia in Duchenne muscular dystrophy (Siegel 1978). However, there are problems in defining this condition purely on the basis of clinical features. Evidence of a possible association with Duchenne muscular dystrophy has been critically reviewed by Willner *et al.* (1984) and by Ellis and Heffron (1985) who conclude that any association is far from proved. Ellis states (F. R. Ellis, personal communication, 1985) that the diagnosis has never been convincingly established on the basis of the now accepted *in vitro* tests in any case of Duchenne muscular dystrophy excepting perhaps the case reported by Brownell *et al.* (1983).

Finally, hyperkalaemia may result from increased muscle breakdown, and succinylcholine and other depolarizing agents are inadvisable due to their intrinsic ability to further raise the serum level of potassium (Ellis 1981).

Respiratory problems are also likely *postoperatively*, especially in boys whose respiratory function is already reduced (Smith and Bush 1985). Retention of bronchial secretions, resulting from weakness of the respiratory muscles and associated weak cough, may lead to pneumonitis. Drugs likely to exaggerate respiratory depression, such as barbiturates, have therefore to be used with caution, and postoperative respiratory care and appropriate physiotherapy are essential.

Most of the operative and postoperative problems described in Duchenne muscular dystrophy have been based on case reports and are therefore somewhat selective. In the majority of patients there are no serious anaesthetic problems (Richards 1972), and in a series of patients undergoing major surgery for the correction of thoracic deformities, most responded favourably. There were no cases of hyperpyrexia, hyperkalaemia, or rhabdomyolysis, but succinylcholine was avoided (Milne and Rosales 1982). It is obviously important that the surgeon and anaesthetist appreciate the problems which can occur and be adequately prepared to deal with them should they arise.

Fractures

Fractures occur not infrequently, usually as a result of falls sustained while the boy is still walking but unsteadily, or due to various accidents later on in the course of the disease when the long bones undergo rarefaction as a result of disuse (p. 120). In the first group immobilization may well result in loss of ambulation, and for this reason fractures should be treated with minimal splintage so as to encourage activity and continued independent mobility. Fractures heal normally and the special orthopaedic problems of fractures of the long bones in Duchenne muscular dystrophy have been reviewed in detail (Siegel 1977*b*; Hsu 1979).

Respiratory problems

Impaired pulmonary function is the major factor in morbidity and mortality in Duchenne muscular dystrophy. Over 90 per cent of deaths result from pulmonary infection and respiratory failure (Vignos 1977*b*). Preservation of respiratory function and adequate treatment of respiratory infections are therefore essential elements of patient management.

At the simplest level parents and relatives should be dissuaded from smoking in the same rooms used by the affected boy. Many advocate vaccination against influenza at the beginning of the winter months although the value, even in healthy individuals, is not certain. The adoption of a correct sitting position should be encouraged. Well-designed respiratory exercises are valuable in helping to maintain good pulmonary function (Di Marco *et al.* 1985). However, these measures alone will not prevent the progressive decrease in pulmonary function. It is doubtful if prophylactic antibiotics have any significant effect and are best reserved for use in treating respiratory infections as they occur.

Regular pulmonary function tests, the simplest being the assessment of vital capacity using a spirometer (Macklem 1986), will indicate the development of significant impairment even before problems arise, and can be a good prognostic indicator (Inkley *et al.* 1974; Vignos 1977*b*; Rideau 1979; Ortaggio *et al.* 1984). Deterioration begins around the time the boy becomes confined to a wheelchair, and measures of pulmonary function (vital capacity, maximum inspiratory and expiratory pressures), instead of increasing with age as they do normally, remain more or less the same for some time and then in the later stages actually decrease. Differences between predicted and observed values therefore become more marked as the disease progresses. However, only in the very late stages does actual respiratory failure occur with changes in blood gases.

Attempts to impede the development of scoliosis have already been discussed, and will certainly have a beneficial effect on respiratory function. Parents can also be instructed in breathing exercises, postural drainage, percussion, and even pharyngeal suction. A 10 minute programme of breathing exercises should become a part of the daily routine, but respiratory muscle training *per se* seems to have little effect on respiratory function (Martin *et al.* 1986).

Any chest infection must be treated vigorously with antibiotics and physiotherapy. If there is any suggestion that respiratory function is already impaired, then hospitalization is indicated. Since deaths from respiratory problems usually occur only in the most advanced stages and not in those less severely affected, Vignos (1977*b*) recommends that physicians should be encouraged to attempt energetic treatment of all patients who are at a grade less than Vignos 9.

Practical considerations in the respiratory care of patients with Duchenne muscular dystrophy have recently been reviewed in considerable detail by Smith *et al.* (1987) who provide an extensive and helpful bibliography an the subject.

Assisted ventilation

As we have seen, impaired respiratory function is the main cause of death in Duchenne muscular dystrophy. Respiratory failure may be sudden, often precipitated by a respiratory infection in a boy whose pulmonary function is already impaired. This poses two questions. Firstly, how can such impairment be detected before serious problems arise? Secondly, what can be done to alleviate this impairment?

Once a boy has become chairbound, or even earlier, there is a strong argument for periodically reviewing his condition. Since respiratory insufficiency is first reflected in nocturnal hypoxia, suggestive symptoms of this should be specifically sought for since they may be overlooked (Smith *et al.* 1989*a*). These include restless sleep, nightmares, morning confusion, headache, and hypersomnolence during the day. Later clear signs of impaired pulmonary function become evident including breathlessness and difficulty with speaking. Sleep hypoventilation can be confirmed by overnight oximetry, and impaired pulmonary function by determining the vital capacity and comparing the result with normal values for boys of the same age.

The use of drugs, such as protriptyline, to reduce sleep hypoxia are not helpful because of their anticholinergic side-effects and possible hazards in patients with an incipient cardiomyopathy (Smith *et al.* 1989*b*, 1991).

At present the only way of alleviating impaired respiratory function is by *assisted ventilation* using some form of portable ventilator. This involves either intermittent positive pressure with a nasal tube, mouth adaptor, or facial mask, or the use of a body shell or cuirass. The nasal tube seems to be preferred by most boys (Heckmatt *et al.* 1990). At first this is only necessary at night and can transform a boy's life. But unfortunately pulmonary function often continues to deteriorate, necessitating longer periods of ventilation and eventually, after a few years, a trachestomy may have to be considered (Baydur *et al.* 1990; Mohr and Hill 1990). But this then raises serious problems of maintenance and nursing care. Nevertheless, in recent times many boy's in their twenties and even thirties are now being managed in this way. After all, is this any different from individuals with a high cervical lesion consequent on an accident who, if they survive, have to be managed in this way? A valuable and informative discussion document, *Respiratory insufficiency in neuromuscular disorders*, was published in 1990 by EADMA (The Netherlands), copies of which are available (see Appendix H for the address). The topic has also been the subject of a recent international conference (Make 1991) and so there is clearly much interest in this matter.

Cardiac problems

In less than 10 per cent of patients death occurs suddenly, presumably as a consequence of the associated cardiomyopathy. Long-term prophylactic treatment with cardiac glycosides (digitoxin) although once considered efficacious, has since been shown to have no therapeutic value (Fowler *et al* 1965). Verapamil is often used to control a variety of arrhythmias in otherwise normal individuals but is contra-indicated in Duchenne muscular dystrophy because it may precipitate respiratory failure (Zalman *et al.* 1983), and heart block (Emery and Skinner 1983).

nce from several sources of left ventricular
ly leads to symptoms *per se*. On the other
ction, as a result of anoxia and pulmonary
rbidity and mortality (Ishihara *et al.*, 1991)
on of hypoxaemia (Yotsukura *et al.* 1988). In
ardiac involvement may require conventional
liuretics with some indications that this may
1990*b*).

Psychological problems

Most boys give every impression of being well adapted and of having come to terms with their disability. In fact one expert has said:

... it is worthwhile to emphasise that the Duchenne muscular dystrophy patient, after some initial frustration, is really not suffering, has above all no pain, and is on the contrary often quite content or at least acceptingly resigned after he becomes wheelchair-bound.   (Zellweger 1975)

It would, however, be entirely wrong to assume that affected boys are emotionally and psychologically unscathed by their disease. In reviewing the rather scant older literature, as well as the results of her own studies, Staples (1977) concluded that emotional problems do occur and that, not unexpectedly, affected boys tend to be more introverted than normal children. In-depth assessment, however, may require some very careful and direct questioning in order to elicit feelings on matters such as isolation, dependency, lack of privacy, and sexual needs (Taft 1973). Two more recent studies have looked at these matters in some detail (Buchanan *et al.* 1979; Pullen 1984).

The emotional reaction of a boy to his disease varies from individual to individual and from family to family. Paramount may be a feeling of isolation because of his physical disability and perhaps also intellectual impairment. Recognition that his peers are physically and perhaps sometimes intellectually superior may well lead to withdrawal and depression. As the disease advances his dependency on others, and lack of personal privacy will cause more stress. A proportion may feel physically unattractive. Although some apparently deny that their inability to find sexual satisfaction is a cause of distress (Morgan 1975), others no doubt do, particularly because their physical disability may preclude any relief they might obtain from masturbation. Later, they have to face the imminence of premature death. According to Staples (1977) many accept the concept of premature death without disquiet. However, some develop a major depressive disorder (Fitzpatrick *et al.*

1986) or serious behavioural problems as a reaction to their illness (Buchanan *et al*. 1979). The more emotionally disturbed tend to come from families with marked conflicts and the behaviour of the parents and normal sibs will influence that of the affected boy. An interesting 'family drawing test' may be useful in evaluating interpersonal relationships within the family of an affected boy (Siegel and Kornfeld 1980). The problems are made worse if he is ill-informed about the disease. He is more likely to be emotionally stable and better adapted to his problems if the home environment is stable, there is marital harmony, and the parents are perceived as being close to each other, and there are open and frequent discussions about his problems with a frank expression of feelings. All too often there is little communication within families about the disorder (Fitzpatrick and Barry 1986).

The parents also have to face a great many problems, and again frank discussions between themselves as well as with health professionals can only be beneficial. Quite apart from the emotional problems associated with coping (p. 254), there are others of a more social nature which will also produce psychological reactions. Physical handicap, especially when associated with mental handicap, may be viewed as a social stigma and source of embarrassment. As the physical incapacity increases, there will be a restriction on the family's freedom and activities. The parents might find little time or opportunity to be together or to have a holiday. The husband may feel neglected or rejected because of the mother's necessary involvement with their affected son. Coupled with the fear of also having another affected child, serious psychosexual problems may arise. In one survey of 25 families (Buchanan *et al*. 1979), over half had serious marital problems and a quarter had become divorced. On the other hand, in some families the affected child has the effect of actually bringing the parents closer together.

Finally, unaffected sibs are not excluded from the emotional problems which may arise within the family. Overprotection and pampering of an affected boy may result in jealousy and resentment among sibs. Older sisters may adopt a maternal or protective role, yet at the same time harbour increasing concern about their possibly having an affected son.

Pullen (1984) recognizes seven stages in the evolution of a genetic disease within a family, each being associated with different emotional and psychological responses in different members of the family:

   (*i*) Positive family history
  (*ii*) Abnormality noticed by parents
 (*iii*) Abnormality confirmed by family practitioner
  (*iv*) Diagnosis first made/coping process begins
   (*v*) Resolution/adaptation
  (*vi*) Chronic handicap/progression
 (*vii*) Death/grieving

At stage (*i*) (when there is a family history of Duchenne muscular dystrophy), those who see themselves as being at risk of having an affected son are likely to be anxious and concerned. With new improved methods of carrier detection in some cases reassurance is now possible. Otherwise the medical and genetic aspects of the problem will need to be discussed in detail, perhaps on several occasions, until an acceptable course of action is reached. All-too-often there is a considerable delay between when the parents first noticed that something appeared to be wrong with their son and this is agreed by the family practitioner and then the diagnosis is established. Most couples interviewed find this period of uncertainty one of the most trying and unsettling (Firth 1983). Increased awareness by family practitioners of the possibility of muscular dystrophy should help reduce this problem in future. Stage (*iv*) involves the emotional reaction to the diagnosis and the beginning of the coping process (p. 254). Stages (*v*) and (*vi*) involve the reactions of the patient and his parents and sibs to the disease. Parents must be encouraged to take time off and have regular times set aside for themselves. Organizations, such as the Muscular Dystrophy Group in Britain, through local set-ups, can provide support and advice and help to reduce feelings of isolation. Open and frank discussions between all members of the family should be encouraged, including the affected boy himself. As Pullen, a psychiatrist experienced in this field, has stated

> . . . The physically handicapped child must be allowed to talk about his frustrations, disappointments, depression and anxieties for the future. Many people, including parents, do not allow the child to talk about these areas for fear of putting ideas into his head. The ideas certainly are there already but most children are denied the opportunity of communicating them to others. This may make them feel more isolated and abnormal because it prevents others from empathizing accurately with their position.
> (Pullen, 1984 p. 122)

About a third of parents we have interviewed had great difficulty in talking to each other about the disease.

Finally, at stage (*vii*) parents again should be encouraged to talk honestly
a   eir distress, despair, and perhaps anger.
T   uscular dystrophy are discussed in detail
i   ounselling should not end with the death
o   able to close relatives until grieving has
p   of loss and the attendant grief will ever
c   however, there is often a sense of relief
a   oncern. This is natural and not a reason
f

Educational and social needs

The first question to be answered is whether an affected boy may require special schooling? In a few cases associated with severe mental handicap this may be indicated when the parents find management difficult. In most cases, however, boys can derive considerable benefit by attending a normal school where the teachers can be very helpful once the problem has been explained. Cohen (1977) has listed many of the problems which may affect a boy's educational ability: progressive motor difficulties make acquisition of new skills more difficult; frequent absence from school often occurs with declining physical condition; and affected boys tire easily and may lack initiative and motivation.

Attention should focus on a boy's positive abilities. A proportion will be academically orientated. But their physical incapacity by the time they reach senior school can present a serious problem, and further education and employment prospects are severely limited. In Britain the Open University Courses on television have been a boon to many highly intelligent boys. But others will be more artistically inclined. Over the years I have made a collection of drawings and paintings by my patients, and their skill and ability is frequently a source of admiration.

As the disease progresses and boys become confined to a wheelchair, day schools which cater specially for the physically handicapped can be an attractive proposition. In such an environment they will feel less isolated and more able to share feelings and emotions with fellow sufferers. Most parents prefer to have their child in a day school with other handicapped children rather than in an institution away from home (Zellweger 1975).

At home consideration should be given to the time when he will be unable to walk unaided and appropriate plans made. Ramps to take a wheelchair may be required. A ground floor bedroom/study is ideal, with TV, hi-fi, and other devices of his choosing. In this way he will have a place which he can consider his private sanctum to entertain friends and be on his own if he chooses.

There are a vast array of aids, including wheelchairs, available for the physically handicapped. In Britain some of these can be obtained through the National Health Service at no cost to the family. It would not be appropriate to deal with these matters here. However, there are several publications which are of considerable practical value and provide information not only on aids but also addresses of where to seek help and advice:

With a little help by Philippa Harpin. A series of detailed guides concerned with such matters as clothing, home adaptations, wheelchairs, etc. Addresses of suppliers and helpful organizations are included. Published by the Muscular Dystrophy Group of Great Britain, 7–11 Prescott Place, London SW4 6BS.

The muscular dystrophy handbook. This includes useful information about professional services (including education, leisure, holidays, transport, etc.). Published by the Muscular Dystrophy Group of Great Britain.

Sign post. A directory of where to go for help, advice and information, and *Powered wheelchairs*, a buyer's guide. Published by the Research Institute for Consumer Affairs, 14 Buckingham Street, London WC2N 6DS.

The disability information trust, published a number of booklets on various aids for the handicapped (p. 270), obtainable from Marlborough Lodge, Nuffield Orthopaedic Centre, Oxford OX3 7LD.

Drug therapy

The assessment of the possible therapeutic benefits of a drug in Duchenne muscular dystrophy presents a number of problems. Which have to be considered. Very few drug trials in the past have been properly designed.

Early drug trials

Over the last 50 years there have been many drug trials in Duchenne muscular dystrophy. Some of the drugs which have been tried and the basis for their use are summarized in Table 13.3. Many of the early studies were ill designed and often an initial study claiming benefits for a particular drug was subsequently refuted by a better designed and better controlled study.

Table 13.3 *Drugs used in various therapeutic trials in Duchenne muscular dystrophy*

Drug	Basis for use	First reported trial
Allopurinol	Increases nucleotide formation believed to be depleted in dystrophic muscle	1976
Amino acids	Deficiency of muscle proteins	1953
Anabolic steroids	Anabolic effect	1955
Aspirin, propranolol, etc.	Counteract proposed defect in biogenic amine metabolism	1977
Calcium blockers	Reduce muscle intracellular calcium	1982
Catecholamines	Counteract proposed defect in muscle sympathetic innervation	1930
Coenzyme Q	Possible benefit in murine dystrophy	1974
Dantrolene	Inhibit release of calcium from sarcoplasmic reticulum	1983
Digitalis and other cardiac glycosides	Prevent progressive cardiomyopathy	1963
Glycine	Believed to stimulate muscle creatine synthesis	1932

Table 13.3 *Contd.*

Drug	Basis for use	First reported trial
Growth hormone	Anabolic effect	1973
Growth hormone inhibitor	Growth hormone deficiency ameliorates disease	1984
Ketoacids	Reduce muscle protein degradation	1982
Leucine	Increases protein synthesis	1984
Nucleotides (e.g. Laevadosin)	Replacement of nucleotides believed to be depleted in dystrophic muscle	1960
Oestrogens	Anabolic effect	1972
Pancreatic extract	Possible benefit in murine dystrophy	1976
Penicillamine	Possible benefit in avian dystrophy	1977
Prednisolone	Anabolic effect	1974
Protease inhibitors	Possible benefit in murine dystrophy	1984
Superoxide dismutase	Removal of superoxide radicals associated with membrane damage	1980
Testosterone	Anabolic effect	1955
Thyroxine	Thyroxine depresses SCK	1964
Vasodilators	Counteract proposed defect in muscle microcirculation	1963
Vitamins		
B6	Vitamin B6 deficient rats develop myopathy	1940
E	Vitamin E deficient animals develop a myopathy	1940
Zinc	Membrane 'stabilizer'	1986

Evaluation of drug trials

Dubowitz and Heckmatt (1980) have presented a detailed and critical review of the many therapeutic trials in Duchenne muscular dystropy. They derived a system of awarding a 'quality score' for each report, with a point for each of the following criteria: careful selection and definition of cases; adequate controls; objective ('blind') study; assessment other than by simple clinical ratings; and for a trial lasting longer than two years. Of 34 published trials they analysed, not one was awarded five points, and in half there was no score at all, which means that even the definition of the cases studied was

Table 13.4 *Scoring of 34 drug trials in Duchenne muscular dystrophy (1940–79), (data from Dubowitz and Heckmatt (1980))*

Score	Number of trials
0	17
1	7
2	3
3	3
4	4
5	0

not clear (Table 13.4). Dubowitz and Heckmatt consider that no trial with a score of less than three should be taken seriously otherwise there is the danger of raising false hopes in both the patient and his family.

Design of drug trials

There are a number of general points to be considered in designing a drug trial in Duchenne muscular dystrophy. Patients must be *carefully selected* on the basis of accepted clinical, biochemical, and histological diagnostic criteria for the disease. The inclusion of patients with Becker muscular dystrophy, for example, might give the mistaken impression of slowing the course of the disease. The patients should also be old enough and intelligent enough to cooperate and yet still be ambulant. Ideally they should therefore be aged between 5 and 10 years. The trial should be 'blind', unless the nature of the treatment (e.g. surgery), or the occurrence of unusual side-effects makes this impossible. Ideally it should be *double-blind* with neither the patient and his family, nor the investigator, knowing who is taking the drug and who is taking a placebo. It may be difficult to convince parents of the value of this method because if they already believe the drug could be effective it would mean in some cases denying the possible benefits of treatment for the duration of the trial. For this reason a *cross-over* double-blind study has an advantage, and also requires fewer patients. Others have used 'natural history controls' for comparisons, that is data collected from known cases over a period of time (Mendell *et al.* 1987). The placebo must have the same appearance, texture, and taste as the drug. Boys become adept at recognizing the one from the other on the basis of slight differences in taste or texture. Furthermore the effects of the drug may take some time to wear off (the so-called 'wash-out' effect) and so vitiate the results of a cross-over study.

If there are likely to be clear side-effects this would invalidate a double-blind study, and if they could be serious then a very carefully monitored *pilot study* should be carried out initially.

Table 13.5 *Methods for assessing the possible beneficial
effects of a drug in Duchenne muscular dystrophy*

1. *Muscle strength*
   MRC grading (0–5)
   Ergometry (kg)
2. *Functional ability*
   Swinyard grade (1–8)
   Vignos grade (1–10)
   Hammersmith motor ability score (0–40)
   'CIDD' grade for upper limbs (1–6)
3. *Biochemical*
   SCK
   Urinary creatine/creatinine, 3-methylhistidine, dimethylarginines
4. *Muscle pathology and dystrophin*

The possible beneficial effects may be *assessed* in regard to prolonged survival, prolonged ambulation, or the slowed or arrested progression of muscle weakness. Since changes in muscle strength will be evident first, most emphasis has been placed on this aspect of the problem (Table 13.5). Details of the scoring and grading systems are given in Appendices B–F. Because there is a subjective element in determining muscle strength, and to some extent functional ability, these are best assessed by one examiner. There is also value in using an ergometer (myometer, dynamometer). One which we favoured is a hand-held, sensitive, dead-beat electronic device produced by Penny and Giles Transducers Limited (Christchurch, Dorset, England). The unit has a pressure pad and a digital read-out display which indicates the maximum force applied by the examiner in resisting the actual contraction of the patient's muscles. The operating range is 0.1 to 30 kg and has a repeatability error of less than 1 per cent (Fig. 13.10). The power of each of the major muscle groups is measured and summed for both sides of the body. Other similar instruments are also available (Edwards and McDonnell 1974).

In recent years several investigators have measured various biochemical parameters as a means of assessing any possible improvement. Urinary excretion studies are obviously more acceptable than repeated blood sampling though the former require to be very carefully controlled for age, sex, and diet. There is little value in repeated muscle biopsies though at the end of a trial of a drug which seemed beneficial, muscle pathology could be compared with the findings before the trial was commenced.

Statistical considerations

A drug trial should be designed in such a way as to avoid errors of suggesting a beneficial effect when none exists, or alternatively concluding there is no

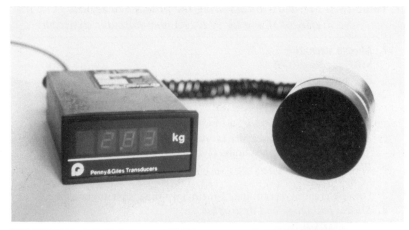

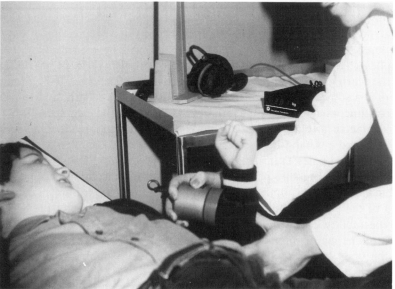

Fig. 13.10 Hand-held ergometer (*above*), and being used to assess the strength of the elbow flexors in an affected boy (*below*).

effect when in fact the drug arrests or slows the disease process. To detect a therapeutic effect which is small, such as a gradual slowing of the disease process, requires a prolonged trial involving a large number of patients. Conversely, a marked therapeutic effect would be detectable in a shorter time and would need fewer individuals. In this regard a helpful parameter to be determined is the so-called *power* of the trial. If the rate of decline in untreated boys is r_1 (with a standard deviation of s.d.), and in treated boys is r_2 then the *standard difference* (delta, Δ) is:

$$\frac{r_1 - r_2}{s.d.}$$

The power of a trial is the probability of detecting a difference in the two rates which is statistically significant ($P < 0.05$) and can be calculated for different numbers of individuals and for trials of different durations. Based on data from 114 untreated boys with Duchenne muscular dystrophy followed for a year, power curves have been derived by Brooke *et al.* (1983). These investigators found that the rate of decline in untreated boys was 0.4 units (of muscle strength) per year (s.d. 0.39). If after a year a drug slowed the disease to 25 per cent of its original rate of progression, then:

$$\Delta = \frac{0.4 - 0.1}{0.39}$$

$$= 0.77$$

To detect such a difference with a 95 per cent probability would require

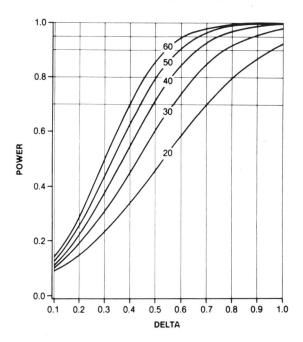

Fig. 13.11 Power curves ($P < 0.05$, one-tail) for drug trials lasting a year for various values of the standard difference (Delta). (From Brooke *et al.* (1983) with permission.)

a study involving at least 40 individuals in each group. On the other hand if a drug actually arrested the progression of the disease then about 25 individuals in each group would be required (Fig.13.11).

The 'power' of therapeutic trials in Duchenne muscular dystrophy is discussed further by Stern (1984). By using more than one set of measurements, the power of a trial study can be increased, thereby decreasing the number of individuals needed and/or the duration of the trial. However, the rate of progression is clearly *not* the same in all boys (Ziter *et al.* 1977; Cohen *et al.* 1982). It might therefore be best to consider each boy as being his own control by comparing rates of progression before and after treatment. Alternatively groups of boys may be compared who, prior to a trial, showed similar rates of progression.

Taking into account the 'power' of a study, the criteria of a good trial in Duchenne muscular dystrophy should be:

• Inclusion only of patients with a clearly established diagnosis of the disease
• Carefully matched control group
• 'Blind' study
• Assessment by several different methods
• Determination of an acceptable 'power' level and therefore the number of individuals to be studied and the duration of the trial.

Table 13.6 *Numbers (rounded off) of individuals (controls and treated) required in a randomized trial where there is a 95 per cent probability ('power') of detecting a significant difference ($P < 0.05$; $P < 0.01$) for various values of Δ, and in each case are roughly four times the required number for a cross-over trial*

	One tail		Two-tail	
Δ	$P < 0.05$	$P < 0.01$	$P < 0.05$	$P < 0.01$
0.1	2165	3154	2599	3563
0.2	541	788	650	891
0.4	135	197	162	223
0.6	60	88	72	99
0.8	34	49	41	56
1.0	22	31	26	36
1.2	15	22	18	25
1.4	11	16	13	18
1.6	8	12	10	14
1.8	7	10	8	11
2.0	5	8	6	9

The assumption underlying the discussion so far is that quite a large number of patients will be involved in a study. Each individual investigator, however, is unlikely to have access to many patients and therefore collaboration between different centres is necessary, to produce data for a so-called 'multi-centre trial'. Uniformity is then essential, both in the design and execution of the trial, particularly with regard to clinical assessment of the possible effects of a drug. The alternative is to study smaller groups of patients but then, as we have seen, only a comparatively large effect would be detected (Table 13.6).

In 1984 a colloquium was held in Bangor, Pennsylvania, sponsored by the Muscular Dystrophy Association of America which addressed many of the problems involved in drug trials in Duchenne muscular dystrophy. The proceedings have been published in full (*Muscle and Nerve* Vol. 8, pp. 451-92, 1985) and provide varied and useful insights into these problems.

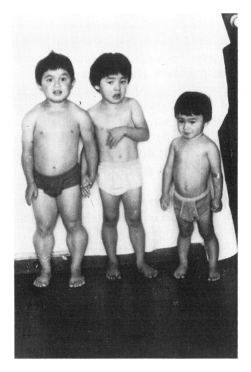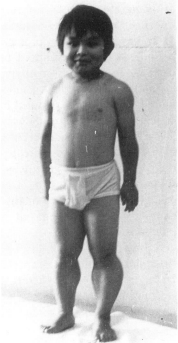

Fig. 13.12 (*Left*) a boy with Duchenne muscular dystrophy and growth hormone deficiency aged 13, and his two younger affected brothers aged 5 and 3. (*Right*) proband aged 18. (Reproduced by kind permission of Dr Mayana Zatz.)

Recent drug trials

The first edition of this book included a lengthy discussion of the possible value of treatment with growth hormone inhibitors. This emanated from the report of a family (Zatz *et al*. 1981*b*) with Duchenne muscular dystrophy in which the eldest affected boy was much less severely affected than his brothers but who also suffered from growth hormone deficiency (Fig. 13.12). Furthermore, since the muscular dystrophy gene is not expressed in genotypic dwarf-dystrophic mice (Totsuka *et al*. 1983) this led to the suggestion that treatment with growth hormone inhibitors might be effective in Duchenne dystrophy. Unfortunately this has not proved to be so. However, these observations do raise a number of intriguing questions regarding the role of growth hormone in the evolution of the disease process.

But more interesting is the possible value of steroids. Early studies were not convincing but more recent work is encouraging. There are several reasons for believing they might have a beneficial effect. An affected boy showed a remarkable improvement in muscle strength after renal transplantation which the authors (Démos *et al*. 1976) attributed to the effects of the drugs need to suppress graft rejection (azathioprine and prednisolone). More directly, the results of several recent drug trials using prednisone (Table 13.7), have shown an improvement in muscle strength (at least over a limited period) with a concomitant increase in urinary creatinine excretion and decrease in urinary 3-methylhistidine excretion. And as discussed earlier (p. 208), such treatment is associated with a decrease in muscle T cells and muscle fibres focally invaded by lymphocytes which suggests the possibility of immunosuppression. However, though prednisone increases dystrophin levels in normal muscle in culture (Sklar and Brown 1991), it has no effect on muscle dystrophin in treated boys which of course would be expected if there is an extensive gene deletion. In view of the side effects of prolonged steriod therapy however, Dubowitz (1991*b*) has suggested that a low dosage pulsed therapy might prove most beneficial. There is certainly a need for further trials of prednisone or perhaps even more effective immunosuppressants.

A fascinating possibility recently suggested by Hoffman and Gorospe (personal communication, 1992) is a model implicating *mast cells* as a major factor in fibrosis and therefore in the pathogenesis of the disease. Drugs which stabilize mast cell activity might therefore also be considered in future as possibly being of therapeutic value.

Myoblast transfer

Early in 1989 Partridge and colleagues (Partridge *et al*. 1989) published a paper in which they showed that the injection of normal myoblasts into the

Table 13.7 Trials of Prednisone (and Deflazacort* which has fewer side-effects) in the treatment of Duchenne muscular dystrophy. Therapeutic value graded as +, +/−, − (no effect).

| Treated Patients | | Controls | Duration | Therapeutic value | Reference |
No.	Age				
14	3–10	−	1–28 mths	+	Drachman et al. (1974)
7	6–9	+	24 mths	−	Siegel et al. (1974)
33	5–15	+	6 mths	+	Brooke et al. (1987)
16	3–10	+	1–11 yrs	+	DeSilva et al. (1987)
103	5–15	+	6 mths	+ (in first 3 mths)	Mendell et al. (1989)
103	5–15	+	6 mths	+ (with *daily* therapy)	Fenichel et al. (1990)
34	5–15	+	6 mths	+ (0.75 mg/kg/d)	Griggs et al. (1991)
33	5–15	+	6 mths	+ / − (0.30 mg/kg/d) (but fewer side-effects)	Griggs et al. (1991)
92	5–15	+	15–39 mths	+ ($\geqslant$ 0.65 mg/kg/d better than < 0.65 mg/kg/d)	Fenichel et al. (1991)
14	5–11	+	9 mths	+ (in first 6 mths)	Mesa et al. (1991)*

muscle of dystrophic *mdx* mice rendered many of the fibres in the vicinity of the injection dystrophin positive. Presumably the normal myoblasts fused with the host muscle fibres. Subsequently, Law and colleagues (1990) reported having obtained similar results in humans. At the present time several groups (including Helen Blau of San Francisco, George Karpati of Montreal, and Jacques Tremblay of Quebec) are investigating the possible therapeutic value of this approach in Duchenne dystrophy.

This is certainly an exciting and novel development which is currently attracting a great deal of interest from medical scientists (Griggs and Karpati 1990; Kakulas *et al.* 1992). But there are a number of problems. The original work involved *mdx*/nude mice, thus avoiding problems of immune rejection. But such an approach is not applicable to humans where problems of graft rejection have to be considered. A sib donor is more likely to be HLA compatible with the patient, though for obvious reasons fathers have so far been used most often, and concomitant immunosuppressive therapy may be necessary, though some have questioned this. Theoretically it might also be expected that when there is normally no dystrophin the treated patient could mount an immune reaction against any synthesized dystrophin since this could be viewed by the treated host's immune system as a 'foreign' protein. It would also be expected that treatment might well require multiple injections into different muscle groups if it is to be effective and conceivably might have to be repeated. There are quite formidable problems of producing cultured myoblasts in sufficient quantities for such treatment. Furthermore, myoblast transfer would not affect cardiac muscle or any central nervous system involvement. Finally, in manifesting carriers where a 'mosaic' of dystrophin-positive fibres occurs naturally (p. 241), their muscle strength does not improve with age but generally deteriorates.

But despite all these problems and reservations, there is evidence that injections of normal myoblasts into patients does lead to a local increase in dystrophin-positive muscle fibres, as well as to dystrophin synthesis as evidenced by the presence of dystrophin mRNA (Gussoni *et al.* 1992). But the real question is, does myoblast transfer have any therapeutic value?

Studies carried out so far have each involved around 10–20 boys, ranging in age from 5–12 years. The muscles injected have included the extensor digitorum brevis of the foot, biceps brachii, tibialis anterior or other leg muscles. The number of cells injected at any one time has ranged from around 10×10^6 to 5×10^9. And though a cell suspension is less susceptible to graft rejection than actual muscle tissue and some investigators have not used immunosuppression, others have (for example, cyclosporin). Such a wide variety of experimental techniques makes comparing results from different studies very difficult. For example, immunosuppression itself could have a beneficial effect and any improvement could be due to this alone rather than myoblast transfer.

It does seem that the technique is feasible, is tolerated well, and is a safe procedure (Huard *et al.* 1992). However, though some remain optimistic (Law *et al.* 1992), on present evidence most consider its therapeutic value (as shown by significantly increased muscle power) very doubtful in Duchenne muscular dystrophy (Rossiter *et al.* 1992), as well as in McArdle's disease (Karpati *et al.* 1992).

Gene therapy

Much has been written on the possibility of treating hereditary diseases by gene therapy, and various strategies are being considered using different delivery systems, including viral vectors (for example, DNA adenoviruses or RNA retroviruses) and direct gene transfer. The technical problems are considerable and have recently been reviewed, for example, in Desnick (1991), Friedmann (1991), Miller (1992), and Gros (1992).

In the case of Duchenne muscular dystrophy, problems are compounded by the immense size of the dystrophin gene which has to be transferred. However, there is the possibility that a functional 'minigene', perhaps only half the size of the normal gene, may suffice for nearly normal muscle function (Love *et al.* 1991; Wells *et al.* 1992). Furthermore, a viral transfer system may not be necessary. Wolff and colleagues (1990) have found that injection of plasmid DNA or RNA directly into mouse skeletal muscle can result in significant expression of reporter genes in muscle cells and no special delivery system is necessary. With regard to the transfer of the dystrophin gene, a human dystrophin plasmid cDNA can be expressed in transfected cell cultures (Dickson *et al.* 1991; Lee *et al.* 1991) as well as in *mdx* mouse muscle after being injected intramuscularly (Acsadi *et al.* 1991*a*). But the latter was very inefficient, with only about 1 per cent of muscle fibres expressing dystrophin. To be clinically effective the efficiency of the system would have to be increased considerably. But the technique certainly offers a method of possibly correcting the gene defect directly. Furthermore, reporter genes are also expressed in myocardial cells if injected directly into the myocardium (Lin *et al.* 1990; Acsadi *et al.* 1991*b*). But in this case foreign gene expression in heart muscle lasted only a few weeks, so again there is a need for improvements in the system if it is to be clinically of any value. But this approach of direct gene therapy does offer hope of possibly correcting myocardial dysfunction in Duchenne muscular dystrophy though, as in myoblast transfer, multiple and repeated injections may be necessary and any central nervous system involvement would be unaffected by this regime. Perhaps a neurotropic virus (such as herpes simplex virus type I: HSV-I) might have to be considered as a possible vector for delivering a gene to the central nervous system (Davies 1992). Nevertheless, there is, I believe, a place for some cautious optimism.

Finally, it has always to be borne in mind that an effective treatment could result from a chance observation. The history of medicine is replete with many such examples. An effective therapy might be found which does not necessarily depend on curing the basic genetic defect. As Sir Andrew Huxley (1980) has said in the case of myasthenia gravis:

> . . . effective anti-cholinesterase therapy was introduced long before the autoimmune basis of the failure of neuromuscular transmission was known, and at the present time treatment designed to combat the autoimmune attack on the end-plates is used without knowing the original reason for the disturbance of the immune system. . . . Rational therapy can just as well be based on an understanding of intermediate steps in the disease process as on a discovery of the nature of the fundamental defect.

Comprehensive management

Duchenne muscular dystrophy is a relatively rare condition, only about a hundred new cases being born each year in the United Kingdom. For this reason, if for no other, family practitioners may not be fully conversant with the disease. Since family practitioners provide primary care for such children it is essential that they be aware of the existence of the disease so that patients and their families are referred to appropriate specialists as soon as possible and delays in reaching the correct diagnosis are reduced to a minimum. Such awareness may be increased by providing instruction on genetic disorders in medical schools and later in postgraduate refresher courses. In Britain many services for the physically handicapped are provided by Statute. However, for the individual case these services are sometimes inadequate because of poor organization and lack of coordination and communication between health and welfare services (Thomas *et al.* 1985). The problem is particularly acute at the period of transition from childhood to adolescence at the time when affected boys are beginning to require increased medical, social, and educational services. Voluntary agencies can provide help in the form of information on what services are available and how they can be obtained. The Muscular Dystrophy Group of Great Britain and Northern Ireland finances several Family Care Officers, each being attached to a unit with particular interests in muscular dystrophy and related disorders. They are often trained nurses or social workers whose function is to maintain contact with patients and their families, to provide advice on welfare, social, and educational services, and in general help families cope with their various problems.

The value of total comprehensive management in Duchenne muscular dystrophy has been argued strongly in Krog (1982), and in order to provide such comprehensive care for the patient and his family there is a need for regional centres for muscular dystrophy in large population areas. Here a team specializing in the disease is able to provide, or have local access to, all the medical and surgical expertise as well as genetic and welfare services needed for comprehensive management. The emphasis is therefore on a team approach (Russman 1984). Patient care could be shared between the centre and local paediatricians, and joint clinics could be held in peripheral hospitals. However, all patients should be notified to, and preferably be assessed at regular intervals by the regional centre. There are a number of arguments to support this idea. A regional centre would concentrate expertise and so reduce the need for patients and families to travel to different hospitals for medical and other services. The members of the centre would also benefit from close relationships with other professionals with related interests. The inclusion of laboratory facilities for enzyme assays and DNA studies would enhance the value of such centres. The inclusion of research facilities as well would ensure that investigators do not work in isolation. But perhaps the most cogent argument is that patients are more likely to benefit f a team with particular expertise in the dis s with Duchenne muscular dystrophy having d it has even been suggested they may have Dunn 1982), which also seems to be the effect nely cystic fibrosis (Anon. 1986). Only by the forts of everyone concerned, will effective evention of further cases be achieved, and an

Summary and conclusions

Although Duchenne muscular dystrophy is not yet curable, it is not untreatable and there are many ways to improve the quality of life of affected boys. Paramount is the maintenance of good general health with emphasis on good nutrition and weight control, the prevention of deformities, and the preservation of respiratory function. The development of deformities can be delayed by passive exercises and various orthoses. Scoliosis is a particularly serious problem because the progressive thoracic deformity restricts adequate pulmonary ventilation and aggravates respiratory problems resulting from weakness of the intercostal muscles. The development of scoliosis can be limited by fitting appropriate moulded back supports, but more effectively by prolonging ambulation and surgical fixation of the spine. However, there can be serious operative risks associated with this disorder which include occasionally cardiac arrest and, more commonly, increased muscle breakdown with myoglobinuria. However, these dangers have been mostly based on case reports and are therefore somewhat selective. In the majority of patients there are few serious anaesthetic or postoperative problems though the anaesthetist and surgeon need to be prepared against these eventualities.

Impaired pulmonary function is the major factor in morbidity and mortality, over 90 per cent of deaths being due to pulmonary infection and respiratory failure. The preservation of respiratory function can be achieved to an extent by impeding the development of scoliosis and regular breathing exercises with postural drainage. All respiratory infections must be treated vigorously and often will need brief hospitalization. In the later stages of the disease assisted ventilation can be helpful and may prolong life for some years.

The psychological effects of the disease on the patient himself as well as on his parents and unaffected sibs cannot be ignored. Open and frequent discussions between all those concerned, including the health care professionals, should be encouraged. The educational needs of affected boys can also raise problems — for those who are severely handicapped and may require special care, and for those who are highly intelligent and may aspire to further education at a time when they are severely physically handicapped. At the beginning most boys will attend normal schools but later special day schools catering for the physically handicapped may have to be considered.

There is at present no effective treatment. However, in recent years there has been considerable interest in the design of drug trials in this disease, the criteria for a good trial being: the inclusion of patients in whom the diagnosis has been fully established; a carefully matched control group; 'blind' assessment by several different methods; and consideration of the number of individuals required and the duration of the study to demonstrate a significant effect ('power' of the trial).

Currently the possibility that prednisone may have a beneficial effect in retarding the progression of the disease is being investigated. Myoblast transfer and gene therapy are also being considere as possible means of correcting the deficiency of muscle dystrophin. There are therefore good reasons for entertaining cautious optimism that an effective treatment for Duchenne muscular dystrophy may be found in the not too distant future.

Finally, comprehensive management through a team approach is advocated. The team should ideally be concentrated in a regional centre for muscular dystrophy where all aspects of management can be coordinated for the benefit of the patient and his family.

Appendices

Appendix A. Duchenne's obituary (*Lancet* 1875)

DUCHENNE (DE BOULOGNE).
(From our Paris Correspondent.)

DUCHENNE (DE BOULOGNE), whose death you noticed in your last issue, was born in 1806, and consequently died at the age of about seventy. After having graduated he began practice in Boulogne-sur-Mer, his native place, but soon found this field too narrow for his restless and inventive mind, and for the experiments which he was already conducting, and so he left for Paris, where, during thirty-three years, he led a life of incessant scientific labour.

In 1847 he presented his first memoir to the Academy of Sciences, and up to within a month previous to his death he continued to publish, either in the Transactions of the two Academies or in the *Archives de Médecine*, the results of his experiments and observations. Amongst the most important of his researches are those on the muscular system; the isolated action and synergy of muscles. His studies on the muscles of the face, and on their office in the mechanism and expression of the human visage, are remarkable, and are familiar in France to artists as well as to medical men. But it was especially in his researches on the nervous centres, on the various forms of paralysis, on congenital or developed deformities, that his great qualities of observation manifested themselves. His name will ever be coupled with the history of progressive muscular atrophy, locomotor ataxy (to which Trousseau proposed that the name of 'Duchenne's disease' should be given), glosso-labio-laryngeal paralysis, and, generally, the microscopical anatomy and pathology of the nervous system. His right of priority to the description of certain forms of nervous diseases has been disputed, and with justice; as, for instance, in the case of locomotor ataxy, where Romberg certainly had the precedence. But at the same time, it may be stated that all Duchenne's descriptions and discoveries were original, and the result of his own labours. The writings of Romberg and other foreign *savants* were at the time unknown in France, not only to Duchenne, but even to the best men having a knowledge of foreign languages.

A great many of his researches were carried on by means of electricity, and in turn they threw light on the uses of this powerful agent, and to Duchenne will redound the honour of having methodically applied electricity to physiological and pathological investigations, and of having scientifically used it for the treatment of disease.

His features were familiar to all who visited habitually the wards of the Paris hospitals. Every morning Duchenne was to be seen in one or other of the hospitals, studying cases, examining specimens, drawing his photographs of microscopical appearances, in which he was extraordinarily skilful. For a long time Duchenne's invariable presence in the wards, his incessant moving about, his ardent interrogation of patients, caused him to be looked upon with a somewhat suspicious and anxious eye by many of the hospital physicians. But his consummate experience of disease, his wonderful keenness and ability in making out a diagnosis in cases of paralysis, the sincerity and earnestness of his manner, the honesty of his proceedings, the authority which he gained by the publication of his original researches, the services which he rendered daily in the wards of the hospitals, brought him the esteem and appreciation of all, and made him a welcome guest everywhere.

He was no orator, and could never have given a lecture on any subject, but he was wonderful at the patient's bedside. Dexterous and nimble in handling his patient, sharp and sensible in his questioning, most striking in the way he got up his data, made out the disease, and gave practical demonstrations of the surety of his diagnosis. Amongst the various instances of this last quality which were related in the hospitals about Duchenne was the fact of his taking patients accounted to be paraplegic out of their beds, and of causing a man to get on their shoulders without their giving way in the slightest.

His patience was extraordinary. He would pursue the investigation of a case for years, never losing sight of it, and following the patient in his peregrinations from hospital to hospital and from house to house, often affording help and means of subsistence.

It may be said of Duchenne that under many adverse circumstances — the suspicions of *confrères*, the disputes as to priority, the difficulty of finding a field of study and experiment, as he had no hospital appointment — his reputation has come out clear and bright, as an honest, hardworking, acute, and ingenious observer, an original discoverer, a skilful professional man, and a kind-hearted, benevolent gentleman.

His various writings have been gathered, and are included in the following important works: — 'Traité de l'Electrisation Localisée' (third edition); 'Le Mécanisme de la Physionomie Humaine'; 'La Physiologie des Mouvements Démontrée à l'aide de l'Expérimentation Electrique'; 'Anatomie du Système Nerveux', 'Orthopédie Physiologique.'

Appendix B. MRC grading of muscle strength (MRC, 1943)

	Grade
No contraction	0
Flicker or trace of contraction only	1
Active movement with gravity eliminated	2
Active movement against gravity	3
Active movement against gravity and resistance	4
Normal power	5

Appendix C. Swinyard grade (Swinyard *et al.* 1957)

	Grade
Walks with waddling gait and marked lordosis. Elevation activities adequate (climbs stairs and curbs without assistance).	1
Walks with waddling gait and marked lordosis. Elevation activities deficient (needs support for curbs and stairs).	2
Walks with waddling gait and marked lordosis. Cannot negotiate curbs or stairs but can achieve erect posture from standard height chair.	3
Walks with waddling gait and marked lordosis. Unable to rise from a standard height chair.	4
Wheelchair independence. Good posture in the chair; can perform all activities of daily living from chair.	5
Wheelchair with dependence. Can roll chair but needs assistance in bed and wheelchair activities.	6
Wheelchair with dependence and back support. Can roll the chair only a short distance; needs back support for good chair position.	7
Bed patient. Can do no activities of daily living without maximum assistance.	8

Appendix D. Vignos grade (Archibald and Vignos 1959)

	Grade
Walks and climbs stairs without assistance.	1
Walks and climbs stairs with aid of railing.	2
Walks and climbs stairs slowly with aid of railing (over 25 seconds for eight standard steps).	3
Walks but cannot climb stairs.	4
Walks unassisted but cannot climb stairs or get out of chair.	5
Walks only with assistance or with braces.	6
In wheelchair. Sits erect, can roll chair and perform bed and wheelchair activities of daily living.	7
In wheelchair. Sits erect. Unable to perform bed and chair activities without assistance.	8
In wheelchair. Sits erect only with support. Able to do only minimal activities of daily living.	9
In bed. Can do no activities of daily living without assistance.	10

Appendix E. Hammersmith motor ability score (Scott *et al*. 1982)

All movements are attempted and scored:
    2 for every completed movement
    1 for help and/or reinforcement
    0 if unable to achieve the movement
    Total possible score = 40
1. Lifts head.
2. Supine to prone over right.
3. Supine to prone over left.
4. Prone to supine over right.
5. Prone to supine over left.
6. Gets to sitting.
7. Sitting.
8. Gets to standing.
9. Standing.
10. Standing on heels.
11. Standing on toes.
12. Stands on right leg.
13. Stands on left leg.
14. Hops on right leg.
15. Hops on left leg.
16. Gets off chair.
17. Climbing step right leg.
18. Descending step right leg.
19. Climbing step left leg.
20. Descending step left leg.

Appendix F. Clinical investigation of Duchenne dystrophy (CIDD) group. Grade for upper limb function (Brooke *et al.* 1983)

	Grade
Starting with arms at the sides, patient can abduct the arms in a full circle until they touch above the head.	1
Can raise arms above head only by flexing the elbow (i.e. shortening the circumference of the movement), or by using accessory muscles.	2
Cannot raise hands above head but can raise an 8 oz glass of water to mouth (using both hands if necessary).	3
Can raise hands to mouth but cannot raise an 8 oz glass of water to mouth.	4
Cannot raise hand to mouth but can use hands to hold pen or pick up pennies from table.	5
Cannot raise hands to mouth and has no useful function of hands.	6

Appendix G. Intragenic RFLPs. (Reproduced by kind permission of Dr Roger Mountford and Dr Andrew Read.)

Probe	Enzyme	Location	Allele frequency
* DYS I	—	brain prom	− (PIC = 0.61)
* DYS II	—	brain prom	− (PIC = 0.77)
* DYS III	—	brain prom	− (PIC = 0.59)
* 841Q	MaeIII	muscle prom	0.74/0.26
* NM72/73	—	Intron 1	− (PIC = 0.57)
* OA34/35	—	Intron 1	− (PIC = 0.25)
Cf27a	PvuII	Exon 2	0.51/0.49
J-47	MspI	Intron 3	0.33/0.67
XJ1.1	TaqI	Intron 7	0.28/0.72
XJ1.2	BclI	Intron 7	0.70/0.30
XJ2.3	TaqI	Intron 7	0.30/0.70
* pERT 87–1	BstNI	Intron 12	0.65/0.35
pERT 87–1	XmnI	Intron 12	0.69/0.31
pERT 87–1	MspI	Intron 12	0.35/0.65
pERT 87–1	EcoRV	Intron 12	0.65/0.35
* pERT 87–8	TaqI	Intron 13	0.26/0.74
pERT 87–8	BstXI	Intron 13	0.64/0.36
pERT 87–8	XmnI	Intron 13	? ?
* pERT 87–15	TaqI	Intron 17	0.33/0.67
* pERT 87–15	Xmnl	Intron 17	0.32/0.68
* pERT 87–15	BamHI	Intron 17	0.38/0.62
Cf27	XmnI	Exon 1–11	? / ?
Ca1b	BgIII	Exon 20	0.37/0.63
* Ca1a	PstI	Intron 24	0.69/0.31
Ca1a	BgIII	Exon 20/27	0.68/0.32
Cf23b	BclI	Exon 28/39	0.51/0.49
Cf23a or b	EcoRV	Exon 30/46	? / ?
Cf23a	BgIII	Exon 38/41	0.30/0.70
Cf23a	XmnI	Exon 42/43	0.54/0.46
* Cf23a	TaqI	Intron 38	0.32/0.68
J-Bir	BamHI	Intron 39/44	0.21/0.79
* STR44	—	Intron 44	− (PIC = 0.87)
p20	MspI	Intron 44	0.60/0.40
p20	EcoRV	Intron 44	0.40/0.60
p20	BstXI	Intron 44	0.67/0.33
p20	HindIII	Intron 44	? ?
* Exon 45 (SSCP)	—	Exon 45	0.66/0.34
* STR45	—	Intron 45	− (PIC = 0.89)
Cf56a	BanI	Exon 48	0.62/0.25/0.13
* Exon 48	MseI	Exon 48	0.26/0.74
* STR49	—	Intron 49	− (PIC = 0.93)

Probe	Enzyme	Location	Allele frequency
* STR50	–	Intron 59	– (PIC = 0.72)
Cf56a	PstI	Exon 51	0.15/0.85
Cf56a	TaqI	Exon 51	0.80/0.20
* DMD1	–	Intron 55/57	– (PIC = 0.50)
CF77	XmnI	Exon 53/59	0.30/0.70
Cf77	EcoRV	Exon 53/59	0.72/0.28
Cf77	PvuII	Exon 53/59	0.13/0.87
probe 10	XbaI	Exon 59/64	0.29/0.71
* J66	PstI	Intron 60	0.18/0.69/0.13
probe 11–14	TaqI	Exon 64/70	0.16/0.84
* MP1P	–	Untranslated regn	0.89/0.11
* 3/CA rpt	–	Untranslated regn	– (PIC = 0.46)

* PCR markers.

Appendix H. Muscular dystrophy associations and groups in various countries

Argentina
CIDIM
Zapiola 740 CP 1426
Buenos Aires
Argentina

Australia
Muscular Dystrophy Association
  of SA Inc
GPO Box 414
Adelaide SA 5001
Australia

Muscular Dystrophy Association
  of NSW
GPO Box 9932
Sydney 2001
Australia

Muscular Dystrophy Association
  of Queensland
PO Box 518
Sunnybank QLD 4109
Australia

Muscular Dystrophy Association
  of Victoria
PO Box 182
Ascot Vale VIC 3032
Australia

Muscular Dystrophy Association
  of Tasmania
Flat 4, 16 Hill Street
Bellerive TAS 7018
Australia

Muscular Dystrophy Association
  of ACT
PO Box 117
Campbell
Australian Capital Territory 2601
Australia

Muscular Dystrophy Research
  Association of Western Australia
PO Box 328
West Perth WA 6005
Australia

Austria
Österreichische Gesellschaft zur
  Bekämpfung der
  Muskelkrankheiten
Wahringer Görtel 18–20
Postfach 23
A-1097 Wien
Austria

Belgium
Ligue Nationale Belge contre la
  Myopathie et la Myasthenie
115 Bld. de Waterloo
10000 Bruxelles
Belgium

Brazil
Associação Brasileira de Distrofia
  Muscular
Rua do Matão 277
Edificio da Biologia
Cidade Universitária
CEP 05499
São Paulo
Brazil

Canada
Muscular Dystrophy Association
  of Canada
150 Eglinton Avenue E
Suite 400
Toronto M3P 1E8
Canada

Muscular Dystrophy Association
of Canada
Ms Elona Brown
460 O'Connor Street
Suite 215
Ottawa
Ontario K1S 511S
Canada

Society for Muscular Dystrophy
Information
PO Box 479
Bridgewater
Nova Scotia B4V 2X6
Canada

Cyprus
Muscular Dystrophy Association
of Cyprus
PO Box 3462
Nicosa
Cyprus

Czechoslovakia
Svaz Invalidu V CSSR
Zakladni Organizace Muskularnih
Dystrofiku
Petyrkova 1953
14900 Praha-4-Chodov
Czechoslovakia

Denmark
Muskelsvindfonden
Vestervang 41
DK-8000 Aarhus C
Denmark

Finland
Lihastautiliitto R. Y. De
Muskelhandikappades Forbund
R. F.
Lantinen Pitkakatu 35
SF-20100 Turku
Finland

France
Association Française contre les
Myopathies (AFM)
13 Place de Rungis
75013 Paris
France

Germany
Deutsche Gesellschaft zur Bekämp-
fung der Muskelkrankheiten
(DGBM)
Rennerstrasse 4
D-7800 Freiburg
Germany

India
Indian Muscular Dystrophy
Association (IMDA)
21–136 Batchupet
Machilipatnam
521 001 (A.P.)
India

Ireland
Muscular Dystrophy Ireland
Carmichael House, North
Brunswick Street
Dublin 7
Ireland

Israel
Muscle Disease Association of
Israel
PO Box 1491
61014 Tel Aviv
Israel

Italy
Unione Italiana Lotta alla
Distrofia Musculare (UILDM)
Via Gozzadani 7
20148 Milano M1
Italy

Unione Italiana Lotta alla
  Distrofia Musculare (UILDM)
Via P.P. Vergerio 17
I-35126 Padavo
Italy

Japan
Muscular Dystrophy Association
  of Japan
2-2-8 Nishi-waseda
Shinjuku-ku
Tokyo 162
Japan

National Centre for Nervous,
  Mental and Muscular Disorders
Kodaira
Tokyo 187
Japan

Malta
Muscular Dystrophy Group of
  Malta
Griza Road
Griza
Malta

The Netherlands
European Alliance of Muscular
  Dystrophy Associations
  (EAMDA)
European Neuromuscular Center
Lt. Gen. van Heutszlaan 6
NL-3743 JN Baarn
The Netherlands

Verenigning Spierziekten
  Nederland (VSN)
Lt. Gen. van Heutszlaan 6
NL-3743 JN Baarn
The Netherlands

New Zealand
Muscular Dystrophy Association
  of New Zealand
PO Box 23-047
Papatoetoe
Auckland
New Zealand

Norway
Foreningen for Muskelsyke
Post 116 Kjelsas
0411 Oslo 4
Norway

Pakistan
Ma Ayshe Memorial Centre
SNPA-22, Block 7/8
Nr. Commercial Area
KMCHS
Karachi
Pakistan

South Africa
Muscular Dystrophy Research
  Foundation of South Africa
PO Box 5446
Johannesburg 2000
South Africa

Spain
Associación Española de
  Enfermedades Musculares
Apartado de Correos 14.170
ES-08080 Barcelona
Spain

Sweden
Swedish National Association for
  Disabled Children and Young
  People (RBU)
David Bagares Gt. 3
S-111 38 Stockholm
Sweden

Neurologiskt Handikappades
  Riksforbund (NHR)
Kungsgatan 32
S-111 35 Stockholm
Sweden

Switzerland
Schweizerische Gesellschaft für
  Muskelkrankheiten (SGMK)
PO Box 85
CH-8053 Zurich
Switzerland

Turkey
Association of Muscle Disorders
Kas Hastaliklari Dernegi
Hatboyu no. 12
Yesilköy, Istanbul
Turkey

United Kingdom
Muscular Dystrophy Group of
  Great Britain and Northern
  Ireland
Nattrass House,
7–11 Prescott Place
London SW4 6BS
United Kingdom

Mobility International
228 Borough High Street
London SE1 1JX
United Kingdom

Motor Neurone Disease
  Association
61 Derngate
Northampton NN1 1UE
United Kingdom

United States of America
Muscular Dystrophy Association
  of America
3561 East Sunrise Drive
Tucson AZ 85718
USA

Uruguay
Asociacion Uruguaya de Aldeas
  Infantiles SOS
Montevideo
Uruguay

Yugoslavia
Savez Distroficara Jugoslavije
Ul. Radomira Vujovica 3
11000 Beograd
Yugoslavia

Savez Distroficara Bosne i
  Hercegovine
Lenjinova 6a
61000 Ljubljana
Yugoslavia

References

Abbadi, N., Philippe, C., Chery, M., and Gilgenkrantz, S. (1991). Inactivation en 'miroir' du chromosome X chez des jumelles monozygotes dont une est atteinte de myopathie de Duchenne. In *Proc. 4ème Colloque National sur les Maladies Neuro-Musculaire*, Montpellier, 24–28 June 1991, p. 79, No. 281 (Abstract). Association Française contre les Myopathies, Paris.

Abbs, S. and Bobrow, M. (1992). Analysis of quantitative PCR for the diagnosis of deletion and duplication carriers in the dystrophin gene. *Journal of Medical Genetics* **29**, 191–6.

——, Roberts, R. G., Mathew, C. G., Bentley, D. R., and Bobrow, M. (1990). Accurate assessment of intragenic recombination frequency within the Duchenne muscular dystrophy gene. *Genomics* **7**, 602–6.

——, Yau, S. C., Clark, S., Mathew, C. G., and Bobrow, M. (1991). A convenient multiplex PCR system for the detection of dystrophin gene deletions: a comparative analysis with cDNA hybridisation shows mistypings by both methods. *Journal of Medical Genetics* **28**, 304–11.

Acsadi, G., Dickson, G., Love. D. R., *et al.* (1991*a*). Human dystrophin expression in mdx mice after intramuscular injection of DNA constructs. *Nature* **352**, 815–18.

——, Jiao, S., Jani, A., Duke, D., Williams, P., Chong, W., and Wolff, J. A. (1991*b*). Direct gene transfer and expression into rat heart in vivo. *The New Biologist* **3**, 71–81.

Adams, R. D. (1975). *Diseases of muscle—a study in pathology*, (3rd edn). Harper & Row, Hagerstown, Maryland.

Adriaenssens, K. and Vermeiren, G. (1980). Simple electrophoretic technique for creatine kinase MM isozyme in neonatal Duchenne muscular disease screening using dried blood samples. *Clinica chimica Acta* **105**, 99–103.

Afifi, A. K., Bergman, R. A., and Zellweger, H. (1973). A possible role for electron microscopy in detection of carriers of Duchenne type muscular dystrophy. *Journal of Neurology, Neurosurgery and Psychiatry* **36**, 643–50.

Aguilar, L., Lisker, R., and Ramos, G. G. (1978). Unusual inheritance of Becker type muscular dystrophy. *Journal of Medical Genetics* **15**, 116–18.

Ahmad, M., Sanderson, J. E., Dubowitz, V., *et al.* (1978). Echocardiographic assessment of left ventricular function in Duchenne's muscular dystrophy. *British Heart Journal* **40**, 734–40.

Al-Qudah, A. A., Kobayashi, J., Chuang, S., *et al.* (1990). Etiology of intellectual impairment in Duchenne muscular dystrophy. *Pediatric Neurology* **6**, 57–9.

Allard, P., Duhaime, M., Thiry, P. S., and Drouin, G. (1981). Use of gait simulation in the evaluation of a spring-loaded knee joint orthosis for Duchenne muscular dystrophy patients. *Medical and Biological Engineering and Computing* **19**, 165–70.

Allen, J. E. and Rodgin, D. W. (1960). Mental retardation in association with progressive muscular dystrophy. *American Journal of Diseases of Children* **100**, 208–11.

Allen, N. R. (1973). Hearing acuity in patients with muscular dystrophy. *Developmental Medicine and Child Neurology* **15**, 500-5.

Allsop, K. G. and Ziter, F. A. (1981). Loss of strength and functional decline in Duchenne's dystrophy. *Archives of Neurology* **38**, 406-11.

Anand, R. and Emery, A. E. H. (1980). Calcium stimulated enzyme efflux from human skeletal muscle. *Research Communications in Chemical Pathology and Pharmacology* **28**, 541-50.

Anderson, M. D. S., Kunkel, L. M., and Khurana, T. S. (1992). Dystrophin mRNA in lyophilized tissue. *Nature* **355**, 778.

Angelini, C., Beggs, A. H., Hoffman, E. P., Fanin, M., and Kunkel, L. M. (1990). Enormous dystrophin in a patient with Becker muscular dystrophy. *Neurology* **40**, 808-12.

Anon. (1984). Psychological sequelae of female sterilization. *Lancet* **ii**, 144-5.

—— (1986). Regional centres for cystic fibrosis. *Lancet* **i**, 514.

Appleton, R. E., Bushby, K., Gardner-Medwin, D., *et al.* (1991). Head circumference and intellectual performance of patients with Duchenne muscular dystrophy. *Developmental Medicine and Child Neurology* **33**, 884-90.

Appleyard, S. T., Dunn, M. J., Dubowitz, V., and Rose, M. L. (1985). Increased expression of HLA ABC class I antigens by muscle fibres in Duchenne muscular dystrophy, inflammatory myopathy and other neuromuscular disorders. *Lancet* **i**, 361-33.

Aprin, H., Bowen, J. R., MacEwen, G. D., and Hall, J. E. (1982). Spine fusion in patients with spinal muscular atrophy. *Journal of Bone and Joint Surgery* **64A**, 1179-87.

Arahata, K. and Engel, A. G. (1982). Monoclonal antibody analysis of the mononuclear cell in muscle biopsy. *Annals of Neurology* **12**, 79 (Abstract).

——, Ishiura, S., Ishiguro, T., *et al.* (1988). Immunostaining of skeletal and cardiac muscle surface membrane with antibody against Duchenne muscular dystrophy peptide. *Nature* **333**, 861-3.

——, Ishihara, T., Kamakura, K., *et al.* (1989*a*). Mosaic expression of dystrophin in symptomatic carriers of Duchenne's muscular dystrophy. *New England Journal of Medicine* **320**, 138-42.

——, Hoffman, E. P., Kunkel, L. M., *et al.* (1989*b*). Dystrophin diagnosis: Comparison of dystrophin abnormalities by immunofluorescence and immunoblot analyses. *Proceedings of the National Academy of Sciences USA* **86**, 7154-8.

——, Beggs, A. H., Honda, H., *et al.* (1991). Preservation of the C-terminus of dystrophin molecule in the skeletal muscle from Becker muscular dystrophy. *Journal of the Neurological Sciences* **101**, 148-56.

Araki, S., Uchino, M., and Kumamoto, T. (1987). Prevalence studies of multiple sclerosis, myasthenia gravis, and myopathies in Kumamoto District, Japan. *Neuroepidemiology* **6**, 120-9.

Archibald, K. C. and Vignos, P. J. (1959). A study of contractures in muscular dystrophy. *Archives of Physical and Medical Rehabilitation* **40**, 150-7.

Armstrong, P. and Keevil, S. F. (1991). Magnetic resonance imaging. *British Medical Journal* **303**, 35-40, 105-9.

Armstrong, R. M. and Appel, S. H. (1981). Neuromuscular disorders. *Current Neurology* **3**, 17-42.

Askanas, V., Engel, W. K., and Kobayashi, T. (1985). Thyrotropin-releasing hormone enhances motor neuron-evoked contractions of cultured human muscle.

Annals of Neurology **18**, 716–19.

——, Martinuzzi, A., Engel, W. K., *et al.* (1987). Accumulation of CK-MM is impaired in innervated and contracting cultured muscle fibers of Duchenne muscular dystrophy patients. *Life Sciences* **41**, 927–33.

Asmussen, M. A. and Clegg, M. T. (1985). Multiallelic restriction fragment polymorphisms in genetic counseling: population genetic considerations. *Human Heredity* **35**, 129–42.

Averill, D. R. (1980). Diseases of the muscle. *Veterinary Clinics of North America* **10**, 223–34.

Averyanov, Y. N., Bogomazov, E. A., and Logunova, L. V. (1977). Duchenne muscular dystrophy in a girl with chromosomal mosaicism 45, X/46, XX. (Russian). *Zhurnal Nevropatologii i Psikhiatrii Imeni S. S. Korsakova* **77**, 1449–52.

Aymé, S., Pelissier, J, F., Garnier, J. M., Mattei, J. F., and Giraud, F. (1979). Duchenne type muscular dystrophy and consanguinity: difficulties in pedigree analysis. *Journal of Medical Genetics* **16**, 393–5.

——, Aurran, Y., Gouvernet, J., Mattei, J. F., and Giraud, F. (1982). GENTIC: a computerized medical genetic case record system. *American Journal of Medical Genetics* **11**, 43–51.

Bach, J. R., Zeelenberg, A. P., and Winter, C. (1990). Wheelchair-mounted robot manipulators. Long term use by patients with Duchenne muscular dystrophy. *American Journal of Physical and Medical Rehabilitation* **69**, 55–9.

Bakker, E., Hofker, M. H., Goor, N., *et al.* (1985). Prenatal diagnosis and carrier detection of Duchenne muscular dystrophy with closely linked RFLPs. *Lancet* i. 655–8.

——, Van Broeckhoven, C., Bonten, E. J., *et al.* (1987). Germline mosaicism and Duchenne muscular dystrophy mutations. *Nature* **329**, 554–8.

——, Veenema, H., Den Dunnen, J. T., *et al.* (1989). Germinal mosaicism increases the recurrence risk for 'new' Duchenne muscular dystrophy mutations. *Journal of Medical Genetics* **26**, 553–9.

Ballard, F. J., Tomas, F. M., and Stern, L. M. (1979). Increased turnover of muscle contractile proteins in Duchenne muscular dystrophy as assessed by 3-methylhistidine and creatinine excretion. *Clinical Science* **56**, 347–52.

Bank, W. J., Rowland, L. P., and Ipsen, J. (1971). Amino acids of plasma and urine in diseases of muscle. *Archives of Neurology* **24**, 176–86.

Baraitser, M. (1985). *The genetics of neurological disorders*, (2nd edn). Oxford University Press.

Barbujani, G., Russo, A., Danieli, G. A., *et al.* (1990). Segregation analysis of 1885 DMD families: significant departure from the expected proportion of sporadic cases. *Human Genetics* **84**, 522–6.

Baricordi, O. R., Sensi, A., Balboni, A., *et al.* (1989). Impairment of capping in lymphoblastoid cell lines of Duchenne patients indicates an intrinsic cellular defect. *Human Genetics* **83**, 217–19.

Barkhaus, P. E. and Gilchrist, J. M. (1989). Duchenne muscular dystrophy manifesting carriers. *Archives of Neurology* **46**, 673–5.

Barnea, E., Zuk, D., Simantov, R., Nudel, U., and Yaffe, D. (1990). Specificity of expression of the muscle and brain dystrophin gene promoters in muscle and brain cells. *Neuron* **5**, 881–8.

Barohn, R. J., Levine, E. J., Olson, J. O., and Mendell, J. R. (1988). Gastric hypomotility in Duchenne's muscular dystrophy. *New England Journal of Medicine* **319**, 15–18.

Bartlett, R. J., *et al.* (1988). Duchenne muscular dystrophy: high frequency of deletions. Neurology **38**, 1-4.

Bartley, J. A., Miller, D. K., Hayford, J. T., and McCabe, E. R. B. (1982). Concordance of X-linked glycerol kinase deficiency with X-linked congenital adrenal hypoplasia. *Lancet* **ii**, 733-6.

——, Patil, S., Davenport, S., Goldstein, D., and Pickens, J. (1986). Duchenne muscular dystrophy, glycerol kinase deficiency and adrenal insufficiency associated with Xp21 interstitial deletion. *Journal of Pediatrics* **108**, 189-92.

Barwick, D. D., Osselton, J. W., and Walton, J. N. (1965). Electroencephalographic studies in hereditary myopathy. *Journal of Neurology, Neurosurgery and Psychiatry* **28**, 109-14.

Bassöe, H. H. (1956). Familial congenital muscular dystrophy with gonadal dysgenesis. *Journal of Clinical Endocrinology* **16**, 1614-21.

Baur, X., Witt T. N., Pongratz, D., *et al.* (1987). Autosomal dominantes Humero-Peroneales Syndrom mit frühzeitigen Kontrakturen und Kardiomyopathie (Emery-Dreifuss-Syndrom). *Klinische Wochenschrift* **65**, 738-45.

Bawle, E., Tyrkus, M., Lipman, S., and Bozimowski, D. (1984). Aarskog syndrome: full male and female expression associated with an X-autosome translocation. *American Journal of Medical Genetics* **17**, 595-602.

Baydur, A., Gilgoff, I., Prentice, W., Carlson, M., and Fischer, D. A. (1990). Decline in respiratory function and experience with long-term assisted ventilation in advanced Duchenne's muscular dystrophy. *Chest* **97**, 884-9.

Becker, P. E. (1953). *Dystrophia Musculorum Progressiva*. Thieme, Stuttgart.

—— (1957). Neue Ergebnisse der Genetik der Muskeldystrophien. *Acta Genetica (Basel)* **7**, 303-10.

—— (1962). Two new families of benign sex-linked recessive muscular dystrophy. *Revue Canadienne de Biologie* **21**, 551-66.

—— (1964). Myopathien. In *Humangenetik: Ein kurzes Handbuch in fünf Bänden*, (ed. P. E. Becker), Vol. 3, Pt. 1. Thieme, Stuttgart.

—— (1972). Neues zur Genetik und Klassifikation der Muskeldystrophien. *Humangenetik* **17**, 1-22.

—— (1980). Epidemiology of Duchenne muscular dystrophy in South-West Germany. In *Muscular dystrophy research: advances and new trends*, (ed. C. Angelini, G. A. Danieli, and D. Fontanari), pp. 149-56. Excerpta Medica, Amsterdam.

—— and Kiener, F. (1955). Eine neue X-chromosomale Muskeldystrophie. *Archiv fur Psychiatric und Nervenkrankheiten* **193**, 427-48.

Beckmann, J. S., Richard, I., Hillaire, D., *et al.* (1991). A gene for limb-girdle muscular dystrophy maps to chromosome 15 by linkage. *Comptes Rendus de l'Academie des Sciences, Serie III, Sciences de la Vie (Paris)* **312**, 141-8.

Beckmann, R. and Scheuerbrandt, G. (1976). Screening auf erhöhte CK-aktivitäten. *Der Kinderarzt* **7**, 1267-72.

Beeson, D. and Golbus, M. S. (1985). Decision making: Whether or not to have prenatal diagnosis and abortion for X-linked conditions. *American Journal of Medical Genetics* **20**, 107-14.

Beggs, A. H. and Kunkel, L. M. (1990). Improved diagnosis of Duchenne/Becker muscular dystrophy. *Journal of Clinical Investigation* **85**, 613-19.

——, Hoffman, E. P., Snyder, J. R., *et al.* (1991). Exploring the molecular basis for variability among patients with Becker muscular dystrophy: dystrophin gene and protein studies. *American Journal of Human Genetics* **49**, 54-67.

——, Neumann, P. E., Arahata, K., *et al.* (1992). Possible influences on the expression of X chromosome-linked dystrophin abnormalities by heterozygosity for autosomal recessive Fukuyama congenital muscular dystrophy. *Proceedings of the National Academy of Sciences USA* **89**, 623–7.

Bell, C. (1830). *The nervous system of the human body: as explained in a series of papers read before the Royal Society of London.* Adam and Charles Black, Edinburgh.

Bell, J. (1943). On pseudohypertrophic and allied types of progressive muscular dystrophy. In *Treasury of human inheritance*, Vol. 4, Pt. 4. Cambridge University Press, London.

Ben Hamida, M., Fardeau, M., and Attia, N. (1983). Severe childhood muscular dystrophy affecting both sexes and frequent in Tunisia. *Muscle and Nerve* **6**, 469–80.

Berg, B. O. and Conte, F. (1974). Duchenne muscular dystrophy in a female with a structurally abnormal X-chromosome. *Neurology* **24**, 356 (Abstract).

Berlit, P. and Stegaru-Hellring, B. (1991). The heart in muscular dystrophy: an electrocardiographic and ultrasound study of 20 patients. *European Archives of Psychiatry and Clinical Neuroscience* **241**, 177–80.

Berthillier, G., Eichenberger, D., Carrier, H. N., Guibaud, P., and Got, R. (1982). Carnitine metabolism in early stages of Duchenne muscular dystrophy. *Clinica Chimica Acta* **122**, 369–75.

Bertorini, T. E. and Igarashi, M. (1985). Postpoliomyelitis muscle pseudohypertrophy. *Muscle and Nerve* **8**, 644–9.

——, Bhattacharya, S. K., Palmieri, G. M. A., Chesney, C. M., Pifer, D., and Baker, B. (1982). Muscle calcium and magnesium content in Duchenne muscular dystrophy. *Neurology* **32**, 1088–92.

——, Cornelio, F., Bhattacharya, S. K., Palmieri, G. M. A., Dones, I., Dworzak, F., and Brambati, B. (1984). Calcium and magnesium content in fetuses at risk and prenecrotic Duchenne muscular dystrophy. *Neurology* **34**, 1436–40.

Bethlem, J. (1970). *Muscle pathology – introduction and atlas.* Elsevier/North Holland, Amsterdam.

Bevans, M. (1945). Changes in the musculature of the gastrointestinal tract and in the myocardium in progressive muscular dystrophy. *Archives of Pathology* **40**, 225–38.

Biddison, J. H., Dembo, D. H., Spalt, H., Hayes, M. G., and LeDoux, C. W. (1979). Familial occurrence of mitral valve prolapse in X-linked muscular dystrophy. *Circulation* **59**, 1299–1304.

Bies, R. D., Phelps, S. F., Cortez, M. D., Roberts, R., Caskey, C. T., and Chamberlain, J. S. (1992). Human and murine dystrophin mRNA transcripts are differentially expressed during skeletal muscle, heart and brain development. *Nucleic Acids Research* **20**, 1725–31.

Billard, C., Signoret, J. L., Jambaque, I., *et al.* (1991). Etude des fonctions cognatives (langage et mémoire) dans la dystrophie musculaire de Duchenne (DMD). In *Proc. 4ème Colloque National sur les Maladies Neuro-Musculaire*, Montpellier, 24–28 June, 1991. No. 271 (Abstract). Association Française contre les Myopathies, Paris.

Bjerglund Nielsen, L. and Nielsen, I. M. (1984). Turner's syndrome and Duchenne muscular dystrophy in a girl with an X;autosome translocation. *Annales de Génétique* **27**, 173–7.

——, Jacobsen, B. B., Nielsen, I. M., and Tabor, A. (1983). X;autosome translocation in a girl with muscular dystrophy. *Clinical Genetics* **23**, 242 (Abstract).

Bkaily, G., Jasmin, G., Tautu, C., *et al.* (1990). A tetrodotoxin- and Mn^{2+}-insensitive Na^+ current in Duchenne muscular dystrophy. *Muscle and Nerve* **13**, 939–48.

Black, F. W. (1973). Intellectual ability as related to age and stage of disease in muscular dystrophy: a brief note. *Journal of Psychology* **84**, 333–4.

Blake, D. J., Love, D. R., Tinsley, J., *et al.* (1992). Characterization of a 4.8 kb transcript from the Duchenne muscular dystrophy locus expressed in Schwannoma cells. *Human Molecular Genetics* **1**, 103–9.

Blum, D. and Brauman, J. (1975). Serum enzymes in the neonatal period. *Biology of the Neonate* **26**, 53–7.

Blumberg, B. (1984). The emotional implications of prenatal diagnosis. In *Psychological aspects of genetic counselling*, (ed. A. E. H. Emery and I. M. Pullen), pp. 201–17. Academic Press, London.

Blyth, H. and Pugh, R. J. (1959). Muscular dystrophy in childhood: the genetic aspect. *Annals of Human Genetics* **23**, 127–63.

Bodensteiner, J. B. and Engel, A. G. (1978). Intracellular calcium accumulation in Duchenne dystrophy and other myopathies: a study of 567,000 muscle fibres in 114 biopsies. *Neurology* **28**, 439–46.

Bodrug, S. E., Roberson, J. R., Weiss, L., *et al.* (1990). Prenatal identification of a girl with a t(X;4) (p 2l;q 35) translocation: molecular characterisation, paternal origin, and association with muscular dystrophy. *Journal of Medical Genetics* **27**, 426–32.

Boelter, W. D., Burt, B. A., Spector, E. B., Hinton, D. R., Pavlova, Z., and Fujimoto, A. (1990). Dystrophin protein and RFLP analysis for fetal diagnosis and carrier confirmation of Duchenne muscular dystrophy. *Prenatal Diagnosis* **10**, 703–15.

Boltshauser, E., Steinmann, B., Meyer, A., and Jerusalem, F. (1980). Anaesthesia-induced rhabdomyolysis in Duchenne muscular dystrophy. *British Journal of Anaesthesia* **52**, 559.

Bonilla, E., Samitt, C. E., Miranda, A. F., *et al.* (1988*a*). Duchenne muscular dystrophy: deficiency of dystrophin at the muscle cell surface. *Cell* **54**, 447–52.

——, Schmidt, B., Samitt, C. E., *et al.* (1988*b*). Normal and dystrophin-deficient muscle fibers in carriers of the gene for Duchenne muscular dystrophy. *American Journal of Pathology* **133**, 440–5.

——, Younger, D. S., Chang, H. W., *et al.* (1990). Partial dystrophin deficiency in monozygous twin carriers of the Duchenne gene discordant for clinical myopathy. *Neurology* **40**, 1267–70.

Bonsett, C. A. (1969). *Studies of pseudohypertrophic muscular dystrophy*. Thomas, Springfield.

Bortolini, E. R. and Zatz, M. (1986). Investigation on genetic heterogeneity in Duchenne muscular dystrophy. *American Journal of Medical Genetics* **24**, 111–17.

——, da Silva, D. M., Chequer, R. S., *et al.* (1986). Duchenne muscular dystrophy in a girl with a 45, X/46, XX/47, XXX chromosome constitution. *American Journal of Medical Genetics* **25**, 239–43.

Bossingham, D. H., Williams, E., and Nichols, P. J. R. (1977). *Severe childhood neuromuscular disease—the management of Duchenne muscular dystrophy and spinal muscular atrophy*. Muscular Dystrophy Group of Great Britain, London.

Boyd, Y. and Buckle, V. J. (1986). Cytogenetic heterogeneity of translocations associated with Duchenne muscular dystrophy. *Clinical Genetics* **29**, 108–15.

Bradley, R., McKerrell, R. E., and Barnard, E. A (1988). Neuromuscular diseases in animals. In *Disorders of voluntary muscle*, (5th edn), (ed. J. N. Walton), pp. 910–80. Churchill Livingstone, Edinburgh.

Bradley, W. G. and Fulthorpe, J. J. (1978). Studies of sarcolemmal integrity in myopathic muscle. *Neurology* **28**, 670–7.

——, Hudgson, P., Larson, P. F., Papapetropoulos, T. A., and Jenkison, M. (1972). Structural changes in the early stages of Duchenne muscular dystrophy. *Journal of Neurology, Neurosurgery and Psychiatry* **35**, 451–5.

——, Jenkison, M., and Montgomery, A. (1975*a*). The significance of neural abnormalities in muscular dystrophy. In *Recent advances in myology*, (ed. W. G. Bradley, D. Gardner-Medwin, and J. N. Walton), pp. 116–24. Excerpta Medica, Amsterdam.

——, O'Brien, M. D., Walder, D. N., Murchison, D., Johnson, M., and Newell, D. J. (1975*b*). Failure to confirm a vascular cause of muscular dystrophy. *Archives of Neurology* **32**, 466–73.

——, Jones, M. Z., Mussini, J. M., and Fawcett, P. R. W. (1978). Becker-type muscular dystrophy. *Muscle and Nerve* **1**, 111–32.

Brooke, M. H. and Kaiser, K. K. (1970). Muscle fiber types: how many and what kind? *Archives of Neurology* **23**, 369–79.

——, Carroll, J. E., and Ringel, S. P. (1979). Congenital hypotonia revisited. *Muscle and Nerve* **2**, 84–100.

——, Fenichel, G. M., Griggs, R. C., *et al.* (1983). Clinical investigation in Duchenne dystrophy: 2. Determination of the 'power' of therapeutic trials based on the natural history. *Muscle and Nerve* **6**, 91–103.

——, Fenichel, G. M., Griggs, R. C., *et al.* (1987). Clinical investigation of Duchenne muscular dystrophy: interesting results in a trial of prednisone. *Archives of Neurology* **44**, 812–17.

Brooks, A. P. and Emery, A. E. H. (1977). The incidence of Duchenne muscular dystrophy in the South-East of Scotland. *Clinical Genetics* **11**, 290–4.

Brown, C. S., Thomas, N. S. T., Sarfarazi, M., *et al.* (1985). Genetic linkage relationships of seven DNA probes with Duchenne and Becker muscular dystrophy. *Human Genetics* **71**, 62–74.

Brownell, A. K. W., Paasuke, R. T., Elash, A., *et al.* (1983). Malignant hyperthermia in Duchenne muscular dystrophy. *Anaesthesiology* **58**, 180–2.

Brumback, R. A. and Leech, R. W. (1984). *Color atlas of muscle histochemistry*. PSG Publishing, Littleton, Mass.

Buchanan, D. C., Labarbera, C. J., Roelofs, R., and Olson, W. (1979). Reactions of families to children with Duchenne muscular dystrophy. *General Hospital Psychiatry* **1**, 262–9.

Bucher, K., Ionasescu, V., and Hanson, J. (1980). Frequency of new mutants among boys with Duchenne muscular dystrophy. *American Journal of Medical Genetics* **7**, 27–34.

Buchthal, F. (1957). *An introduction to electromyography*. Gyldendal, Copenhagen.

—— and Clemmesen, S. (1941). On the differentiation of muscle atrophy by electromyography. *Acta Psychiatrica et Neurologica Scandinavica* **16**, 143–81.

—— and Olsen, P. Z. (1970). Electromyography and muscle biopsy in infantile spinal muscular atrophy. *Brain* 93, 15-30.

—— and Pinelli, P. (1951). Analysis of motor action potentials as a diagnostic aid in neuromuscular disorders. *Acta Medica Scandinavica* 142 (Suppl. 266), 315-27.

—— and Rosenfalck, P. (1963). Electrophysiological aspects of myopathy with particular reference to progressive muscular dystrophy. In *Muscular dystrophy in man and animals*, (ed. G. H. Bourne and M. N. Golarz), pp. 193-262. Hafner, New York, and Karger, Basel.

Bulfield, G., Siller, W. G., Wight, P. A. L., and Moore, K. J. (1984). X chromosome-linked muscular dystrophy (*mdx*) in the mouse. *Proceedings of the National Academy of Sciences USA* 81, 1189-92.

Buller, A., Eccles, J. C., and Eccles, R. M. (1960). Interactions between motor neurones and muscles in respect of the characteristic speeds of their responses. *Journal of Physiology* 150, 417-39.

Bullock, D. G., McSweeney, F. M., Whitehead, T. P., and Edwards, J. H. (1979). Serum creatine kinase activity and carrier status for Duchenne muscular dystrophy. *Lancet* ii, 1370.

Bulman, D. E., Murphy, E. G., Zubrzycka-Gaarn, E. E., *et al.* (1991). Differentiation of Duchenne and Becker muscular dystrophy phenotypes with amino- and carboxy-terminal antisera specific for dystrophin. *American Journal of Human Genetics* 48, 295-304.

——, Pillers, D. M., Weleber, R. G., *et al.* (1992). Dystrophin isoform expression in the outer plexiform layer of human retina is required for normal function. *Science* (In press.)

Bundey, S. (1978). Calculation of genetic risks in Duchenne muscular dystrophy by geneticists in the United Kingdom. *Journal of Medical Genetics* 15, 249-53.

—— (1981). A genetic study of Duchenne muscular dystrophy in the West Midlands. *Journal of Medical Genetics* 18, 1-7.

—— (1992). *Genetics and neurology*, (2nd edn). Churchill Livingstone, Edinburgh.

—— and Ebdy, J. (1982). Fetal sexing in possible carriers for Duchenne muscular dystrophy. *Prenatal Diagnosis* 2, 1-6.

——, Crawley, J. M., Edwards, J. H., and Westhead, R. A. (1979*a*). Serum creatine kinase levels in pubertal, mature, pregnant, and postmenopausal women. *Journal of Medical Genetics* 16, 117-21.

——, Edwards, J. H., and Insley, J. (1979*b*). Carrier detection in Duchenne muscular dystrophy. *Lancet* i, 881.

Burghes, A. H. M., Logan, C., Hu, X., Belfall, B., Worton, R. G., and Ray, P. N. (1987). A cDNA clone from the Duchenne/Becker muscular dystrophy gene. *Nature* 328, 434-7.

Burn, J., Povey, S., Boyd, Y., Munro, E. A., West, L., Harper, K., and Thomas, D. (1986). Duchenne muscular dystrophy in one of monozygotic twin girls. *Journal of Medical Genetics* 23, 494-500.

Bush, A. and Dubowitz, V. (1991). Fatal rhabdomyolysis complicating general anaesthesia in a child with Becker muscular dystrophy. *Neuromuscular Disorders* 1, 201-4.

Bushby, K. M. D. and Gardner-Medwin, D. (1992). The clinical, genetic and dystrophin characteristics of Becker muscular dystrophy. 1. Natural history. *Journal of Neurology* (In press.)

——, Thambyayah, M., and Gardner-Medwin, D. (1991*a*). Prevalence and incidence of Becker muscular dystrophy. *Lancet* **337**, 1022-4.

——, Cleghorn, N. J., Curtis, A., *et al.* (1991*b*). Identification of a mutation in the promoter region of the dystrophin gene in a patient with atypical Becker muscular dystrophy. *Human Genetics* **88**, 195-9.

——, Gardner-Medwin, D., Nicholson, L. V. B., *et al.* (1992). The clinical, genetic and dystrophin characteristics of Becker muscular dystrophy. 2. Correlation of phenotype with genetic and protein abnormalities. *Journal of Neurology* (In press.)

Buzello, W. and Huttarsch, H. (1988). Muscle relaxation in patients with Duchenne's muscular dystrophy. *British Journal of Anaesthesia* **60**, 228-31.

Byers, T. J., Kunkel, L. M., and Watkins, S. C. (1991). The subcellular distribution of dystrophin in mouse skeletal, cardiac, and smooth muscle. *Journal of Cell Biology* **115**, 411-21.

Call, G. and Ziter, F. A. (1985). Failure to thrive in Duchenne muscular dystrophy. *Journal of Pediatrics* **106**, 939-41.

Campbell, K. P. and Kahl, S. D. (1989). Association of dystrophin and an integral membrane glycoprotein. *Nature* **338**, 259-62.

Cammann, R., Vehreschild, T., and Ernst, K. (1974). Eine neue Sippe von X-chromosomaler benigner Muskeldystrophie mit Frühkontrakturen (Emery-Dreifuss). *Psychiatrie, Neurologie und Medizinische Psychologie* **26**, 431-8.

Canki, N., Dutrillaux, B., and Tivadar, I. (1979). Dystrophie musculaire de Duchenne chez une petite fille porteuse d'une translocation t(X;3) (p 2l;q 13) *de novo*. *Annales de Génétique* **22**, 35-9.

Carpenter, S. and Karpati, G. (1984). *Pathology of skeletal muscle*. Churchill Livingstone, Edinburgh.

Carr, E. F. and Oppé, T. E. (1971). The birth of an abnormal child: telling the parents. *Lancet* **ii**, 1075-7.

Carroll, J. E., Villadiego, A., and Brooke, M. H. (1983). Increased long chain acyl CoA in Duchenne muscular dystrophy. *Neurology* **33**, 1507-10.

Carry, M. R., Ringel, S. P., and Starcevich, J. M. (1986). Distribution of capillaries in normal and diseased muscle. *Muscle and Nerve* **9**, 445-54.

Carter, C. O. (1979). Carrier detection in Duchenne muscular dystrophy. *Lancet* **i**, 979.

——, Roberts, J. A. F., Evans, K. A., and Buck, A. R. (1971). Genetic clinic: a follow up. *Lancet* **i**, 281-5.

Carter, N., Jeffery, S., Shiels, A., Edwards, Y., Tipler, T., and Hopkinson, D. A. (1979). Characterization of human carbonic anhydrase III from skeletal muscle. *Biochemical Genetics* **17**, 837-54.

Carter, N. D., Heath, R., and Jeffery, S. (1980). Serum carbonic anhydrase III in Duchenne dystrophy. *Lancet* **ii**, 542.

——, Morgan, J. E., Monaco, A. P., *et al.* (1990). Dystrophin expression and genotypic analysis of two cases of benign X linked myopathy (McLeod's syndrome). *Journal of Medical Genetics* **27**, 345-7.

Caskey, C. T. (1991). American Society of Human Genetics Presidential Address, October 18, 1990. *American Journal of Human Genetics* **49**, 911-16.

——, Nussbaum, R. L., Cohan, L. C., and Pollack, L. (1980). Sporadic occurrence of Duchenne muscular dystrophy: evidence for new mutation. *Clinical Genetics* **18**, 329-41.

Cattanach, B. M. (1975). Control of chromosome inactivation. *Annual Review of Genetics* **9**, 1-18.

—— and Williams, C. E. (1972). Evidence of non-random X chromosome activity in the mouse. *Genetical Research* **19**, 229-40.

Cattelaens, N., Gerckens, U., Steudel, A., and Grube, E. (1990). Kardiomyopathie bei progressiver Muskeldystrophie. *Deutsche Medizinische Wochenschrift* **115**, 1507-10.

Cavanagh, N. P. C. and Preece, M. A. (1981). Calf hypertrophy and asymmetry in female carriers of X-linked Duchenne muscular dystrophy: an over-diagnosed clinical manifestation. *Clinical Genetics* **20**, 168-72.

Cestan, R. and Lejonne. (1902). Une myopathie avec rétractions familiales. *Nouvelle Iconographie de la Salpêtrière* **15**, 38-52.

Chakrabarti, A. and Pearce, J. M. S. (1981). Scapuloperoneal syndrome with cardiomyopathy: report of a family with autosomal dominant inheritance and unusual features. *Journal of Neurology, Neurosurgery and Psychiatry* **44**, 1146-52.

Chalkiadis, G. A. and Branch, K. G. (1990). Cardiac arrest after isoflurane anaesthesia in a patient with Duchenne's muscular dystrophy. *Anaesthesia* **45**, 22-5.

Chamberlain, J. S., Gibbs, R. A., Ranier, J. E., Nguyen, P. N., and Caskey, C. T. (1988). Deletion screening of the Duchenne muscular dystrophy locus via multiplex DNA amplification. *Nucleic Acids Research* **16**, 11141-56.

——, Gibbs, R. A., Ranier, J. E., and Caskey, C. T. (1991). Detection of gene deletions using multiplex polymerase chain reactions. In *Methods in molecular biology, Vol. 9: Protocols in human molecular genetics*, (ed. C. Mathew), pp. 299-312. Humana Press, Clifton, NJ.

——, Chamberlain, J. R., Fenwick, R. G., *et al.* (1992). Diagnosis of Duchenne and Becker muscular dystrophy by polymerase chain reaction: a multicenter study. *Journal of the American Medical Assocation* **267**, 2609-15.

Charash, L. I., Wolf, S. G., Kutscher, A. H., Lovelace, R. E., and Hale, M. S. (ed.) (1983). *Psychological aspects of muscular dystrophy and allied diseases*. Thomas, Springfield.

——, Lovelace, R. E., Leach, C. F., Kutscher, A. H., Goldberg, J., and Roye, D. P., Jr. (ed.) (1991). *Muscular dystrophy and other neuromuscular diseases: psychosocial issues*. Haworth Press, New York.

Cheeseman, E. A., Kilpatrick, S. J., Stevenson, A. C., and Smith, C. A. B. (1958). The sex ratio of mutation rates of sex-linked recessive genes in man with particular reference to Duchenne type muscular dystrophy. *Annals of Human Genetics* **22**, 235-43.

Chelly, J., Marlhens, F., Le Marec, B., *et al.* (1986). *De novo* DNA microdeletion in a girl with Turner syndrome and Duchenne muscular dystrophy. *Human Genetics* **74**, 193-6.

——, Kaplan, J.-C., Maire, P., *et al.* (1988). Transcription of the dystrophin gene in human muscle and non-muscle tissues. *Nature* **333**, 858-60.

——, Concordet, J.-P., Kaplan, J-C., and Kahn, A. (1989). Illegitimate transcription: transcription of any gene in any cell type. *Proceedings of the National Academy of Sciences, USA* **86**, 2617-21.

——, Gilgenkrantz, H., Lambert M., *et al.* (1990a). Effect of dystrophin gene deletions on mRNA levels and processing in Duchenne and Becker muscular dystrophies. *Cell* **63**, 1239-48.

——, Hamard, G., Koulakoff, A., *et al.* (1990*b*). Dystrophin gene transcribed from different promoters in neuronal and glial cells. *Nature* **344**, 64–5.

——, Gilgenkrantz, H., Lambert, M., *et al.* (1991). The dystrophin transcripts in DMD and BMD patients with gene deletion. In *Muscular dystrophy research: from molecular diagnosis toward therapy*, (ed. C. Angelini, G. A. Danieli, and D. Fontanari), pp. 147–56. Excerpta Medica, Amsterdam.

Chen, J., Denton, M. J., Morgan, G., Pearn, J. H., and Mackinlay, A. G. (1988). The use of field-inversion gel electrophoresis for deletion detection in Duchenne muscular dystrophy. *American Journal of Human Genetics* **42**, 777–80.

Chevron, M-P., Tuffery, S., Echenne, B., Demaille, J., and Claustres, M. (1992). Becker muscular dystrophy: demonstration of the carrier status of a female by immunoblotting and immunostaining. *Neuromuscular Disorders* **2**, 47–50.

Chutkow, J. G., Hyser, C. L., Edwards, J. A., Heffner, R. R., and Czyrny, J. J. (1987). Monozygotic female twin carriers discordant for the clinical manifestations of Duchenne muscular dystrophy. *Neurology* **37**, 1147–51.

Clark, A. G. (1985). The use of multiple restriction fragment length polymorphisms in prenatal risk estimation. *American Journal of Human Genetics* **37**, 60–72.

Clayton, J. F. (1986). A computer programme to calculate risk in X linked disorders using multiple marker loci. *Journal of Medical Genetics* **23**, 35–9.

Clayton, J. and Emery, A. E. H. (1984). DNA probes in Duchenne muscular dystrophy. *Lancet* **ii**, 1151–2.

Clemens, P. R., Fenwick, R. G., Chamberlain, J. S., *et al.* (1991). Carrier detection and prenatal diagnosis in Duchenne and Becker muscular dystrophy families, using dinucleotide repeat polymorphisms. *American Journal of Human Genetics* **49**, 951–60.

Clerk, A., Rodillo, E., Heckmatt, J. Z., Dubowitz, V., Strong, P. N., and Sewry, C. A. (1991). Characterisation of dystrophin in carriers of Duchenne muscular dystrophy. *Journal of the Neurological Sciences* **102**, 197–205.

——, Strong, P. N., and Sewry, C. A. (1992). Characterisation of dystrophin during development of human skeletal muscle. *Development* **114**, 395–402.

Cochrane, G. M. (ed.) (1990*a*). *Personal care*, (6th edn). Oxfordshire Health Authority, Oxford.

—— (ed.) (1990*b*). *Communication*, (7th edn). Oxfordshire Health Authority, Oxford.

—— and Wilson, A. K. (ed.) (1990). *Hoists and lifts*, (2nd edn). Oxfordshire Health Authority, Oxford.

—— and Wilson, A. K. (ed.) (1991). *Walking aids*, (2nd edn). Disability Information Trust, Oxford.

Coërs, C. and Woolf, A. L. (1959). *The innervation of muscle – a biopsy study*. Blackwell, Oxford.

Cohen, A. (1977). Education of children with muscular dystrophy. In *Muscular dystrophy 1976*, (ed. G. C. Robin and G. Falewski de Leon), pp. 139–41. Karger, Basel.

Cohen, H. J., Molnar, G. E., and Taft, L. T. (1968). The genetic relationship of progressive muscular dystrophy (Duchenne type) and mental retardation. *Developmental Medicine and Child Neurology* **10**, 754–65.

Cohen, L., Morgan, J., Babbs, R., Gilula, Z., Karrison, T., and Meier, P. (1982). A statistical analysis of the loss of muscle strength in Duchenne's muscular dystrophy. *Research Communications in Chemical Pathology and Pharmacology* **37**, 123–38.

Cohn, D. H., Starman, B. J., Blumberg, B., and Byers, P. H. (1990). Recurrence of lethal osteogenesis imperfecta due to parental mosaicism for a dominant mutation in a human type I collagen gene (COL1A1). *American Journal of Human Genetics* **46**, 591-601.

Cole, C. G., Walker, A., Coyne, A., *et al.* (1988). Prenatal testing for Duchenne and Becker muscular dystrophy. *Lancet* **i**, 262-5.

Conomy, J. P. (1970). Late-onset slowly progressive sex-linked recessive muscular dystrophy. *Military Medicine* **135**, 471-5.

Conte, G. and Gioja, L. (1836). Scrofola del sistema muscolare. *Annali Clinici dell' Ospedale degli Incurabili di Napoli* **2**, 66-79.

Cooke, A., Lanyon, W. G., Wilcox, D. E., *et al.* (1990). Analysis of Scottish Duchenne and Becker muscular dystrophy families with dystrophin cDNA probes. *Journal of Medical Genetics* **27**, 292-7.

Cooper, B. J., Winand, N. J., Stedman, H., *et al.* (1988). The homologue of the Duchenne locus is defective in X-linked muscular dystrophy of dogs. *Nature* **334**, 154-6.

——, Gallagher, E. A., Smith, C. A., Valentine, B. A., and Winand, N. J. (1990). Mosaic expression of dystrophin in carriers of canine X-linked muscular dystrophy. *Laboratory Investigation* **62**, 171-8.

Cordone, G., Venzano, V., Rossi, G., Cavallero, G., and Minetti, C. (1984). Valutazione critica della variazione della CK serica dopo sforzo nell'identificazione delle portatrici di distrofia muscolare di Duchenne. *Pediatria Medica e Chirurgica* **6**, 819-22.

Cornelio, F. and Dones, I. (1984). Muscle fiber degeneration and necrosis in muscular dystrophy and other muscle diseases: cytochemical and immunocytochemical data. *Annals of Neurology* **16**, 694-701.

——, Dworzak, F., Morandi, L., Fedrizzi, E., Balestrini, M. R., and Gondoni, L. (1982). Functional evaluation of Duchenne muscular dystrophy: proposal for a protocol. *Italian Journal of Neurological Sciences* **4**, 323-30.

Cosmos, E. and Butler, J. (1980). Animal models of muscle diseases, Part III: Compilation of therapeutic trials for hereditary muscular dystrophy. *Muscle and Nerve* **3**, 427-35.

——, Butler, J., Mazliah, J., and Allard, E. P. (1980). Animal models of muscle diseases, Part II: Murine dystrophy. *Muscle and Nerve* **3**, 350-9.

Covone, A. E., Lerone, M., and Romeo, G. (1991). Genotype-phenotype correlation and germline mosaicism in DMD/BMD patients with deletions of the dystrophin gene. *Human Genetics* **87**, 353-60.

Cowan, J., Macdessi, J., Stark, A., and Morgan, G. (1980). Incidence of Duchenne muscular dystrophy in New South Wales and the Australian Capital Territory. *Journal of Medical Genetics* **17**, 245-9.

Crisp, D. E., Ziter, F. A., and Bray, P. F. (1982). Diagnostic delay in Duchenne's muscular dystrophy. *Journal of the American Medical Association* **247**, 478-80.

Critchley, M. (1949). *Sir William Gowers (1845-1915) — biographical appreciation.* Heinemann, London.

Cross, G. S., Speer, A., Rosenthal, A., *et al.* (1987). Deletions of fetal and adult muscle cDNA in Duchenne and Becker muscular dystrophy patients. *EMBO Journal* **6**, 3277-83.

Cullen, M. J. and Mastaglia, F. L. (1980). Morphological changes in dystrophic muscle. *British Medical Bulletin* **36**, 145-52.

——, Hudgson, P., and Mastaglia, F. L. (1988). Ultrastructural studies of diseased muscle. In *Disorders of voluntary muscle*, (5th edn), (ed. J. N. Walton), pp. 284–344. Churchill Livingstone, Edinburgh.

——, Walsh, J., Nicholson, L. V. B., *et al.* (1991). Immunogold labelling of dystrophin in human muscle, using an antibody to the last 17 amino acids of the C-terminus. *Neuromuscular Disorders* **1**, 113–19.

Curnutte, J. T., Hopkins, P. J., Kuhl, W., and Beutler, E. (1992). Studying X inactivation. *Lancet* **339**, 749.

Cuthbertson, R. A. (1977). *Duchenne de Boulogne, his life, his times and the significance of his work, with special reference to his study of mechanism of human facial expression*. Thesis, University of Melbourne.

Dangain, J. and Vrbova, G. (1984). Muscle development in *mdx* mutant mice. *Muscle and Nerve* **7**, 700–4.

Danieli, G. A. (1984). Studies on the prevalence of the Duchenne muscular dystrophy genotype at birth. In *Research into the origin and treatment of muscular dystrophy*, (ed. L. P. ten Kate, P. L. Pearson, and A. M. Stadhouders), pp. 17–32. Excerpta Medica, Amsterdam.

—— and Barbujani, G. (1984). Duchenne muscular dystrophy – frequency of sporadic cases. *Human Genetics* **67**, 252–6.

——, Mostacciuolo, M. L., Bonfante, A., and Angelini, C. (1977). Duchenne muscular dystrophy – a population study. *Human Genetics* **35**, 225–31.

——, Mostacciuolo, M. L., Pilotto, G., Angelini, C., and Bonfante, A. (1980). Duchenne muscular dystrophy – data from family studies. *Human Genetics* **54**, 63–8.

Danilowicz, D., Rutkowski, M., Myung, D., and Schively, D. (1980). Echocardiography in Duchenne muscular dystrophy. *Muscle and Nerve* **3**, 298–303.

Darras, B. T. and Francke, U. (1987). A partial deletion of the muscular dystrophy gene transmitted twice by an unaffected male. *Nature* **329**, 556–8.

—— and Francke, U. (1988). Normal human genomic restriction-fragment patterns and polymorphisms revealed by hybridization with the entire dystrophin cDNA. *American Journal of Human Genetics* **43**, 612–19.

——, Harper, J. F., and Francke, U. (1987). Prenatal diagnosis and detection of carriers with DNA probes in Duchenne's muscular dystrophy. *New England Journal of Medicine* **316**, 985–92.

Davie, A. M. and Emery, A. E. H. (1978). Estimation of proportion of new mutants among cases of Duchenne muscular dystrophy. *Journal of Medical Genetics* **15**, 339–45.

Davies, K. (1992). Moving straight to the target. *Nature* **358**, 519.

Davies, K. E., Young, B. D., Elles, R. G., Hill, M. E., and Williamson, R. (1981). Cloning of a representative genomic library of the human X chromosome after sorting by flow cytometry. *Nature* **293**, 374–6.

——, Pearson, P. L., Harper, P. S., *et al.* (1983). Linkage analysis of two cloned DNA sequences flanking the Duchenne muscular dystrophy locus on the short arm of the human X chromosome. *Nucleic Acids Research* **11**, 2303–12.

——, Briand, P., Ionasescu, V., *et al.* (1985*a*). Gene for OTC: characterization and linkage to Duchenne muscular dystrophy. *Nucleic Acids Research* **13**, 155–65.

——, Speer, A., Herrmann, F., *et al.* (1985*b*). Human X chromosome markers and Duchenne muscular dystrophy. *Nucleic Acids Research* **13**, 3419–26.

——, Thomas, N. H., Daniels, R. J., and Dubowitz, V. (1991). Molecular studies of spinal muscular atrophy. *Neuromuscular Disorders* **1**, 83–5.

De Coster, W., De Reuck, J., and Thiery, E. (1974). A late autosomal dominant form of limb-girdle muscular dystrophy. A clinical, genetic and morphological study. *European Neurology* **12**, 159-72.

Delaporte, C., Dautreaux, B., Rouche, A., and Fardeau, M. (1990). Changes in surface morphology and basal lamina of cultured muscle cells from Duchenne muscular dystrophy patients. *Journal of the Neurological Sciences* **95**, 77-88.

Dellamonica, C., Collombel, C., Cotte, J., and Addis, P. (1983). Screening for neonatal Duchenne muscular dystrophy by bioluminescence measurement of creatine kinase in a blood sample spotted on paper. *Clinical Chemistry* **29**, 161-3.

Demany, M. A., and Zimmerman, H. A. (1969). Progressive muscular dystrophy: haemodynamic, angiographic and pathologic study of a patient with myocardial involvement. *Circulation* **40**, 377-84.

Démos, J. (1961). Un nouveau problème posé par la myopathie humaine; les troubles des temps de circulation et leur liaison avec l'activité enzymatique sérique. *Bulletin et Mémoires de la Societe Médicine Hôpital (Paris)* **77**, 636-46.

—— and Maroteaux, P. (1961). Mesure des temps de circulation chez 141 sujets normaux par une technique originale. Rôle de la taille de l'enfant sur les temps de circulation de bras à bras. *Revue Française Études Clinique et Biologie* **6**, 773-8.

——, Dreyfus, J. C., Schapira, F., and Schapira, G. (1962). Anomalies biologiques chez les transmetteurs apparement sains de la myopathie. *Revue Canadienne de Biologie* **21**, 587-97.

——, Tuil, D., Berthelon, M., *et al.* (1976). Progressive muscular dystrophy — functional improvement after a renal allograft. *Journal of the Neurological Sciences* **30**, 41-53.

Den Dunnen, J. T., Grootscholten, P. M., Bakker, E., *et al.* (1989). Topography of the Duchenne muscular dystrophy (DMD) gene: FIGE and cDNA analysis of 194 cases reveals 115 deletions and 13 duplications. *American Journal of Human Genetics* **45**, 835-47.

——, Casula, L., Makover, A., *et al.* (1991). Mapping of dystrophin brain promoter: a deletion of this region is compatible with normal intellect. *Neuromuscular Disorders* **1**, 327-31.

——, Grootscholten, P. M., Dauwerse, J. G., *et al.* (1992). Reconstruction of the 2.4 Mb human DMD-gene by homologous YAC recombination. *Human Molecular Genetics* **1**, 19-28.

Dennis, N. R., Evans, K., Clayton, B., and Carter, C. O. (1976). Use of creatine kinase for detecting severe X-linked muscular dystrophy carriers. *British Medical Journal* **2**, 577-9.

Denny-Brown, D. (1949). Interpretation of the electromyogram. *Archives of Neurology and Psychiatry* **61**, 99-128.

Desai, A. D., Jayam, A. V., Banerji, A. P., Kohiyar, F. N., and Ardhapurkar, I. (1969). Study of the central nervous system in Duchenne type of muscular dystrophy. *Neurology, India* **17**, 184-90.

DeSilva, S., Drachman, D. B., Mellits, D., and Kuncl, R. W. (1987). Prednisone treatment in Duchenne muscular dystrophy. *Archives of Neurology* **44**, 818-22.

Desnick, R. J. (ed.) (1991). *Treatment of genetic diseases.* Churchill Livingstone, Edinburgh.

Dickey, R. P., Ziter, F. A., and Smith, R. A. (1984). Emery-Dreifuss muscular dystrophy. *Journal of Pediatrics* **104**, 555-9.

Dickson, G., Love, D. R., Davies, K. E., Wells, K. E., Piper, T. A., and Walsh, F. S. (1991). Human dystrophin gene transfer: production and expression of a functional recombinant DNA-based gene. *Human Genetics* **88**, 53–8.

DiMarco, A. F., Kelling, J. S., DiMarco, M. S., Jacobs, I., Shields, R., and Altose, M. D. (1985). The effects of inspiratory resistive training on respiratory muscle function in patients with muscular dystrophy. *Muscle and Nerve* **8**, 284–90.

DiMauro, S. and Rowland, L. P. (1976). Urinary excretion of carnitine in Duchenne muscular dystrophy. *Archives of Neurology* **33**, 204–5.

——, Angelini, C., and Catani, C. (1967). Enzymes of the glycogen cycle and glycolysis in various human neuromuscular disorders. *Journal of Neurology, Neurosurgery and Psychiatry* **30**, 411–15.

Dominici, P., Bonfiglioli, S., Merlini, L., and Granata, C. (1984). Implicazioni cardiache nella sindrome di Emery–Dreifuss. *Cardiomyology* **3**, 47–52.

Donner, M., Rapola, J., and Somer, H. (1975). Congenital muscular dystrophy: a clinico-pathological and follow-up study of 15 patients. *Neuropädiatrie* **6**, 239–58.

Dorkins, H., Junien, C., Mandel, J. L., *et al.* (1985). Segregation analysis of a marker localised Xp 21.2–Xp 21.3 in Duchenne and Becker muscular dystrophy families. *Human Genetics* **71**, 103–7.

D'Orsogna, L., O'Shea, J. P., and Miller, G. (1988). Cardiomyopathy of Duchenne muscular dystrophy. *Pediatric Cardiology* **9**, 205–13.

Drachman, D. B., Toyka, K. V., and Myer, E. (1974). Prednisone in Duchenne muscular dystrophy. *Lancet* **2**, 1409–12.

Dreifuss, F. E. and Hogan, G. R. (1961). Survival in X-chromosomal muscular dystrophy. *Neurology* **11**, 734–7.

Drennan, J. C. (1984). Surgical management of neuromuscular scoliosis. In *Neuromuscular diseases*, (ed. G. Serratrice *et al.*), pp. 551–6. Raven Press, New York.

Dreyfus, J. C., Schapira, G., Schapira, F., and Démos, J. (1956). Activités enzymatique du muscle humain. Recherches sur la biochimie comparée de l'homme normal et myopathique et du rat. *Clinica Chimica Acta* **1**, 434–49.

——, Schapira, G., and Démos, J. (1960). Étude de la créatine-kinase sérique chez les myopathies et leurs familles. *Revue Française Études Clinique et Biologie* **5**, 384–6.

——, Démos, J., Schapira, F., and Schapira, G. (1962). La lacticodéshydrogénase musculaire chez le myopathie: persistance apparente du type foetal. *Comptes Rendus de l'Academie des Sciences* **254**, 4384–6.

Driessen-Kletter, M. F., Amelink, G. J., Bär, P. R., and van Gijn, J. (1990). Myoglobin is a sensitive marker of increased muscle membrane vulnerability. *Journal of Neurology* **237**, 234–8.

Drummond, L. M. (1979). Creatine phosphokinase levels in the newborn and their use in screening for Duchenne muscular dystrophy. *Archives of Disease in Childhood* **54**, 362–6.

—— and Veale, A. M. O. (1978). Muscular dystrophy screening. *Lancet* **i**, 1258–9.

Du Bois, D. and Du Bois, E. F. (1916). A formula to estimate the approximate surface area if height and weight be known. *Archives of Internal Medicine* **17**, 863–71.

Dubowitz, V. (1960). Progressive muscular dystrophy of the Duchenne type in females and its mode of inheritance. *Brain* **83**, 432–9.

—— (1963a). Some clinical observations on childhood muscular dystrophy. *British Journal of Clinical Practice* **17**, 283–8.

—— (1963*b*). Myopathic changes in a muscular dystrophy carrier. *Journal of Neurology, Neurosurgery and Psychiatry* **26**, 322–5.

—— (1965). Intellectual impairment in muscular dystrophy. *Archives of Disease in Childhood* **40**, 296–301.

—— (1978). *Muscle disorders in childhood*. Saunders, London.

—— (1982). Carrier detection. In *Disorders of the motor unit*, (ed. D. L. Schotland), pp. 858–9. Wiley, Chichester.

—— (1985). *Muscle biopsy – a practical approach*, (2nd edn). Ballière Tindall, London.

—— (1988). *Muscle disorders in childhood*, (2nd edn). Saunders, London.

—— (1989). *A colour atlas of muscle disorders in childhood*. Wolfe Medical Publications, London.

—— (1991*a*). Chaos in classification of the spinal muscular atrophies of childhood. *Neuromuscular Disorders* **1**, 77–80.

—— (1991*b*). Prednisone in Duchenne dystrophy. *Neuromuscular Disorders* **1**, 161–3.

—— and Crome, L. (1969). The central nervous system in Duchenne muscular dystrophy. *Brain* **92**, 805–8.

—— and Heckmatt, J. (1980). Management of muscular dystrophy – pharmacological and physical aspects. *British Medical Bulletin* **36**, 139–44.

——, Hyde, S. A., Scott, O. M., and Goddard, C. (1984). Controlled trial of exercise in Duchenne muscular dystrophy. In *Neuromuscular diseases*, (ed. G. Serratrice *et al.*), pp. 571–5. Raven Press, New York.

Duchenne, G. B. A. (1861). *De l'electrisation localisée et son application à la pathologie et à la thérapeutique*, (2nd edn). Baillière et fils, Paris.

—— (1868). Recherches sur la paralysie musculaire pseudohypertrophique ou paralysie myo-sclérosique. *Archives Génerales de Médecine* **11**, 5–25, 179–209, 305–21, 421–43, 552–88.

Dudley, M. and Gibson, W. C. (1964). Photomicrographic study on the capillary nail beds of muscular dystrophy patients. *Canadian Medical Association Journal* **90**, 1226–8.

Duncan, C. J. (1978). Role of intracellular calcium in promoting muscle damage: a strategy for controlling the dystrophic condition. *Experientia* **34**, 1531–5.

—— (1989). Dystrophin and the integrity of the sarcolemma in Duchenne muscular dystrophy. *Experientia* **45**, 175–7.

Dunger, D. B., Davies, K. E., Pembrey, M., *et al.* (1986). Deletion on the X chromosome detected by direct DNA analysis in one of two unrelated boys with glycerol kinase deficiency, adrenal hypoplasia, and Duchenne muscular dystrophy. *Lancet* **i**, 585–7.

Durnin, R. E., Ziska, J. H., and Zellweger, H. (1971). Observations on the electrocardiogram in Duchenne's progressive muscular dystrophy. *Helvetica Paediatrica Acta* **26**, 331–9.

EAMDA (1984). Registration of patients with neuromuscular diseases in Europe. In *Research into the origin and treatment of muscular dystrophy*, (ed. L. P. ten Kate, P. L. Pearson, and A. M. Stadhouders), pp. 82–7. Excerpta Medica, Amsterdam.

Ebashi, S., Toyokura, Y., Momoi, H., and Sugita, H. (1959). High creatine phosphokinase activity of sera of progressive muscular dystrophy. *Journal of Biochemistry (Tokyo)* **46**, 103–4.

Edwards, J. H. (1989). Familiarity, recessivity and germline mosaicism. *Annals of Human Genetics* **53**, 33–47.

Edwards, R. H. T. (1977). Energy metabolism in normal and dystrophic human muscle. In *Pathogenesis of human muscular dystrophies*, (ed. L. P. Rowland), pp. 415–28. Excerpta Medica, Amsterdam.

—— and McDonnell, M. (1974). Hand-held dynamometer for evaluating voluntary-muscle function. *Lancet* **ii**, 757–8.

——, Young, A., and Wiles, M. (1980). Needle biopsy of skeletal muscle in the diagnosis of myopathy and the clinical study of muscle function and repair. *New England Journal of Medicine* **302**, 261–71.

Edwards, R. J., Watts, D. C., Watts, R. L., and Rodeck, C. H. (1984). Creatine kinase estimation in pure fetal blood samples for the prenatal diagnosis of Duchenne muscular dystrophy. *Prenatal Diagnosis* **4**, 267–77.

Eiholzer, U., Boltshauser, E., Frey, D., *et al.* (1988). Short stature: a common feature in Duchenne muscular dystrophy. *European Journal of Pediatrics* **147**, 602–5.

Ellis, D. A. (1978). Changes in muscle enzymes in Duchenne dystrophy and their possible relations to functional disturbance. In *The biochemistry of myasthenia gravis and muscular dystrophy*, (ed. G. G. Lunt and R. M. Marchbanks), pp. 245–65. Academic Press, London.

—— (1980). Intermediary metabolism of muscle in Duchenne muscular dystrophy. *British Medical Bulletin* **36**, 165–71.

Ellis, F. R. (1981). Muscle disease. In *Inherited disease and anaesthesia*, (ed. F. R. Ellis), pp. 315–36. Elsevier, Amsterdam.

—— and Heffron, J. J. A. (1985). Clinical and biochemical aspects of malignant hyperpyrexia. In *Recent advances in anaesthesia and analgesia*, (ed. R. S. Atkinson and A. P. Adams), pp. 173–207. Churchill Livingstone, Edinburgh.

Ellis, J. M., Nguyen thi Man, Morris, G. E. *et al.* (1990). Specificity of dystrophin analysis improved with monoclonal antibodies. *Lancet* **336**, 881–2.

Emanuel, B. S., Zackai, E. H., and Tucker, S. H. (1983). Further evidence for Xp21 location of Duchenne muscular dystrophy (DMD) locus: X;9 translocation in a female with DMD. *Journal of Medical Genetics* **20**, 461–3.

Emery, A. E. H. (1963). Clinical manifestations in two carriers of Duchenne muscular dystrophy. *Lancet* **i**, 1126–8.

—— (1964a). Hereditary myopathies. *Clinical Orthopaedics and Related Research* **33**, 164–73.

—— (1964b). Electrophoretic pattern of lactic dehydrogenase in carriers and patients with Duchenne muscular dystrophy. *Nature* **201**, 1044–5.

—— (1965a). Carrier detection in sex-linked muscular dystrophy. *Journal de Génétique Humaine* **14**, 318–29.

—— (1965b). Muscle histology in carriers of Duchenne muscular dystrophy. *Journal of Medical Genetics* **2**, 1–7.

—— (1967a). The determination of lactate dehydrogenase isoenzymes in normal human muscle and other tissues. *Biochemical Journal* **105**, 599–604.

—— (1967b). The use of serum creatine kinase for detecting carriers of Duchenne muscular dystrophy. In *Exploratory concepts in muscular dystrophy and related disorders*, (ed. A. T. Milhorat), pp. 90–7. Excerpta Medica, Amsterdam.

—— (1968). Muscle lactate dehydrogenase isoenzymes in hereditary myopathies. *Journal of the Neurological Sciences* **7**, 137–48.

—— (1969*a*). Abnormalities of the electrocardiogram in female carriers of Duchenne muscular dystrophy. *British Medical Journal* **2**, 418–20.

—— (1969*b*). Genetic counselling in X-linked muscular dystrophy. *Journal of the Neurological Sciences* **8**, 579–87.

—— (1971). The nosology of the spinal muscular atrophies. *Journal of Medical Genetics* **8**, 481–95.

—— (1972). Abnormalities of the electrocardiogram in hereditary myopathies. *Journal of Medical Genetics* **9**, 8–12.

—— (1977*a*). Muscle histology and creatine kinase levels in the foetus in Duchenne muscular dystrophy. *Nature* **266**, 472–3.

—— (1977*b*). Genetic considerations in the X-linked muscular dystrophies. In *Pathogenesis of human muscular dystrophies*, (ed. L. P. Rowland), pp. 42–52. Excerpta Medica, Amsterdam.

—— (1980). Duchenne muscular dystrophy. Genetic aspects, carrier detection and antenatal diagnosis. *British Medical Bulletin* **36**, 117–22.

—— (1982). Prevention of Duchenne muscular dystrophy: genetic counselling and prenatal diagnosis. In *New approaches to nerve and muscle disorders: basic and applied contributions*, (ed. A. D. Kidman, J. K. Tomkins, and R. A. Westerman), pp. 332–41. Excerpta Medica, Amsterdam.

—— (1984). Genetic heterogeneity in Duchenne muscular dystrophy. *Journal of Medical Genetics* **21**, 76–7.

—— (1985). *An introduction to recombinant DNA*. Wiley, Chichester.

—— (1986). *Methodology in medical genetics — an introduction to statistical methods*, (2nd edn). Churchill Livingstone, Edinburgh.

—— (1987). X-linked muscular dystrophy with early contractures and cardiomyopathy (Emery-Dreifuss type). *Clinical Genetics* **32**, 360–7.

—— (1988). Genetic aspects of neuromuscular disease. In *Disorders of voluntary muscle*, (5th end), (ed J. N. Walton), pp. 869–90. Churchill Livingstone, Edinburgh.

—— (1989*a*). Emery-Dreifuss muscular dystrophy and other related disorders. *British Medical Bulletin* **45**, 772–87.

—— (1989*b*). Emery-Dreifuss syndrome. *Journal of Medical Genetics* **26**, 637–41.

—— (1990*a*). The muscular dystrophies. In *Principles and practice of medical genetics*, (2nd edn), (ed. A. H. Emery and D. L. Rimoin), Vol. 1, pp. 539–63. Churchill Livingstone, Edinburgh.

—— (1990*b*). Mosaic pattern of dystrophin in DMD. *Pediatric Neurology* **6**, 282.

—— (1991*a*). Population frequencies of inherited neuromuscular diseases — a world survey. *Neuromuscular Disorders* **1**, 19–29.

—— (1991*b*). Clinical and genetic heterogeneity in spinal muscular atrophy — the multiple allele model. *Neuromuscular Disorders* **1**, 307–8.

—— (1991*c*). Genetic registers: problems old and new. In *Molecular genetics in medicine*, (ed. D. F. Roberts and R. Chester), pp. 184–92. Macmillan, Basingstoke.

—— and Burt, D. (1980). Intracellular calcium and pathogenesis and antenatal diagnosis of Duchenne muscular dystrophy. *British Medical Journal* **280**, 355–7.

—— and Dreifuss, F. E. (1966). Unusual type of benign X-linked muscular dystrophy. *Journal of Neurology, Neurosurgery and Psychiatry* **29**, 338–42.

—— and Emery, M. (1993). Edward Meryon and muscular dystrophy (In press).

—— and Holloway, S. (1977). Use of normal daughters' and sisters' creatine kinase levels in estimating heterozygosity in Duchenne muscular dystrophy. *Human Heredity* **27**, 118–26.

—— and Holloway, S. (1982). Familial motor neuron diseases. In *Human motor neuron diseases*, (ed. L. P. Rowland), pp. 139–45. Raven Press, New York.

—— and McGregor, L. (1977). The foetus in Duchenne muscular dystrophy: muscle growth in tissue culture. *Clinical Genetics* **12**, 183–7.

—— and Miller, J. R. (eds) (1976). *Registers for the detection and prevention of genetic disease.* Symposia Specialists, Miami, and Stratton, New York.

—— and Morton, R. (1968). Genetic counselling in lethal X-linked disorders. *Acta Genetica (Basel)* **18**, 534–42.

—— and Pascasio, F. M. (1965). The effects of pregnancy on the concentration of creatine kinase in serum, skeletal muscle, and myometrium. *American Journal of Obstetrics and Gynecology* **91**, 18–22.

—— and Schelling, J. L. (1965). Limb blood flow in patients and carriers of Duchenne muscular dystrophy. *Acta Genetica (Basel)* **15**, 337–44.

—— and Skinner, R. (1976). Clinical studies in benign (Becker type) X-linked muscular dystrophy. *Clinical Genetics* **10**, 189–201.

—— and Skinner, R. (1983). Double-blind controlled trial of a 'calcium blocker' in Duchenne muscular dystrophy. *Cardiomyology* **2**, 13–23.

—— and Smith, C. (1970). Ascertainment and prevention of genetic disease. *British Medical Journal* **3**, 636–7.

—— and Spikesman, A. M. (1970*a*). The existence of a subclinical form of Duchenne muscular dystrophy? In *Muscle diseases*, (ed. J. N. Walton, N. Canal, and G. Scarlato), pp. 424–30. Excerpta Medica, Amsterdam.

—— and Spikesman, A. M. (1970*b*). Evidence against the existence of a subclinical form of X-linked Duchenne muscular dystrophy. *Journal of the Neurological Sciences* **10**, 523–33.

—— and Walton, J. N. (1967). The genetics of muscular dystrophy. *Progress in Medical Genetics* **5**, 116–45.

——, Teasdall, R. D., and Coomes, E. N. (1966). Electromyographic studies in carriers of Duchenne muscular dystrophy. *Bulletin of the Johns Hopkins Hospital* **118**, 439–43.

——, King, B., and Brock, D. J. H. (1971). Leucocyte metabolism in hereditary neuromuscular disorders. *Journal of the Neurological Sciences* **14**, 463–8.

——, Watt, M. S., and Clack, E. R. (1972). The effects of genetic counselling in Duchenne muscular dystrophy. *Clinical Genetics* **3**, 147–150.

——, Anderson, A. R., and Noronha, M. J. (1973*a*). Electromyographic studies in parents of children with spinal muscular atrophy. *Journal of Medical Genetics* **10**, 8–10.

——, Watt, M. S., and Clack, E. (1973*b*). Social effects of genetic counselling. *British Medical Journal* **1**, 724–6.

——, Elliott, D., Moores, M., and Smith, C. (1974). A genetic register system (RAPID). *Journal of Medical Genetics* **11**, 145–51.

——, Hausmanowa-Petrusewicz, I., Davie, A. M., Holloway, S., Skinner, R., and Borkowska, J. (1976*a*). International collaborative study of the spinal muscular atrophies. Part 1. Analysis of clinical and laboratory data. *Journal of the Neurological Sciences* **29**, 83–94.

——, Davie, A. M., Holloway, S., and Skinner, R. (1976*b*). International collaborative study of the spinal muscular atrophies. Part 2. Analysis of genetic data. *Journal of the Neurological Sciences* **30**, 375–84.

——, Brough, C., Crawfurd, M. D'A., Harper, P., Harris, R., and Oakshott, G. (1978). A report on genetic registers. *Journal of Medical Genetics* **15**, 435–42.

——, Burt, D., Dubowitz, V., *et al.* (1979*a*). Antenatal diagnosis of Duchenne muscular dystrophy. *Lancet* **i**, 847–9.

——, Skinner, R., and Holloway, S. (1979*b*). A study of possible heterogeneity in Duchenne muscular dystrophy. *Clinical Genetics* **15**, 444–9.

——, Raeburn, J. A., Skinner, R., Holloway, S., and Lewis, P. (1979*c*). Prospective study of genetic counselling. *British Medical Journal* **1**, 1253–6.

——, Skinner, R., Howden, L. C., and Matthews, M. B. (1982). Verapamil in Duchenne muscular dystrophy. *Lancet* **i**, 559.

Emslie-Smith, A. M., Arahata, K., and Engel, A. G. (1989). Major histocompatibility complex class I antigen expression, immunolocalization of interferon subtypes, and T cell-mediated cytotoxicity in myopathies. *Human Pathology* **20**, 224–31.

Engel, A. G. and Arahata, K. (1986). Mononuclear cells in myopathies. *Human Pathology* **17**, 704–21.

—— and Banker, B. Q. (1986). *Myology*, (2 vols). McGraw Hill, New York.

—— and Biesecker, G. (1982). Complement activation in muscle fiber necrosis: demonstration of the membrane attack complex of complement in necrotic fibers. *Annals of Neurology* **12**, 289–96.

——, Arahata, K., and Biesecker, G. (1984). Mechanisms of muscle fiber destruction. In *Neuromuscular diseases*, (ed. G. Serratrice *et al.*), pp. 137–41. Raven Press, New York.

Engel, W. K. (1970). Selective and nonselective susceptibility of muscle fibre types. A new approach to human neuromuscular diseases. *Archieves of Neurology* **22**, 97–117.

—— (1975). The vascular hypothesis. In *Recent advances in myology*, (ed. W. G. Bradley, D. Gardner-Medwin, and J. N. Walton), pp. 166–73. Excerpta Medica, Amsterdam.

England, S. B., Nicholson, L. V. B., Johnson, M. A., *et al.* (1990). Very mild muscular dystrophy associated with the deletion of 46% of dystrophin. *Nature* **343**, 180–2.

Ennor, A. H. and Rosenberg, H. (1954). Some properties of creatine phosphokinase. *Biochemical Journal* **57**, 203–12.

Erb, W. H. (1884). Über die 'juvenile Form' der progressiven Muskelatrophie und ihre Beziehungen zur sogenannten Pseudohypertrophie der Muskeln. *Deutsches Archiv für Klinische Medizin* **34**, 467–519.

—— (1891). Dystrophia muscularis progressiva—Klinische und pathologisch-anatomische Studien. *Deutsche Zeitschrift für Nervenheilkunde* **1**, 13–261.

Ervasti, J. M. and Campbell, K. P. (1991). Membrane organization of the dystrophin–glycoprotein complex. *Cell* **66**, 1121–31.

——, Ohlendieck, K., Kahl, S. D., *et al.* (1990). Deficiency of glycoprotein component of the dystrophin complex in dystrophic muscle. *Nature* **345**, 315–19.

——, Kahl, S. D., and Campbell, K. P. (1991). Purification of dystrophin from skeletal muscle. *Journal of Biological Chemistry* **266**, 9161–5.

van Essen, A. J. and ten Kate, L. P. (1984). Epidemiologic survey of Duchenne muscular dystrophy in the Netherlands. Preliminary results. In *Research into the origin and treatment of muscular dystrophy*, (ed. L. P. ten Kate, P. L. Pearson, and A. M. Stadhouders), pp. 33–40. Excerpta Medica, Amsterdam.

——, Busch, H. F. M., te Meerman, G. J., and ten Kate, L. P. (1992*a*). Birth and population prevalence of Duchenne muscular dystrophy in the Netherlands. *Human Genetics* **88**, 258–66.

——, Abbs, S., Baiget, M., *et al.* (1992*b*). Parental origin and germline mosaicism of deletions and duplications of the dystrophin gene: a European study. *Human Genetics* **88**, 249–57.

Etiemble, J., Kahn, A., Boivin, P., Bernard, J. F., and Goudemand, M. (1976). Hereditary hemolytic anemia with erythrocyte phosphofructokinase deficiency. Studies of some properties of erythrocytes and muscle enzymes. *Human Genetics* **31**, 83–91.

Evans, C. D. H. and Lacey, J. H. (1986). Toxicity of vitamins: complications of a health movement. *British Medical Journal* **292**, 509–10.

Evans, M. I., Greb, A., Kunkel, L. M., *et al.* (1991). In utero fetal muscle biopsy for the diagnosis of Duchenne muscular dystrophy. *American Journal of Obstetrics and Gynecology* **165**, 728–32.

Fadda, S., Mochi, M., Roncuzzi, L., *et al.* (1985). Definitive localization of Becker muscular dystrophy in Xp by linkage to a cluster of DNA polymorphisms (DXS43 and DXS9). *Human Genetics* **71**, 33–6.

Faganel, J., Lavrič, A., Sršen, V., and Tivadar, I. (1977). Degenerativne živčano-mišićne bolesti u Sloveniji. *Neurologija (Yugoslavia)* **25**, 29–33.

Falcão-Conceição, D. N., Gonçalves-Pimentel, M. M., Baptista, M. L., and Ubatuba, S. (1983*a*). Detection of carriers of X-linked gene for Duchenne muscular dystrophy by levels of creatine kinase and pyruvate kinase. *Journal of the Neurological Sciences* **62**, 171–80.

——, Pereira, M. C. G., Gonçalves, M. M., and Baptista, M. L. (1983*b*). Familial occurrence of heterozygous manifestations in X-linked muscular dystrophies. *Brazilian Journal of Genetics* **6**, 527–38.

Falek, A. (1977). Use of the coping process to achieve psychological homeostasis in genetic counseling. In *Genetic counseling*, (ed. H. A. Lubs and F. de la Cruz), pp. 179–88. Raven Press, New York.

—— (1984). Sequential aspects of coping and other issues in decision making in genetic counseling. In *Psychological aspects of gentic counselling*, (ed. A. E. H. Emery and I. M. Pullen), pp. 23–36. Academic Press, London.

Falewski de Leon, G. H. (1984). Orthotic jackets for scoliosis. In *Neuromuscular diseases*, (ed. G. Serratrice *et al.*), pp. 539–43. Raven Press, New York.

Fanin, M., Danieli, G. A., Vitiello, L., Senter, L., and Angelini, C. (1992). Prevalence of dystrophin-positive fibers in 85 Duchenne muscular dystrophy patients. *Neuromuscular Disorders* **2**, 41–5.

Fardeau, M., Tomé, F. M. S., Collin, H., *et al.* (1990). Présence d'une protéine de type dystrophine au niveau de la jonction neuromusculaire dans la dystrophie musculaire de Duchenne et la souris mutante 'mdx'. *Comptes Rendus de l'Academie des Sciences, Serie III, Sciences de la Vie* **311**, 197–204.

Feener, C. A., Koenig, M., and Kunkel, L. M. (1989). Alternative splicing of human dystrophin mRNA generates isoforms at the carboxy terminus. *Nature* **338**, 509–11.

——, Boyce, F. M., and Kunkel, L. M. (1991). Rapid detection of CA polymorphisms in cloned DNA: application to the 5′ region of the dystrophin gene. *American Journal of Human Genetics* **48**, 621-7.

Feiling, A. (1958). *A history of the Maida Vale Hospital for nervous diseases*. Butterworths, London.

Feingold, J., Feingold, N., and Démos, J. (1971). Gènes majeurs, gènes modificateurs et effets du milieu dans la myopathie de Duchenne de Boulogne. *Annales de Génétique* **14**, 207-11.

Fenichel, G. M., Sul, Y. C., Kilroy, A. W., and Blouin, R. (1982). An autosomal-dominant dystrophy with humeropelvic distribution and cardiomyopathy. *Neurology* **32**, 1399-1401.

——, Mendell, J. R., Moxley, R. T., *et al.* (1990). Prednisone treatment of Duchenne dystrophy. *Journal of the Neurological Sciences* **98** (Suppl.), 421 (Astract).

——, Florence, J. M., Pestronk, A., *et al.* (1991). Long-term benefit from prednisone therapy in Duchenne muscular dystrophy. *Neurology* **41**, 1874-7.

Ferrari, E., Intino, M. T., Perniola, T., and Russo, M. G. (1980). Epidemiology of Duchenne dystrophy and carrier detection in Puglia. Preliminary reports. In *Muscular dystrophy research: advances and new trends*, (ed. C. Angelini, G. A. Danieli, and D. Fontanari), pp. 264-5. Excerpta Medica, Amsterdam.

Ferretti, G., Tangorra, A., and Curatola, G. (1990). Effects of intramembrane particle aggregation on erythrocyte membrane fluidity: an electron spin resonance study in normal and in dystrophic subjects. *Experimental Cell Research* **191**, 14-21.

Ferrier, P., Bamatter, F., and Klein, D. (1965). Muscular dystrophy (Duchenne) in a girl with Turner's syndrome. *Journal of Medical Genetics* **2**, 38-46.

Fiacchino, F., Bricchi, M., Balestrini, M. R., *et al.* (1984). La rabdomiolisi anestesiologica nella distrofia muscolare. Segnalazione di un caso. *Minerva Anestesiologica* **50**, 521-6.

Fidziańska, A., Goebel, H. H., Kosswig, R., and Burck, U. (1984). 'Killer' cells in Duchenne disease: Ultrastructural study. *Neurology* **34**, 295-303.

Fingerman, E., Campisi, J., and Pardee, A. B. (1984). Defective Ca^{2+} metabolism in Duchenne muscular dystrophy: effects on cellular and viral growth. *Proceedings of the National Academy of Sciences USA* **81**, 7617-21.

Firth, M. A. (1983). Diagnosis of Duchenne muscular dystrophy: experiences of parents and sufferers. *British Medical Journal* **286**, 700-1.

—— and Wilkinson, E. J. (1983). Screening the newborn for Duchenne muscular dystrophy: parents' views. *British Medical Journal* **286**, 1933-4.

Fischbeck, K. H., Ritter, A. W., Tirschwell, D. L., *et al.* (1986). Recombination with PERT 87 (DXS 164) in families with X-linked muscular dystrophy. *Lancet* **ii**, 104.

Fisher, E. R., Wassinger, A., Gerneth, J. A., and Danowski, T. S. (1972). Ultrastructural changes in skeletal muscle of muscular dystrophy carriers. *Archives of Pathology* **94**, 456-60.

Fisher, R. A. and Yates, F. (1967). *Statistical tables for biological, agricultural and medical research*, (6th edn). Oliver & Boyd, Edinburgh.

Fitzpatrick, C. and Barry, C. (1986). Communication within families about Duchenne muscular dystrophy. *Developmental Medicine and Child Neurology* **28**, 596-9.

——, Barry, C., and Garvey, C. (1986). Psychiatric disorder among boys with Duchenne muscular dystrophy. *Developmental Medicine and Child Neurology* **28**, 589–95.

Fitzsimons, R. B. and Hoh, J. F. Y. (1981). Embryonic and foetal myosins in human skeletal muscle. The presence of foetal myosins in Duchenne muscular dystrophy and infantile spinal muscular atrophy. *Journal of the Neurological Sciences* **52**, 367–84.

Florek, M. and Karolak, S. (1977). Intelligence level of patients with the Duchenne type of progressive muscular dystrophy (PMD-D). *European Journal of Pediatrics* **126**, 275–82.

Fong, P., Turner, P. R., Denetclaw, W. F., and Steinhardt, R. A. (1990). Increased activity of calcium leak channels in myotubes of Duchenne human and *mdx* mouse origin. *Science* **250**, 673–5.

Forrest, S. M., Cross, G. S., Speer, A., Gardner-Medwin, D., Burn, J., and Davies, K. E. (1987*a*). Preferential deletion of exons in Duchenne and Becker muscular dystrophies. *Nature* **329**, 638–40.

——, Smith, T. J., Cross, G. S., *et al.* (1987*b*). Effective strategy for prenatal prediction of Duchenne and Becker muscular dystrophy. *Lancet* **ii**, 1294–6.

——, Smith, T. J., Cross, G. S., *et al.* (1988). Molecular analysis and diagnosis of Duchenne muscular dystrophy. *Journal of the Royal College of Physicians (London)* **22**, 65–7.

Fowler, W. M. and Nayak, N. N. (1983). Slowly progressive proximal weakness: limb-girdle syndromes. *Archives of Physical and Medical Rehabilitation* **64**, 527–38.

——, Pearson, C. M., Egstrom, G. H., and Gardner, G. W. (1965). Ineffective treatment of muscular dystrophy with an anabolic steroid and other measures. *New England Journal of Medicine* **272**, 875–82.

Francke, U., Ochs, H. D., de Martinville, B., *et al.* (1985). Minor Xp21 chromosome deletion in a male associated with expression of Duchenne muscular dystrophy, chronic granulomatous disease, retinitis pigmentosa, and McLeod syndrome. *American Journal of Human Genetics* **37**, 250–67.

——, Darras, B. T., Hersh, J. H. *et al.* (1989). Brother/sister pairs affected with early-onset, progressive muscular dystrophy: molecular studies reveal etiologic heterogeneity. *American Journal of Human Genetics* **45**, 63–72.

Franco, Jr., A. and Lansman, J. B. (1990). Calcium entry through stretch-inactivated ion channels in *mdx* myotubes. *Nature* **344**, 670–3.

Frankel, K. A. and Rosser, R. J. (1976). The pathology of the heart in progressive muscular dystrophy: epimyocardial fibrosis. *Human Pathology* **7**, 375–86.

Franklin, G. I., Cavanagh, N. P. C., Hughes, B. P., Yasin, R., and Thompson, E. J. (1981). Creatine kinase isoenzymes in altered human muscle cells. I. Comparison of Duchenne muscular dystrophy with other myopathic and neurogenic diseases. *Clinica Chimica Acta* **115**, 179–89.

Fraser, F. C. (1963). Taking the family history. *American Journal of Medicine* **34**, 585–93.

Freeman, R. D. and Pearson, P. H. (1978). Counselling with parents. In *Care of the handicapped child*, (Clinics in Developmental Medicine, No. 67), (ed. J. Apley), pp. 35–47. Heinemann, London.

Frets, P. G., Duivenvoorden, H. J., Niermeijer, M. F., van de Berge, S. M. M., and Galjaard, H. (1990*a*). Factors influencing the reproductive decision after genetic counseling. *American Journal of Medical Genetics* **35**, 496–502.

——, Duivenvoorden, H. J., Verhage, F., Ketzer, E., and Niermeijer, M. F. (1990*b*). Model identifying the reproductive decision after genetic counselling. *American Journal of Medical Genetics* **35**, 503–9.

——, Duivenvoorden, H. J., Verhage, F., Peters-Romeyn, B. M. T., and Niermeijer, M. F. (1991). Analysis of problems in making the reproductive decision after genetic counselling. *Journal of Medical Genetics* **28**, 194–200.

Friedmann, T. (ed.) (1991). *Therapy for genetic disease.* Oxford University Press.

Frouhar, Z. R., Spiro, R., and Lubs, M. L. (1975). Familial carrier manifestations in families with X-linked Duchenne muscular dystrophy. *American Journal of Human Genetics* **27**, 37A (Abstract).

Fu, W. and Barbujani, G. (1990). Segregation and sporadic cases of Duchenne muscular dystrophy in the Henan province, China. *Human Heredity* **40**, 167–72.

Fukuyama, Y., Kawazura, M., and Haruna, H. (1960). A peculiar form of congenital progressive muscular dystrophy: report of 15 cases. *Paediatria, Tokyo* **4**, 5–8.

——, Osawa, M., and Suzuki, H. (1981). Congenital progressive muscular dystrophy of the Fukuyama type – clinical, genetic and pathological considerations. *Brain and Development* **3**, 1–29.

Furukawa, T. and Peter, J. B. (1977). X-linked muscular dystrophy. *Annals of Neurology* **2**, 414–16.

—— and Toyokura, Y. (1977). Congenital, hypotonic-sclerotic muscular dystrophy. *Journal of Medical Genetics* **14**, 426–9.

Gaffney, J. F., Kingston, W. J., Metlay, L. A., *et al.* (1989). Left ventricular thrombus and systemic emboli complicating the cardiomyopathy of Duchenne's muscular dystrophy. *Archives of Neurology* **46**, 1249–52.

Gaines, R. F., Pueschel, S. M., Sassaman, E. A., and Driscoll, J. L. (1982). Effect of exercise on serum creatine kinase in carriers of Duchenne muscular dystrophy. *Journal of Medical Genetics* **19**, 4–7.

Galasko, C. S. B., Delaney, C., and Morris, P. (1992). Spinal stabilisation in Duchenne muscular dystrophy. *Journal of Bone and Joint Surgery* **74B**, 210–14.

Galassi, G., Modena, M. G., Benassi, A., *et al.* (1986). Autosomal-dominant dystrophy with humeroperoneal weakness and cardiopathy: a genetic variant of Emery–Dreifuss disease? *Italian Journal of Neurological Sciences* **7**, 125–32.

Gale, A. N. and Murphy, E. A. (1979). The use of serum creatine phosphokinase in genetic counseling for Duchenne muscular dystrophy. *Journal of Chronic Diseases* **32**, 639–51.

Gardner-Medwin, D. (1970). Mutation rate in Duchenne type of muscular dystrophy. *Journal of Medical Genetics* **7**, 334–7.

—— (1975). The effects of genetic counselling in Duchenne muscular dystrophy. In *Recent advances in myology*, (ed. W. G. Bradley, D. Gardner-Medwin, and J. N. Walton), pp. 474–6. Excerpta Medica, Amsterdam.

—— (1977). Children with genetic muscular disorders. *British Journal of Hospital Medicine* **17**, 314–40.

—— (1982*a*). The natural history of Duchenne muscular dystrophy. In *Topics in child neurology*, (ed. G. B. Wise, M. E. Blaw, and P. G. Procopis), Vol. 2, pp. 17–29. S. P. Medical and Scientific Books, Spectrum Publications, New York.

—— (1982*b*). Uncertainties in the diagnosis of Duchenne muscular dystrophy. *Cardiomyology* **1**, 15–20.

—— (1992). *Duchenne muscular dystrophy. Some questions answered for parents who have just learned about the diagnosis.* Muscular Dystrophy Group of Great Britain and Northern Ireland, London.

—— and Johnston, H. M. (1984). Severe muscular dystrophy in girls. *Journal of the Neurological Sciences* **64**, 79–87.

—— and Sharples, P. (1989). Some studies of the Duchenne and autosomal recessive types of muscular dystrophy. *Brain and Development* **11**, 91–7.

——, Hudgson, P., and Walton, J. N. (1967). Benign spinal muscular atrophy arising in childhood and adolescence. *Journal of the Neurological Sciences* **5**, 121–58.

——, Bundey, S., and Greer, S. (1978). Early diagnosis of Duchenne muscular dystrophy. *Lancet* **i**, 1102.

Gaschen, F. P., Hoffman, E. P., Gorospe, J. R. M., *et al.* (1992). Dystrophin deficiency causes lethal muscle hypertrophy in cats. *Journal of the Neurological Sciences* (In press.)

Gerald, P. S. and Brown, J. A. (1974). Report of the Committee on the genetic constitution of the X chromosome. *Birth Defects Original Article Series* **10**, 29–34.

Gilchrist, J. M. and Leshner, R. T. (1986). Autosomal dominant humeroperoneal myopathy. *Archives of Neurology* **43**, 734–5.

Gilgenkrantz, H., Chelly, J., Lambert, M., Récan, D., Barbot, J. C., van Ommen, G. J. B., and Kaplan, J. C. (1989). Analysis of molecular deletions with cDNA probes in patients with Duchenne and Berker muscular dystrophies. *Genomics* **5**, 574–80.

Gilgenkrantz, S., Tridon, P., Pinel-Briquel, N., Beurey, J., and Weber, M. (1985). Translocation (X;9)(p11;q34) in a girl with incontinentia pigmenti (IP): implications for the regional assigment of the IP locus to Xp11. *Annales de Génétique* **28**, 90–2.

Gillard, E. F., Chamberlain, J. S., Murphy, E. G., *et al.* (1989). Molecular and phenotypic analysis of patients with deletions within the deletion-rich region of the Duchenne muscular dystrophy (DMD) gene. *American Journal of Human Genetics* **45**, 507–20.

Gilroy, J., Cahalan, J. L., Berman, R., and Newman, M. (1963). Cardiac and pulmonary complications in Duchenne's progressive muscular dystrophy. *Circulation* **27**, 484–93.

Ginjaar, I. B., Bakker, E., van Paassen, M. M. B., *et al.* (1991*a*). Immunohistochemical studies show truncated dystrophins in the myotubes of three fetuses at risk for Duchenne muscular dystrophy. *Journal of Medical Genetics* **28**, 505–10.

——, Soffers, S., Moorman, A. F. M., *et al.* (1991*b*). Fetal dystrophin to diagnose carrier status. *Lancet* **338**, 258–9.

Glass, I. A., Nicholson, L. V. B., Watkiss, E., *et al.* (1992). Investigation of a female manifesting Becker muscular dystrophy. *Journal of Medical Genetics* **29**, 578–82.

Golbus, M. S., Conte, F., Schneider, E., and Epstein, C. (1974). Intrauterine diagnosis of genetic defects: results, problems and follow-up of one hundred cases in a prenatal genetic detection center. *American Journal of Obstetrics and Gynecology* **118**, 897–905.

——, Stephens, J. D., Mahoney, M. J., *et al.* (1979). Failure of fetal creatine phosphokinase as a diagnostic indicator of Duchenne muscular dystrophy. *New England Journal of Medicine* **300**, 860–1.

Goldberg, S. J., Stern, L. Z., Feldman, L., Allen, H. D., Sahn, D. J., and Valdes-

Cruz, L. M. (1982). Serial two-dimensional echocardiography in Duchenne muscular dystrophy. *Neurology* **32**, 1101-5.

Gomez, M. R., Engel, A. G., Dewald, G., and Peterson, H. A. (1977). Failure of inactivation of Duchenne dystrophy X-chromosome in one of female identical twins. *Neurology* **27**, 537-41.

Gordon-Taylor, C. and Walls, E. W. (1958). *Sir Charles Bell: his life and times.* E. and S. Livingstone, Edinburgh.

Gorospe, J. R. M., Hoffman, E. P., McQuarrie, P. S. R., and Cardinet, G. H. (1991). Duchenne muscular dystrophy in a wire-haired fox (WHF) terrier: a new dog model with no somatic reversion. Proceedings of the VIIIth International Congress on Human Genetics. *American Journal of Human Genetics* **49** (Suppl.), 97 (Abstract).

Gorza, L., Ausoni, S., and Schiaffino, S. (1991). Re-expression of cardiac troponin T in regenerating muscle fibers of hunan dystrophic muscle. In *Muscular dystrophy research: from molecular diagnosis toward therapy*, (ed. C. Angelini, G. A. Danieli, and D. Fontanari), pp. 213-14. Excerpta Medica, Amsterdam.

Gospe, S. M., Lazaro, R. P., Lava, N. S., Grootscholten, P. M., Scott, M. O., and Fischbeck, K. H. (1989). Familial X-linked myalgia and cramps: A nonprogressive myopathy associated with a deletion in the dystrophin gene. *Neurology* **39**, 1277-80.

Goto, I., Ishimoto, S., Yamada, T., *et al.* (1986). The rigid spine syndrome and Emery–Dreifuss muscular dystrophy. *Clinical Neurology and Neurosurgery* **88**, 293-8.

Gottrand, F., Guillonneau, I., and Carpentier, A. (1991). Segmental colonic transit time in Duchenne dystrophy. *Archives of Disease in Childhood* **66**, 1262.

Gowers, W. R. (1879*a*). Clinical lecture on pseudo-hypertrophic muscular paralysis. *Lancet* **2**, 1-2, 37-9, 73-5, 113-16.

—— (1879*b*). *Pseudo-hypertrophic muscular paralysis — a clinical lecture.* J. and A. Churchill, London.

Granata, C., Merlini, L., Rubbini, L., Bonfiglioli, S., and Mattutini, P. (1984). Tenotomia sottocutanea del tendine di Achille in anestesia locale, nella distrofia muscolare di Duchenne. *Cardiomyology* **3**, 89-96.

Greenberg, C. R., Hamerton, J. L., Nigli, M., and Wrogemann, K. (1987). DNA studies in a family with Duchenne muscular dystrophy and a deletion at Xp2l. *American Journal of Human Genetics* **41**, 128-37.

——, Jacobs, H. K., Halliday, W., *et al.* (1991). Three years' experience with neonatal screening for Duchenne/Becker muscular dystrophy: gene analysis, gene expression, and phenotype prediction. *American Journal of Medical Genetics* **39**, 68-75.

Greenstein, R. M., Reardon, M. P., and Chan, T. S. (1977). An X/autosome translocation in a girl with Duchenne muscular dystrophy (DMD): evidence for DMD gene localization. *Pediatric Research* **11**, 457 (Abstract).

——, Reardon, M. P., Chan, T. S., *et al.* (1980). An (X;11) translocation in a girl with Duchenne muscular dystrophy. *Cytogenetics and Cell Genetics* **27**, 268.

Griffiths, R. D and Edwards, R. H. T. (1988). A new chart for weight control in Duchenne muscular dystrophy. *Archives of Disease in Childhood* **63**, 1256-8.

——, Cady, E. B., Edwards, R. H. T., and Wilkie, D. R. (1985). Muscle energy metabolism in Duchenne dystrophy studied by ^{31}P-NMR: controlled trials show no effect of allopurinol or ribose. *Muscle and Nerve* **8**, 760-7.

Griggs, R. C. and Karpati, G. (eds) (1990). *Myoblast transfer therapy*. Plenum Press, New York.

——, Moxley, R. T. III, Mendell, J. R., *et al.* (1991). Prednisone in Duchenne dystrophy: a randomized, controlled trial defining the time course and dose response. *Archives of Neurology* **48**, 383–8.

Grimm, T. (1981). Neugeborenen-Screening nach Duchennescher Muskeldystrophie. *Monatsschrift Kinderheilkunde* **129**, 414–17.

——, Müller, B., Dreier, M., *et al.* (1989). Hot spot of recombination within DXS164 in the Duchenne muscular dystrophy gene. *American Journal of Human Genetics* **45**, 368–72.

——, Müller, B., Müller, C. R., and Janka, M. (1990). Theoretical considerations on germline mosaicism in Duchenne muscular dystrophy. *Journal of Medical Genetics* **27**, 683–7.

Gros, F. (1992). Gene therapy: present situation and future prospects. *Neuromuscular Disorders* **2**, 75–83.

de Grouchy, J., Lamy, M., Frézal, J., and Garcin, R. (1963). Étude d'un couple de jumeaux monozygotes dont un seul est atteint de myopathie (Forme pseudohypertrophique). *Acta Geneticae Medicae et Gemellologiae (Roma)* **12**, 324–34.

Gudmundsson, K. R. (1968). The prevalence of some neurological diseases in Iceland. *Acta Neurologica Scandinavica* **44**, 57–69.

Guggenheim, M. A., McCabe, E. R. B., Roig, M., *et al.* (1980). Glycerol kinase deficiency with neuromuscular, skeletal, and adrenal abnormalities. *Annals of Neurology* **7**, 441–9.

Guibaud, P., Carrier, H. N., Plauchu, H., Lauras, B., Jolivet, M. J., and Robert, J. M. (1981). Manifestations musculaires précoces cliniques et histopathologiques, chez 14 garçons présentant dans la première année une activité sérique elevée de creatine-phosphokinase. *Journal de Génétique Humaine* **29**, 71–84.

Guilly, P. (1936). *Duchenne de Boulogne*. Baillière, Paris.

Gussoni, E., Pavlath, G. K., Lanctot, A. M., *et al.* (1992). Normal dystrophin transcripts detected in Duchenne muscular dystrophy patients after myoblast transplantation. *Nature* **356**, 435–8.

Gustavii, B., Löfberg, L., and Henriksson, K. G. (1983). Fetal muscle biopsy. *Acta Obstetrica et Gynecologica Scandinavica* **62**, 369–71.

Haldane, J. B. S. (1935). The rate of spontaneous mutation of a human gene. *Journal of Genetics* **31**, 317–26.

—— (1956). Mutation in the sex-linked recessive type of muscular dystrophy. A possible sex difference. *Annals of Human Genetics* **22**, 344–7.

Hall, J. G. (1988). Review and hypotheses: Somatic mosaicism: observations related to clinical genetics. *American Journal of Human Genetics* **43**, 355–63.

Hammond, J., Howard, N. J., Brookwell, R., Purvis-Smith, S., Wilcken, B., and Hoogenraad, N. (1985). Proposed assignment of loci for X-linked adrenal hypoplasia and glycerol kinase genes. *Lancet* **i**, 54.

Hara, H., Nagara, H., Mawatari, S., Kondo, A., and Sato, H. (1987). Emery-Dreifuss muscular dystrophy—an autopsy case. *Journal of the Neurological Sciences* **79**, 23–31.

Harper, P. S. (1982). Carrier detection in Duchenne muscular dystrophy: a critical assessment. In *Disorders of the motor unit*, (ed. D. L. Schotland), pp. 821–44. Wiley, Chichester.

——, O'Brien, T., Murray, J. M., Davies, K. E., Pearson, P., and Williamson, R.

(1983). The use of linked DNA polymorphisms for genotype prediction in families with Duchenne muscular dystrophy. *Journal of Medical Genetics* **20**, 252–4.

Harris, J. B. (ed.) (1979). *Muscular dystrophy and other inherited diseases of skeletal muscle in animals.* Annals of the New York Academy of Sciences, Vol. 317. Academy of Sciences, New York.

—— and Slater, C. R. (1980). Animal models: what is their relevance to the pathogenesis of human muscular dystrophy? *British Medical Bulletin* **36**, 193–7.

Hart, K. A., Hodgson, S., Walker, A., *et al.* (1987). DNA deletions in mild and severe Becker muscular dystrophy. *Human Genetics* **75**, 281–5.

Hassan, Z., Fastabend, C. P., Mohanty, P. K., and Isaacs, E. R. (1979). Atrioventricular block and supraventricular arrhythmias with X-linked muscular dystrophy. *Circulation* **60**, 1365–9.

Hastings, B. A., Groothuis, D. R., and Vick, N. A. (1980). Dominantly inherited pseudohypertrophic muscular dystrophy with internalized capillaries. *Archives of Neurology* **37**, 709–14.

Hausmanowa-Petrusewicz, I. and Borkowska, J. (1978). Intrafamilial variability of X-linked progressive muscular dystrophy. Mild and acute forms of X-linked muscular dystrophy in the same family. *Journal of Neurology* **218**, 43–50.

——, Askanas, W., Badurska, B., *et al.* (1968*a*). Infantile and juvenile spinal muscular atrophy. *Journal of the Neurological Sciences* **6**, 269–87.

——, Prot, J., Niebrój-Dobosz, I., *et al.* (1968*b*). Studies of healthy relatives of patients with Duchenne muscular dystrophy. *Journal of the Neurological Sciences* **7**, 465–80.

——, Wierzbicka, M., Jozwik, A., Szmidt-Salkowska, E., and Borkowska, J. (1982). A nearest neighbour decision rule for EMG detection of carriers of Duchenne muscular dystrophy. *Electromyography and Clinical Neurophysiology* **22**, 445–57.

——, Zaremba, J., Borkowska, J., and Szirkowiec, W. (1984). Chronic proximal spinal muscular atrophy of childhood and adolescence: sex influence. *Journal of Medical Genetics* **21**, 447–50.

Haymond, M. W., Strobel, K. E., and DeVivo, D. C. (1978). Muscle wasting and carbohydrate homeostasis in Duchenne muscular dystrophy. *Neurology* **28**, 1224–31.

Hazama, R., Tsujihata, M., Mori, M., and Mori, K. (1979). Muscular dystrophy in six young girls. *Neurology* **29**, 1486–91.

Heckmatt, J. Z. and Dubowitz, V. (1983). Detecting the Duchenne carrier by ultrasound and computerized tomography. *Lancet* **ii**, 1364.

—— and Dubowitz, V. (1990). Congenital myopathies. In *Principles and practice of medical genetics*, (2nd edn), (ed. A. E. H. Emery and D. L. Rimoin), Vol. 1, pp. 513–37. Churchill Livingstone, Edinburgh.

——, Leeman, S., and Dubowitz, V. (1982). Ultrasound imaging in the diagnosis of muscle disease. *Journal of Pediatrics* **101**, 656–60.

——, Moosa, A., Hutson, C., Maunder-Sewry, C. A., and Dubowitz, V. (1984). Diagnostic needle muscle biopsy: a practical and reliable alternative to open biopsy. *Archives of Disease in Childhood* **59**, 528–32.

——, Dubowitz, V., Hyde, S. A., Florence, J., Gabain, A. C., and Thompson, N. (1985). Prolongation of walking in Duchenne muscular dystrophy with lightweight orthoses: review of 57 cases. *Developmental Medicine and Child Neurology* **27**, 149–54.

——, Rodillo, E., Doherty, M., Willson, K., and Leeman, S. (1989). Quantitative sonography of muscle. *Journal of Child Neurology* **4**, S101–6.

——, Loh, L., and Dubowitz, V. (1990). Night-time nasal ventilation in neuro-muscular disease. *Lancet* **335**, 579–82.

Held, F. W., Groothuis, D. R., Salafsky, I. S., and Vick, N. A. (1980). Autosomal recessive pseudohypertrophic muscular dystrophy: a Duchenne phenocopy. *Neurology* **30**, 402 (Abstract).

Helliwell, T. R., Ellis, J. M., Mountford, R. C., Appleton, R. E., and Morris, G. E. (1992). A truncated dystrophin lacking the C-terminal domains is localized at the muscle membrane. *American Journal of Human Genetics* **50**, 508–14.

Henson, T. E., Muller, J., and DeMyer, W. E. (1967). Hereditary myopathy limited to females. *Archives of Neurology* **17**, 238–47.

Herrmann, F. H. and Spiegler, A. W. J. (1985). *X-linked muscular dystrophies – a bibliography*. University Press, Leipzig.

——, Spiegler, A., and Wiedemann, G. (1982). Muscle provocation test. A sensitive method for discrimination between carriers and non-carriers of Duchenne muscular dystrophy. *Human Genetics* **61**, 102–4.

Herva, R., Kaluzewski, B., and de la Chapelle, A. (1979). Inherited interstitial del. (Xp) with minimal clinical consequences: with a note on the location of genes controlling phenotypic features. *American Journal of Medical Genetics* **3**, 43–58.

Heyck, H. and Laudahn, G. (1969). *Die progressiv-dystrophischen Myopathien*. Springer, Berlin.

——, Laudahn, G., and Lüders, C. J. (1963). Fermentaktivitätsbestimmungen in der gesunden menschlichen Muskulatur und bei Myopathien. II. Enzymaktivitäts-veränderungen im Muskel bei Dystrophia musculorum progressiva. *Klinische Wochenschrift* **41**, 500–9.

Hillier, J., Jones, G. E., Statham, H. E., Witkowski, J. A., and Dubowitz, V. (1985). Cell surface abnormality in clones of skin fibroblasts from a carrier of Duchenne muscular dystrophy. *Journal of Medical Genetics* **22**, 100–3.

Hirano, K., Sakamoto, Y., and Itagaki, Y. (1983). The disability state and urinary excretion of dimethylarginine, glycine and creatine in Duchenne and non-Duchenne muscular dystrophy. *Brain and Development* **5**, 242.

Hirsch-Kauffmann, M., Valet, G., Wieser, J., and Schweiger, M. (1985). Progres-sive muscular dystrophy (Duchenne): biochemical studies by flow-cytometry. *Human Genetics* **69**, 332–6.

Ho, A. D., Reitter, B., Stojakowits, S., Fiehn, W., and Weisser, J. (1980). Capping of lymphocytes for carrier detection in Duchenne muscular dystrophy: techni-cal problems and a review of the literature. *European Journal of Pediatrics* **134**, 211–16.

Ho, M. F., Monaco, A. P., Blonden, L. A. J., *et al.* (1992). Fine mapping of the McLeod locus (XK) to a 150-380-kb region in Xp21. *American Journal of Human Genetics* **50**, 317–30.

Hodgson, S. V., Heckmatt, J. Z., Hughes, E., Crolla, J., Dubowitz, V., and Bobrow, M. (1986*a*). A balanced *de novo* X/autosome translocation in a girl with manifestations of Lowe syndrome. *American Journal of Medical Genetics* **23**, 837–47.

——, Boswinkel, E., Cole, C., *et al.* (1986*b*). A linkage study of Emery-Dreifuss muscular dystrophy. *Human Genetics* **74**, 409–16.

Hodson, A. and Pleasure, D. (1977). Erythrocyte cation-activated adenosine triphosphatases in Duchenne muscular dystrophy. *Journal of the Neurological Sciences* **32**, 361-9.

Hoffman, E. P. (1991). Molecular diagnostics of Duchenne/Becker dystrophy: new additions to a rapidly expanding literature. *Journal of the Neurological Sciences* **101**, 129-32.

—— and Gorospe, J. R. M. (1991). The animal models of Duchenne muscular dystrophy: windows on the pathophysiological consequences of dystrophin deficiency. *Current Topics in Membranes* **38**, 113-54.

—— and Kunkel, L. M. (1989). Dystrophin abnormalities in Duchenne/Becker muscular dystrophy. *Neuron* **2**, 1019-29.

——, Brown, R. H., and Kunkel, L. M. (1987*a*). Dystrophin: the protein product of the Duchenne muscular dystrophy locus. *Cell* **51**, 919-28.

——, Knudson, C. M., Campbell, K. P. *et al.* (1987*b*). Subcellular fractionation of dystrophin to the triads of skeletal muscle. *Nature* **330**, 754-7.

——, Fischbeck, K. H., Brown, R. H., *et al.* (1988). Characterization of dystrophin in muscle-biopsy specimens from patients with Duchenne's or Becker's muscular dystrophy. *New England Journal of Medicine* **318**, 1363-8.

——, Garcia, C. A., Chamberlain, J. S., *et al.* (1991). Is the carboxyl-terminus of dystrophin required for membrane association? A novel, severe case of Duchenne muscular dystrophy. *Annals of Neurology* **30**, 605-10.

——, Arahata, K., Minetti, C., *et al.* (1992). Dystrophinopathy in isolated cases of myopathy in females. *Neurology* **42**, 967-75.

Hogge, W. A., Schonberg, S. A., and Golbus, M. S. (1985). Prenatal diagnosis by chorionic villus sampling: lessons of the first 600 cases. *Prenatal Diagnosis* **5**, 393-400.

Hohlfeld, R. and Toyka, K. V. (1985). Strategies for the modulation of neuro-immunological disease at the level of autoreactive T-lymphocytes. *Journal of Neuroimmunology* **9**, 193-204.

Höhn H. (1987). Duchennesche Muskeldystrophie: Inzidenz und Pravalenz in Unterfranken. Dissertation in the Medical Faculty, University of Wurzburg.

Ho-Kim, M-A., Bédard, A., Vincent, M., and Rogers, P. A. (1991). Dystrophin: a sensitive and reliable immunochemical assay in tissue and cell culture homogenates. *Biochemical and Biophysical Research Communications* **181**, 1164-72.

Hopkins, L. C., Jackson, J. A., and Elsas, L. J. (1981). Emery-Dreifuss humeroperoneal muscular dystrophy: an X-linked myopathy with unusual contractures and bradycardia. *Annals of Neurology* **10**, 230-7.

Horowits, R., Dalakas, M. C., and Podolsky, R. J. (1990). Single skinned muscle fibers in Duchenne muscular dystrophy generate normal force. *Annals of Neurology* **27**, 636-41.

Horvath, B. and Proctor, J. B. (1960). Muscular dystrophy: quantitative studies on the composition of dystrophic muscle. *Research Publications — Association for Research in Nervous and Mental Disease* **38**, 740-66.

Hovstad, L., Løchen, E. A., and Sjaastad, O. (1976). Pneumoencephalographic findings in various primary and secondary muscular disorders. *Acta Neurologica Scandinavica* **53**, 128-36.

Hsia, Y. E. (1974). Choosing my children's genes: genetic counseling. In *Genetic responsibility: on choosing our children's genes*, (ed. M. Lipkin and P. T. Rowley), pp. 43-59. Plenum Press, New York.

Hsu, J. D. (1976). Management of foot deformity in Duchenne's pseudohypertrophic muscular dystrophy. *Orthopedic Clinics of North America* **7**, 979–84.

—— (1979). Extremity fractures in children with neuromuscular disease. *Johns Hopkins Medical Journal* **145**, 89–93.

Hu, X., Burghes, A. H. M., Ray, P. N., Thompson, M. W., Murphy, E. G., and Worton, R. G. (1988). Partial gene duplication in Duchenne and Becker muscular dystrophies. *Journal of Medical Genetics* **25**, 369–76.

——, Burghes, A. H. M., Bulman, D. E., Ray, P. N., and Worton, R. G. (1989). Evidence for mutation by unequal sister chromatid exchange in the Duchenne muscular dystrophy gene. *American Journal of Human Genetics* **44**, 855–63.

Huard, J., Bouchard, J. P., Roy, R., *et al.* (1992). Human myoblast transplantation: preliminary results of 4 cases. *Muscle and Nerve* **15**, 550–60.

Hudgson, P., Pearce, G. W., and Walton, J. N. (1967*a*). Preclinical muscular dystrophy: histopathological changes observed on muscle biopsy. *Brain* **90**, 565–76.

——, Gardner-Medwin, D., Pennington, R. J. T., and Walton, J. N. (1967*b*). Studies of the carrier state in the Duchenne type of muscular dystrophy. Part 1. Effect of exercise on serum creatine kinase activity. *Journal of Neurology, Neurosurgery and Psychiatry* **30**, 416–19.

Hughes, B. P. (1972). Lipid changes in Duchenne muscular dystrophy. *Journal of Neurology, Neurosurgery and Psychiatry* **35**, 658–63.

Hughes, J. T. (1974). *Pathology of muscle*. Lloyd-Luke, London.

Hunsaker, R. H., Fulkerson, P. K., Barry, F. J., Lewis, R. P., Leier, C. V., and Unverferth, D. V. (1982). Cardiac function in Duchenne's muscular dystrophy. Results of 10-year follow-up study and noninvasive tests. *American Journal of Medicine* **73**, 235–8.

Hunter, A. (1992). Familial occurrence of Duchenne dystrophy through paternal lines in four families. *American Journal of Medical Genetics* **42**, 213.

Hunter, S. (1980). The heart in muscular dystrophy. *British Medical Bulletin* **36**, 133–4.

Hurko, O., Hoffman, E. P., McKee, L., *et al.* (1989). Dystrophin analysis in clonal myoblasts derived from a Duchenne muscular dystrophy carrier. *American Journal of Human Genetics* **44**, 820–6.

Hurse, P. V. and Kakulas, B. A. (1974). Genetic counselling in neuromuscular diseases in Western Australia. *Proceedings of the Australian Association of Neurology* **11**, 145–53.

Hutton, E. M. and Thompson, M. W. (1970). Parental age and mutation rate in Duchenne muscular dystrophy. *American Journal of Human Genetics* **22**, 26A (Abstract).

—— and Thompson, M. W. (1976). Carrier detection and genetic counselling in Duchenne muscular dystrophy: a follow up study. *Canadian Medical Association Journal* **115**, 749–52.

Huvos, A. G. and Pruzanski, W. (1967). Smooth muscle involvement in primary muscle disease. II. Progressive muscular dystrophy. *Archives of Pathology* **83**, 234–40.

Huxley, A. F. (1980). Future prospects. *British Medical Bulletin* **36**, 199–200.

Hyde, S. A. (1984). *The parents' guide to the physical management of Duchenne muscular dystrophy*. Muscular Dystrophy Group of Great Britain and Northern Ireland, London.

——, Scott, O. M., Goddard, C. M., and Dubowitz, V. (1982). Prolongation of ambulation in Duchenne muscular dystrophy by appropriate orthoses. *Physiotherapy* **68**, 105–8.

Ibraghimov-Beskrovnaya, O., Ervasti, J. M., Leveille, C. J., *et al.* (1992). Primary structure of dystrophin-associated glycoproteins linking dystrophin to the extracellular matrix. *Nature* **355**, 696–702.

Inkley, S. R., Oldenburg, F. C., and Vignos, P. J. (1974). Pulmonary function in Duchenne muscular dystrophy related to stage of disease. *American Journal of Medicine* **56**, 297–306.

Inoue, R., Miyake, M., Kanazawa, A., Sato, M., and Kakimoto, Y. (1979). Decrease of 3-methylhistidine and increase of N^G, N^G-dimethylarginine in the urine of patients with muscular dystrophy. *Metabolism* **28**, 801–4.

Ionasescu, V. and Ionasescu, R. (1982). Increased collagen synthesis by Duchenne myogenic clones. *Journal of the Neurological Sciences* **54**, 79–87.

——, Zellweger, H., and Cancilla, P. (1978). Fetal serum creatine phosphokinase not a valid predictor of Duchenne muscular dystrophy. *Lancet* **ii**, 1251.

——, Burmeister, L., and Hanson, J. (1980). Discriminant analysis of ribosomal protein synthesis findings in carrier detection of Duchenne muscular dystrophy. *American Journal of Medical Genetics* **5**, 5–12.

Ishihara, T., Kawamura, J., Sasaki, A., and Aoyagi, T. (1991). Relationship between cardiac and pulmonary function in late stage of Duchenne muscular dystrophy patients. *Acta Cardiomiologica* **3**, 357–67.

Ishikawa, K., Shirato, C., Yotsukura, M., Ishihara, T., Tamura, T., and Inoue, M. (1982). Sequential changes in high frequency notches on QRS complexes in progressive muscular dystrophy of the Duchenne type—a 3-year follow-up study. *Journal of Electrocardiology* **15**, 23–30.

Jackson, C. E. and Strehler, D. A. (1968). Limb-girdle muscular dystrophy: clinical manifestations and detection of preclinical disease. *Pediatrics* **41**, 495–502.

Jackson, M. J., Brooke, M. H., Kaiser, K., *et al.* (1991). Creatine kinase and prostaglandin E_2 release from isolated Duchenne muscle. *Neurology* **41**, 101–4.

Jackson, R. C., Taylor, B. D., Zellweger, H., and Bianchine, J. W. (1974). Muscular dystrophy: Duchenne type and Becker type within a kindred. *American Journal of Human Genetics* **26**, 44A (Abstract).

Jacobs, P. A., Hunt, P. A., Mayer, M., and Bart, R. D. (1981). Duchenne muscular dystrophy (DMD) in a female with an X/autosome translocation: further evidence that the DMD locus is at Xp21. *American Journal of Human Genetics* **33**, 513–18.

Jaffe, K. M., McDonald, C. M., Ingman, E., and Haas, J. (1990). Symptoms of upper gastrointestinal dysfunction in Duchenne muscular dystrophy: case-control study. *Archives of Physical and Medical Rehabilitation* **71**, 742–4.

Jagadha, V. and Becker, L. E. (1988). Brain morphology in Duchenne muscular dystrophy: a Golgi study. *Pediatric Neurology* **4**, 87–92.

Jalbert, P., Mouriquand, C., Beaudoing, A., and Jaillard, M. (1966). Myopathie progressive de type Duchenne et mosaique XO/XX/XXX: consideration sur la genèse de la fibre musculaire striée. *Annales de Génétique* **9**, 104–8.

James J. I. P., Zorab, P. A., and Wynne-Davies, R. (1976). *Scoliosis*, (2nd edn). Churchill Livingstone, Edinburgh.

Jeanpierre, M. (1992). Germinal mosaicism and risk calculation in X-linked diseases. *American Journal of Human Genetics* **50**, 960–7.

Jedrzejowska-Kulakowska, H., Hausmanowa-Petrusewicz, I., Gawlik, Z., Rafalowska, J., and Slucka, C. (1968). Zweryfikowany sekcyjnie przypadek postepujacej dystrofii mieśniowej typu Duchenne'a. *Neuropatologia Polska* **6**, 71-85.

Jellett, L. B., Kennedy, M. C., and Goldblatt, E. (1974). Duchenne pseudohypertrophic muscular dystrophy: a clinical and electrocardiographic study of patients and female carriers. *Australian and New Zealand Journal of Medicine* **4**, 41-7.

Jerusalem, F. and Zierz, S. (1991). *Muskelerkrankungen: Klinik — Therapie — Pathologie*. Thieme, Stuttgart.

——, Engel, A. G., and Gomez, M. R. (1974). Duchenne dystrophy. I. Morphometric study of the muscle microvasculature. *Brain* **97**, 115-22.

Johnson, E. W., Reynolds, H. T., and Stauch, D. (1985). Duchenne muscular dystrophy: a case with prolonged survival. *Archives of Physical and Medical Rehabilitation* **66**, 260-1.

Johnson, M. A., Polgar, J., Weightman, D., and Appleton, D. (1973). Data on the distribution of fibre types in thirty-six human muscles — an autopsy study. *Journal of the Neurological Sciences* **18**, 111-29.

Johnston, A. W. and McKay, E. (1986). X-linked muscular dystrophy with contractures. *Journal of Medical Genetics* **23**, 591-5.

Johnston, P. G. and Cattanach, B. M. (1981). Controlling elements in the mouse. IV. Evidence of non-random X-inactivation. *Genetical Research* **37**, 151-60.

Jones, G. E. and Witkowski, J. A. (1983). A cell surface abnormality in Duchenne muscular dystrophy: intercellular adhesiveness of skin fibroblasts from patients and carriers. *Human Genetics* **63**, 232-7.

Jørgensen, A. L., Philip, J., Raskind, W. H., *et al.* (1992). Different patterns of X inactivation in MZ twins discordant for red-green colour-vision deficiency. *American Journal of Human Genetics* **52**, 291-8.

Kääriäinen, H., Lindlöf, M., Somer, H., and de la Chapelle, A. (1990). Genetic counselling in Duchenne and Becker muscular dystrophy is problematic when carrier studies give controversial results. *Clinical Genetics* **37**, 179-87.

Kaeser, H. E. (1965). Scapuloperoneal muscular atrophy. *Brain* **88**, 407-18.

Kakulas, B. A. and Adams, R. D. (1985). *Diseases of muscle. Pathological foundations of clinical myology*, (4th edn). Harper and Row, Philadelphia.

—— and Hurse, P. V. (1977). The muscular dystrophies: results of carrier detection and genetic counselling in Western Australia. *Records of the Adelaide Children's Hospital* **1**, 232-43.

——, Howell, J. M., and Roses, A. D. (eds) (1992). *Duchenne muscular dystrophy. Animal models and genetic manipulation*. Raven Press, New York.

Kamakura, K., Kawai, M., Arahata, K., *et al.* (1990). A manifesting carrier of Duchenne muscular dystrophy with severe myocardial symptoms. *Journal of Neurology* **237**, 483-5.

Kamoshita, S., Konishi, Y., Segawa, M., and Fukuyama, Y. (1976). Congenital muscular dystrophy as a disease of the central nervous system. *Archives of Neurology* **33**, 513-16.

Kanamori, M., Morton, N. E., Fujiki, K., *et al.* (1987). Genetic epidemiology of Duchenne muscular dystrophy in Japan: classical segregation analysis. *Genetic Epidemiology* **4**, 425-32.

Kaplan, L. C. and Elias, E. R. (1986). Diagnosis of muscular dystrophy in patients referred for evaluation of language delay. *Developmental Medicine and Child Neurology* **28**, 110 (Abstract).

Kapur, S., Higgins, J. V., Delp, K., and Rogers, B. (1987). Menkes syndrome in a girl with X-autosome translocation. *American Journal of Medical Genetics* **26**, 503–10.

Kar, N. C. and Pearson, C. M. (1972*a*). Acyl phosphatase in normal and diseased human muscle. *Clinica Chimica Acta* **40**, 262–5.

—— and Pearson, C. M. (1972*b*). Acid, neutral and alkaline cathepsins in normal and diseased human muscle. *Enzyme* **13**, 188–96.

—— and Pearson, C. M. (1973). Muscle adenylic acid deaminase activity. Selective decrease in early-onset Duchenne muscular dystrophy. *Neurology* **23**, 478–82.

—— and Pearson, C. M. (1977). Hydrolytic enzymes and human muscular dystrophy. In *Pathogenesis of human muscular dystrophies*, (ed. L. P. Rowland), pp. 387–94. Excerpta Medica, Amsterdam.

—— and Pearson, C. M. (1980). Methylthioadenosine nucleosidase in normal and dystrophic human muscle. *Clinica Chimica Acta* **108**, 465–8.

Karagan, N. J. and Sorensen, J. P. (1981). Intellectual functioning in non-Duchenne muscular dystrophy. *Neurology* **31**, 448–52.

—— and Zellweger, H. U. (1978). Early verbal disability in children with Duchenne muscular dystrophy. *Developmental Medicine and Child Neurology* **20**, 435–41.

——, Richman, L. C., and Sorensen, J. P. (1980). Analysis of verbal disability in Duchenne muscular dystrophy. *Journal of Nervous and Mental Disease* **168**, 419–23.

Karpati, G. (1990). Possible treatment of Duchenne muscular dystrophy by non-dystrophic myoblast implantation into dystrophic muscles. In *Pathogenesis and therapy of Duchenne and Becker muscular dystrophy*, (ed. B. A. Kakulas and F. L. Mastaglia), pp. 59–63. Raven Press, New York.

—— and Carpenter, S. (1986). Small-caliber skeletal muscle fibers do not suffer deleterious consequences of dystrophic gene expression. *American Journal of Medical Genetics* **25**, 653–8.

——, Zubrzycka-Gaarn, E. E., Carpenter, S., Bulman, D. E., Ray, P. N., and Worton, R. G. (1990). Age-related conversion of dystrophin-negative to -positive fiber segments of skeletal but not cardiac muscle fibers in heterozygote mdx mice. *Journal of Neuropathology and Experimental Neurology* **49**, 96–105.

——, Johnston, W., Ajdukovic, G., *et al.* (1992). Myoblast transfer (MT) in McArdle's disease (McD). *Neurology* **42** (Suppl. 3), 829S (Abstract).

ten Kate, L. P. and van Essen, A. J. (1992). Duchenne muscular dystrophy inherited through paternal lines. *American Journal of Medical Genetics* **42**, 214.

Kawai, H., Adachi, K., Kimura, C., *et al.* (1990). Secretion and clinical significance of atrial natriuretic peptide in patients with muscular dystrophy. *Archives of Neurology* **47**, 900–4.

Kawai, M., Kunimoto, M., Motoyoshi, Y., Kuwata, T., and Nakano, I. (1985). Computed tomography in Duchenne type muscular dystrophy — morphological stages based on the computed tomographical findings. *Clinical Neurology* **25**, 578–90. (Japanese with detailed abstract in English.)

Kazakov, V. M., Bogorodinsky, D. K., and Skorometz, A. A. (1976). The myogenic scapulo-peroneal syndrome. Muscular dystrophy in the K kindred: clinical study and genetics. *Clinical Genetics* **10**, 41–50.

Kean, V. M., MacLeod, H. L., Thompson, M. W., Ray, P. N., Verellen-Dumoulin, C., and Worton, R. G. (1986). Paternal inheritance of translocation chromosomes in a t(X;21) patient with X-linked muscular dystrophy. *Journal of Medical Genetics* **23**, 491–3.

Kelly, A. M. and Blau, H. M. (ed.) (1992). *Neuromuscular Development and Disease*. Raven Press, New York.

Kessler, S. (1979). The psychological foundations of genetic counseling. In *Genetic counseling—psychological dimensions*, (ed. S. Kessler), pp. 17–33. Academic Press, New York.

Khurana, T. S., Watkins, S. C., Chafey, P., *et al.* (1991). Immunolocalization and developmental expression of dystrophin related protein in skeletal muscle. *Neuromuscular Disorders* **1**, 185–94.

Kiepiela, P., Dawood, A. A., Moosa, A., *et al.* (1988). Evaluation of immunoregulatory cells in Duchenne muscular dystrophy and spinal muscular atrophy among African and Indian patients. *Journal of the Neurological Sciences* **84**, 247–55.

Kimura, S., Mitsuda, T., Misugi, N., *et al.* (1986). Clinical features in a girl with Duchenne muscular dystrophy with an X-autosome translocation; (X;4)(p21;q26). *Brain and Development* **8**, 619–23.

King, B. and Emery, A. E. H. (1973). Leucocyte fatty acid oxidation in hereditary neuromuscular disorders. *Journal of the Neurological Sciences* **20**, 297–302.

——, Spikesman, A., and Emery, A. E. H. (1972). The effect of pregnancy on serum levels of creatine kinase. *Clinica Chimica Acta* **36**, 267–9.

Kingston, H. M., Thomas, N. S. T., Pearson, P. L., Sarfarazi, M., and Harper, P. S. (1983). Genetic linkage between Becker muscular dystrophy and a polymorphic DNA sequence on the short arm of the X chromosome. *Journal of Medical Genetics* **20**, 255–8.

——, Sarfarazi, M., Thomas, N. S. T., and Harper, P. S. (1984). Localisation of the Becker muscular dystrophy gene on the short arm of the X chromosome by linkage to cloned DNA sequences. *Human Genetics* **67**, 6–17.

Kissel, J. T., Burrow, K. L., Rammohan, K. W., *et al.* (1991). Mononuclear cell analysis of muscle biopsies in prednisone-treated and untreated Duchenne muscular dystrophy. *Neurology* **41**, 667–72.

Klamut, H. J., Gangopadhyay, S. B., Worton, R. G., and Ray, P. N. (1990). Molecular and functional analysis of the muscle-specific promoter region of the Duchenne muscular dystrophy gene. *Molecular and Cellular Biology* **10**, 193–205.

Klein, C. J., Coovert, D. D., Bulman, D. E., Ray, P. N., Mendell, J. R., and Burghes, A. H. M. (1992). Somatic reversion/suppression in Duchenne muscular dystrophy (DMD): evidence supporting a frame-restoring mechanism in rare dystrophin-positive fibers. *American Journal of Human Genetics* **50**, 950–9.

Kleine, T. O. (1970). Evidence for the release of enzymes from different organs in Duchenne's muscular dystrophy. *Clinica Chimica Acta* **29**, 227–31.

Klip, A., Elder, B., Ruiz-Funes, H. P., Buchwald, M., and Grinstein, S. (1985). The free cytoplasmic Ca^{2+} levels in Duchenne muscular dystrophy lymphocytes. *Muscle and Nerve* **8**, 317–20.

Kloepfer, H. W. and Emery, A. E. H. (1969). Genetic aspects of neuromuscular disease. In *Disorders of voluntary muscle*, (2nd edn), (ed. J. N. Walton), pp. 683–712. Churchill Livingstone, Edinburgh.

Koehler, J. (1977). Blood vessel structure in Duchenne muscular dystrophy. I. Light and electron microscopic observations in resting muscle. *Neurology* **27**, 861–8.

Koenig, M., Hoffman, E. P., Bertelson, C. J., Monaco, A. P., Feener, C., and Kunkel, L. M. (1987). Complete cloning of the Duchenne muscular dystrophy (DMD) cDNA and preliminary genomic organization of the DMD gene in normal and affected individuals. *Cell* **50**, 509–17.

——, Monaco, A. P., and Kunkel, L. M. (1988). The complete sequence of dystrophin predicts a rod-shaped cytoskeletal protein. *Cell* **53**, 219–28.

——, Beggs, A. H., Moyer, M., *et al.* (1989). The molecular basis for Duchenne versus Becker muscular dystrophy: correlation of severity with type of deletion. *American Journal of Human Genetics* **45**, 498–506.

Koh, J., Bartlett, R. J., Pericak-Vance, M. A., *et al.* (1987). Inherited deletion at Duchenne dystrophy locus in normal male. *Lancet* **ii**, 1154–5.

Konagaya, M., Takayanagi, T., Kamiya, T., and Takamatsu, S. (1982). Genetic linkage study of Duchenne muscular dystrophy and haemophilia A. *Neurology* **32**, 1046–9.

Konno, Y., Ohno, S., Akita, Y., Saito, F., Yamamoto, K., Furusho, T., and Suzuki, K. (1989). Detection of deletions in DNA by slot-blot hybridization: application to Duchenne muscular dystrophy gene. *Biomedical Research* **10**, 65–9.

Kott, E., Golan, A., Don, R., and Bernstein, B. (1973). Muscular dystrophy: the relative frequency in the different ethnic groups in Israel. *Confinia Neurologica* **35**, 177–85.

Kousseff, B. (1981). Linkage between chronic granulomatous disease and Duchenne's muscular dystrophy. *American Journal of Diseases of Children* **135**, 1149.

Kozicka, A., Prot, J., and Wasilewski, R. (1971). Mental retardation in patients with Duchenne progressive muscular dystrophy. *Journal of the Neurological Sciences* **14**, 209–13.

Krendel, D. A. and Jannun, D. R. (1987). A dominantly inherited myopathy with contractures, heart failure ahd marked variability of expression. *Neurology* **37** (Suppl. 1), 208–9.

Krog. E. (ed.) (1982). *Total management in muscular dystrophy*. Muskelsvind-fonden, Copenhagen.

Krstić, R. V. (1978). *Die Gewebe des Menschen und der Säugetiere*. Springer, Berlin.

Kryschowa, N. and Abowjan, W. (1934). Zur Frage der Heredität der Pseudohyper-trophie Duchenne. *Zeitschrift für die gesamte Neurologie und Psychiatrie* **150**, 421–6.

Kuby, S. A., Noda, L., and Lardy, H. A. (1954). Adenosinetriphosphate-creatine transphosphorylase. *Journal of Biological Chemistry* **209**, 191–201.

Kugelberg, E. (1947). Electromyograms in muscular disorders. *Journal of Neurology, Neurosurgery and Psychiatry* **10**(NS), 122–33.

—— and Welander, L. (1956). Heredofamilial juvenile muscular atrophy simulating muscular dystrophy. *Archives of Neurology and Psychiatry* **75**, 500–9.

Kuhn, E. and Rüdel, R. (1990). Wilhelm Heinrich Erb (1840-1921). *Muscle and Nerve* **13**, 567–9.

——, Fiehn, W., Schröder, J. M., Assmus, H. A., and Wagner, A. (1979). Early myocardial disease and cramping myalgia in Becker-type muscular dystrophy: a kindred. *Neurology* **29**, 1144–9.

Kunath, B. (1983). Bericht über die Erfassung von progressiven Muskeldystrophien im Bezirk Dresden. Proceedings of a scientific meeting 'Genetische Defekte', Neubrandenburg 14, 1983.

Kunkel, L. M., Monaco, A. P., Middlesworth, W., Ochs, H. D., and Latt, S. A. (1985). Specific cloning of DNA fragments absent from the DNA of a male patient with an X chromosome deletion. *Proceedings of the National Academy of Sciences, USA* **82**, 4778–82.

——, Hejtmancik, J. F., Caskey, C. T., *et al.* (1986). Analysis of deletions in DNA from patients with Becker and Duchenne muscular dystrophy. *Nature* **322**, 73–7.

Kurland, L. T. (1958). Descriptive epidemiology of selected neurologic and myopathic disorders with particular reference to a survey in Rochester, Minnesota. *Journal of Chronic Diseases* **8**, 378–418.

Kuroiwa, Y. and Miyazaki, T. (1967). Epidemiological study of myopathy in Japan. In *Exploratory concepts in muscular dystrophy and related disorders*, (ed. A. T. Milhorat), pp. 98–102. Excerpta Medica, Amsterdam.

Laing, N. G., Siddique, T., Bartlett, R., *et al.* (1989). Duchenne muscular dystrophy: detection of deletion carriers by spectrophotometric densitometry. *Clinical Genetics* **35**, 393–8.

——, Layton, M. G., Johnsen, R. D., *et al.* (1992). Two distinct mutations in a single dystrophin gene: chance occurrence or premutation? *American Journal of Medical Genetics* **42**, 688–92.

Lalouel, J. M. and White, R. (1990). Analysis of genetic linkage. In *Principles and practice of medical genetics*, (Vol. 1), (2nd edn), (ed. A. E. H. Emery and D. L. Rimoin), pp. 149–64. Churchill Livingstone, Edinburgh.

Lamy, M. and de Grouchy, J. (1954). L'hérédité de la myopathie (formes basses). *Journal de Génétique Humaine* **3**, 219–61.

Landon, D. N. (1982). Skeletal muscle — normal morphology, development and innervation. In *Skeletal muscle pathology*, (ed. F. L. Mastaglia and J. N. Walton), pp. 1–87. Churchill Livingstone, Edinburgh.

Lane, R. J. M. and Roses, A. D. (1981). Variations of serum creatine kinase levels with age in normal females: implications for genetic counselling in Duchenne muscular dystrophy. *Clinica Chimica Acta* **113**, 75–86.

——, Gardner-Medwin, D., and Roses, A. D. (1980). Electrocardiographic abnormalities in carriers of Duchenne muscular dystrophy. *Neurology* **30**, 497–501.

——, Robinow, M., and Roses, A. D. (1983). The genetic status of mothers of isolated cases of Duchenne muscular dystrophy. *Journal of Medical Genetics* **20**, 1–11.

Lang, H., Donner, M., Ignatius, J., *et al.* (1989). Epidemiology of muscular disorders in Finland (in Finnish). In *Lihastautien kehittyva tutkimus ja hoito*, (ed. H. Lang). Kiasma, Turku.

Larsen, U. T., Juhl B., Hein-Sørensen, O., and de Fine Olivarius, B. (1989). Complications during anaesthesia in patients with Duchenne's muscular dystrophy (a retrospective study). *Canadian Journal of Anaesthesia* **36**, 418–22.

La Spada, A. R., Wilson, E. M., Lubahn, D. B., *et al.* (1991). Androgen receptor gene mutations in X-linked spinal and bulbar muscular atrophy. *Nature* **352**, 77–9.

Laurent, C., Biemont, M. C., and Dutrillaux, B. (1975). Sur quatre nouveaux cas de translocation du chromosome X chez l'homme. *Humangenetik* **26**, 35–46.

Law, P. K., Bertorini, T. E., Goodwin, T. G., *et al.* (1990). Dystrophin production induced by myoblast transfer therapy in Duchenne muscular dystrophy. *Lancet* **336**, 114–15.

——, Goodwin, T. G., Fang, Q., *et al.* (1992). Feasibility, safety, and efficacy of myoblast transfer therapy on Duchenne muscular dystrophy boys. *Cell Transplantation* **1**, 235–44.

Lawrence, E. F., Brown, B., and Hopkins, I. J. (1973). Pseudohypertrophic muscular dystrophy of childhood: an epidemiological survey in Victoria.

Australian and New Zealand Journal of Medicine **3**, 142–51.

Lazzeroni, E., Favaro, L., and Botti, G. (1989). Dilated cardiomyopathy with regional myocardial hypoperfusion in Becker's muscular dystrophy. *International Journal of Cardiology* **22**, 126–9.

Lebenthal, E. Shochet, S. B., Adam, A., *et al.* (1970). Arthrogryposis multiplex congenita: twenty-three cases in an Arab kindred. *Pediatrics* **46**, 891–9.

Lebo, R. V., Olney, R. K., and Golbus, M. S. (1990). Somatic mosaicism at the Duchenne locus. *American Journal of Medical Genetics* **37**, 187–90.

Lecky, B. R. F., MacKenzie, J. M., Read, A. P., and Wilcox, D. E. (1991). X-linked and FSH dystrophies in one family. *Neuromuscular Disorders* **1**, 275–8.

Lee, C. C., Pearlman, J. A., Chamberlain, J. S., and Caskey, C. T. (1991). Expression of recombinant dystrophin and its localization to the cell membrane. *Nature* **349**, 334–6.

Lehesjoki, A-E., Sankila, E-M., Miao, J., *et al.* (1990). X linked neonatal myotubular myopathy: one recombination detected with four polymorphic DNA markers from Xq28. *Journal of Medical Genetics* **27**, 288–91.

Leibowitz, D. and Dubowitz, V. (1981). Intellect and behaviour in Duchenne muscular dystrophy. *Developmental Medicine and Child Neurology* **23**, 577–90.

Lenman, J. A. R. and Ritchie, A. E. (1970). *Clinical electromyography.* Pitman, London.

Leon, S. H., Schuffler, M. D., Kettler, M., and Rohrmann, C. A. (1986). Chronic intestinal pseudoobstruction as a complication of Duchenne's muscular dystrophy. *Gastroenterology* **90**, 455–9.

Leonard, C. O., Chase, G. A., and Childs, B. (1972). Genetic counseling: a consumer's view. *New England Journal of Medicine* **287**, 433–9.

Leth, A., Wulff, K., Corfitsen, M., and Elmgreen, J. (1985). Progressive muscular dystrophy in Denmark. Natural history, prevalence and incidence. *Acta Paediatrica Scandinavica* **74**, 881–5.

Lev, A. A., Feener, C. C., Kunkel, L. M., and Brown, Jr., R. H. (1987). Expression of the Duchenne's muscular dystrophy gene in cultured muscle cells. *Journal of Biological Chemistry* **262**, 15817–20.

Levene, P. A. and Kristeller, L. (1909). Factors regulating the creatinin output in man. *American Journal of Physiology* **24**, 45–65.

Levin, R. N. and Narahara, K. A. (1985). Right axis deviation and anterior wall thallium-201 defect in Becker's muscular dystrophy. *American Journal of Cardiology* **56**, 203–4.

Levinson, B., Kenwrick, S., Lakich, D., Hammonds, Jr. G., and Gitschier, J. (1990). A transcribed gene in an intron of the human factor VIII gene. *Genomics* **7**, 1–11.

Levison, H. (1951). *Dystrophia musculorum progressiva.* Munksgaard, Copenhagen.

Lewis, A. J. and Besant, D. F. (1962). Muscular dystrophy in infancy. Report of 2 cases in siblings with diaphragmatic weakness. *Journal of Pediatrics* **60**, 376–84.

Lichter, P., Chang Tang, C-J., Call, K., *et al.* (1990). High-resolution mapping of human chromosome 11 by in situ hybridization with cosmid clones. *Science* **247**, 64–9.

Lidov, H. G. W., Byers, T. J., Watkins, S. C., and Kunkel, L. M. (1990). Localization of dystrophin to postsynaptic regions of central nervous system cortical neurons. *Nature* **348**, 725–8.

Liechti-Gallati, S., Schneider, V., Mullis, P., and Moser, H. (1990). RFLPs for Duchenne muscular dystrophy cDNA clones 9 and 10. *American Journal of Hunan Genetics* **46**, 1090-4.

——, Müller, B., Grimm, T., *et al.* (1991). X-linked centronuclear myopathy: mapping the gene to Xq28. *Neuromuscular Disorders* **1**, 239-45.

Lilienthal, J. L., Zierler, K. L., Folk, B. P., Buka, R., and Riley, M. J. (1950). A reference base and system for analysis of muscle constituents. *Journal of Biological Chemistry* **182**, 501-8.

Lin, H., Parmacek, M. S., Morle, G., Bolling, S., and Leiden, J. M. (1990). Expression of recombinant genes in myocardium in vivo after direct injection of DNA. *Circulation* **82**, 2217-21.

Lindenbaum, R. H., Clarke, G., Patel, C., Moncrieff, M., and Hughes, J. T. (1979). Muscular dystrophy in an X;1 translocation female suggests that Duchenne locus is on X chromosome short arm. *Journal of Medical Genetics* **16**, 389-92.

Lindgren, V., de Martinville, B., Horwich, A. L., Rosenberg, L. E., and Francke, U. (1984). Human ornithine transcarbamylase locus mapped to band Xp21.1 near the Duchenne muscular dystrophy locus. *Science* **226**, 698-700.

Lindlöf, M., Kiuru, A., Kääriäinen, H., *et al.* (1989). Gene deletions in X-linked muscular dystrophy. *American Journal of Human Genetics* **44**, 496-503.

Little, W. J. (1853). *On the nature and treatment of the deformities of the human frame: being a course of lectures delivered at the Royal Orthopaedic Hospital in 1843*, pp. 14-16. Longman, Brown, Green and Longmans, London.

Livingstone, I. R., Gardner-Medwin, D., Pennington, R. J. T., and Walton, J. N. (1982). Serum creatine kinase and pyruvate kinase activities in normal adolescent females. *Journal of the Neurological Sciences* **54**, 349-52.

Lloyd, S. J. and Emery, A. E. H. (1981). A possible circulating plasma factor in Duchenne muscular dystrophy. *Clinica Chimica Acta* **112**, 85-90.

——, Emery, A. E. H., and Brown, J. N. (1981). Erythrocyte membrane studies. *Neurology* **31**, 1371.

——, Skinner, R., and Emery, A. E. H. (1982). Neonatal screening for Duchenne muscular dystrophy (DMD) using a fluorimetric electrophoretic assay for creatine kinase (CK) in dried blood samples. *Proceedings of the Vth International Congress on Neuromuscular Diseases*, Abstract No. 34. Marseilles.

Lord, J., Behrman, B., Varzos, N., *et al.* (1990). Scoliosis associated with Duchenne muscular dystrophy. *Archives of Physical and Medical Rehabilitation* **71**, 13-17.

Lössner, J. and Wagner, A. (ed.) (1987). *Beiträge zur klinischen Myologie*. Hirzel, Leipzig.

——, Kühn, H. J., and Ruchholtz, U. (1982). Hämopexin und Muskeldystrophie. Zur Carrierdiagnostik der Duchenne-Form. *Psychiatrie, Neurologie und Medizinische Psychologie* **34**, 53-9.

Lou, M. F. (1979). Human muscular dystrophy: elevation of urinary dimethylarginines. *Science* **203**, 668-70.

Loughman, W. D., Mitchell, J. A., Mosher, D. C., and Epstein, C. J. (1980). GENFILES: a computerized medical genetics information network. I. An overview. *American Journal of Medical Genetics* **7**, 243-50.

Love, D. R., Hill, D. F., Dickson, G., *et al.* (1989). An autosomal transcript in skeletal muscle with homology to dystrophin. *Nature* **339**, 55-8.

——, Flint, T. J., Marsden, R. S., *et al.* (1990). Characterization of deletions in the dystrophin gene giving mild phenotypes. *American Journal of Medical Genetics* **37**, 136–42.

——, Flint, T. J., Genet, S. A., Middleton-Price, H. R., and Davies, K. E. (1991). Becker muscular dystrophy patient with a large intragenic dystrophin deletion: implications for functional minigenes and gene therapy. *Journal of Medical Genetics* **28**, 860–4.

Lowenstein, A. S., Arbeit, S. R., and Rubin, I. L. (1962). Cardiac involvement in progressive muscular dystrophy. An electrocardiographic and ballistocardiographic study. *American Journal of Cardiology* **9**, 528–33.

Lubinsky, M. S. and Hall, J. G. (1991). Genomic imprinting, monozygous twinning, and X inactivation. *Lancet* **337**, 1288.

Lubs, M. L. (1974). Hemophilia A and Duchenne muscular dystrophy in Colorado. *American Journal of Human Genetics* **26**, 56A (Abstract).

Lucci, B. (1980). Incidence, prevalence and mutation rate of Duchenne muscular dystrophy in the province of Reggio Emilia. In *Muscular dystrophy research: advances and new trends*, (ed. C. Angelini, G. A. Danieli, and D. Fontanari), pp. 289–90. Excerpta Medica, Amsterdam.

——, Pegoraro, E., Fanin, M., Hoffman, E., and Angelini, C. (1990). Myoglobinuria and very mild late onset dystrophy in the same family due to dystrophin abnormality. *Journal of the Neurological Sciences* **98** (Suppl.), 227 (Abstract).

——, Bortotto, L., Ferlini, A., *et al.* (1991). Clinical, cytogenetical and molecular findings in an X-autosomal translocated female with Becker muscular dystrophy and mental retardation. In *Muscular dystrophy research: from molecular diagnosis toward therapy*, (ed. C. Angelini, G. A. Danieli, and D. Fontanari), pp. 227–8. Excerpta Medica, Amsterdam.

Lucy, J. A. (1980). Is there a membrane defect in muscle and other cells? *British Medical Bulletin* **36**, 187–92.

Lunt, P. W., Cumming, W. J. K., Kingston, H., *et al.* (1989). DNA probes in differential diagnosis of Becker muscular dystrophy and spinal muscular atrophy. *Lancet* **i**, 46–7.

Lupski, J. R., Garcia, C. A., Zoghbi, H. Y., *et al.* (1991). Discordance of muscular dystrophy in monozygotic female twins. *American Journal of Medical Genetics* **40**, 354–64.

Luque, E. R. (1982). Segmental spinal instrumentation for correction of scoliosis. *Clinical Orthopaedics and Related Research* **163**, 192–8.

Luthra, M. G., Stern, L. Z., and Kim, H. D. (1979). $(Ca^{++} + Mg^{++})$-ATPase of red cells in Duchenne and myotonic dystrophy: effect of soluble cytoplasmic activator. *Neurology* **29**, 835–41.

Mabry, C. C., Roeckel, I. E., Munich, R. L., and Robertson, D. (1965). X-linked pseudohypertrophic muscular dystrophy with a late onset and slow progression. *New England Journal of Medicine* **273**, 1062–70.

McGuire, S. A. and Fischbeck, K. H. (1991). Autosomal recessive Duchenne-like muscular dystrophy: molecular and histochemical results. *Muscle and Nerve* **14**, 1209–12.

McKishnie, J. D., Muir, J. M., and Girvan, D. P. (1983). Anaesthesia induced rhabdomyolysis—a case report. *Canadian Anaesthetists Society Journal* **30**, 295–8.

Macklem, P. T. (1986). Muscular weakness and respiratory function. *New England Journal of Medicine* **314**, 775–6.

McKusick, V. A. (1964). *On the X chromosome of man*. American Institute of Biological Sciences, Washington.

—— (1992). *Mendelian inheritance in man: catalogs of autosomal dominant, autosomal recessive, and X-linked phenotypes*, (10th edn). Johns Hopkins, Baltimore.

MacLeod, P. M., Holden, J., and Masotti, R. (1983). Duchenne muscular dystrophy in a female with an X-autosome translocation. *American Journal of Human Genetics* **35**, 104A (Abstract).

McMenamin, J. B., Becker, L. E., and Murphy, E. G. (1982). Congenital muscular dystrophy: a clinicopathologic report of 24 cases. *Journal of Pediatrics* **100**, 692–7.

Maguire, P. (1984). Training in genetic counselling. In *Psychological aspects of genetic counselling*, (ed. A. E. H. Emery and I. M. Pullen), pp. 219–28. Academic Press, London.

Mair, W. G. P. and Tomé, F. M. S. (1972). *Atlas of the ultrastructure of diseased human muscle*. Churchill Livingstone, Edinburgh.

Make, B. J. (1991). Mechanical ventilation in the home: summary of the 3rd International Conference on Pulmonary Rehabilitation and Home Mechanical Ventilation. *Neuromuscular Disorders* **1**, 229–30.

Malhotra, S. B., Hart, K. A., Klamut, H. J., *et al.* (1988). Frame-shift deletions in patients with Duchenne and Becker muscular dystrophy. *Science* **242**, 755–9.

Marandian, M. H., Ramine, M., Djafarian, M., *et al.* (1977). Association de rétinopathie pigmentaire et de maladie de Duchenne dans une famille. *Annales de Pediatrie* **24**, 789–95.

Markand, O. N., North, R. R., D'Agostino, A. N., and Daly, D. D. (1969). Benign sex-linked muscular dystrophy: clinical and pathological features. *Neurology* **19**, 617–33.

Marsh, G. G. and Munsat, T. L. (1974). Evidence for early impairment of verbal intelligence in Duchenne muscular dystrophy. *Archives of Disease in Childhood* **49**, 118–22.

Marsh, W. L. (1978). Chronic granulomatous disease, the McLeod syndrome, and the Kell blood groups. *Birth Defects Original Article Series* **XIV** (No. 6A), 9–25.

——, Marsh, N. J., Moore, A., Symmans, W. A., Johnson, C. L., and Redman, C. M. (1981). Elevated serum creatine phosphokinase in subjects with McLeod syndrome. *Vox Sanguinis* **40**, 403–11.

Martin, A. J., Stern, L., Yeates, J., Lepp, D., and Little, J. (1986). Respiratory muscle training in Duchenne muscular dystrophy. *Developmental Medicine and Child Neurology* **28**, 314–18.

Martonosi, A. (1989). Calcium regulation in muscle disease: the influence of innervation and activity. *Biochimica et Biophysica Acta* **991**, 155–242.

Mastaglia, F. L. and Walton, J. (ed.) (1982). *Skeletal muscle pathology*. Churchill Livingstone, Edinburgh.

Matsumura, K., Tomé, F. M. S., Collin, H., *et al.* (1992). Deficiency of the 50K dystrophin-associated glycoprotein in severe childhood autosomal recessive muscular dystrophy. *Nature* **359**, 320–2.

Matsuo, M., Masumura, T., Nakajima, T., *et al.* (1990). A very small frame-shifting deletion within exon 19 of the Duchenne muscular dystrophy gene. *Biochemical and Biophysical Research Communications* **170**, 963–7.

Maunder-Sewry, C. A. and Dubowitz, V. (1979). Myonuclear calcium in carriers of

Duchenne muscular dystrophy. An X-ray microanalysis study. *Journal of the Neurological Sciences* **42**, 337–47.

——— and Dubowitz, V. (1981). Needle muscle biopsy for carrier detection in Duchenne muscular dystrophy. Part 1. Light microscopy-histology, histochemistry and quantitation. *Journal of the Neurological Sciences* **49**, 305–24.

———, Gorodetsky, R., Yarom, R., and Dubowitz, V. (1980). Element analysis of skeletal muscle in Duchenne muscular dystrophy using X-ray fluorescence spectrometry. *Muscle and Nerve* **3**, 502–8.

Mauro, A. (ed.) (1979). *Muscle regeneration.* Raven Press, New York.

Mawatari, S. and Katayama, K. (1973). Scapuloperoneal muscular atrophy with cardiopathy. An X-linked recessive trait. *Archives of Neurology* **28**, 55–9.

Mechler, F., Mastaglia, F. L., Haggith, J., and Gardner-Medwin, D. (1980). Adrenergic receptor responses of vascular smooth muscle in Becker muscular dystrophy. A muscle blood flow study using the ^{133}Xe clearance method. *Journal of the Neurological Sciences* **46**, 291–302.

Meltzer, H. Y. (1971). Factors affecting serum creatine phosphokinase levels in the general population: the role of race, activity and age. *Clinica Chimica Acta* **33**, 165–72.

——— and Holy, P. A. (1974). Black–white differences in serum creatine phosphokinase (CPK) activity. *Clinica Chimica Acta* **54**, 215–24.

———, Dorus, E., Grunhaus, L., Davis, J. M., and Belmaker, R. (1978). Genetic control of human plasma creatine phosphokinase activity. *Clinical Genetics* **13**, 321–6.

Mendell, J. R., Higgins, R., Sahenk, Z., and Cosmos, E. (1979). Relevance of genetic animal models of muscular dystrophy to human muscular dystrophies. *Annals of the New York Academy of Sciences* **317**, 409–30.

———, Province, M. A., Moxley, R. T. III., *et al.* (1987). Clinical investigation of Duchenne muscular dystrophy. A methodology for therapeutic trials based on natural history controls. *Archives of Neurology* **44**, 808–11.

———, Moxley, R. T., Griggs, R. C., *et al.* (1989). Randomized, double-blind six-month trial of prednisone in Duchenne's muscular dystrophy. *New England Journal of Medicine* **320**, 1592–7.

Menke, A. and Jockusch, H. (1991). Decreased osmotic stability of dystrophin-less muscle cells from the *mdx* mouse. *Nature* **349**, 69–71.

———, Brinkmeier, H., Naumann, T., Rüdel, R., and Jockusch, H. (1991). Role of dystrophin in cell stability: Differences between DMD and control myotubes detected by osmotic shock treatment. Proceedings of the Annual Meeting of the Deutsche Gesellschaft fur Zellbiologie. *European Journal of Cell Biology* **57** (Suppl. 36), p. 52.

Merchut, M. P., Zdonczyk, D., and Gujrati, M. (1990). Cardiac transplantation in female Emery–Dreifuss muscular dystrophy. *Journal of Neurology* **237**, 316–19.

Merlini, L., Granata, C., Dominici, P., and Bonfiglioli, S. (1986). Emery–Dreifuss muscular dystrophy: Report of five cases in a family and review of the literature. *Muscle and Nerve* **9**, 481–5.

Merritt, A. D., Kang, K. W., Conneally, P. M., Gersting, J. M., and Rigo, T. (1976). MEGADATS: A computer system for family data acquisition, storage and analysis. In *Registers for the detection and prevention of genetic disease*, (ed. A. E. H. Emery and J. R. Miller), pp. 31–49. Stratton Intercontinental, New York.

Meryon, E. (1852). On granular and fatty degeneration of the voluntary muscles. *Medico-Chirurgical Transactions (London)* **35**, 73–84.

—— (1864). *Practical and pathological researches on the various forms of paralysis.* Churchill, London.

Mesa, L. E., Dubrovsky, A. L., Corderi, J., Marco, P., and Flores, D. (1991). Steroids in Duchenne muscular dystrophy—Deflazacort trial. *Neuromuscular Disorders* **1**, 261–6.

Michaels, J., Krol, R. B., Bach, J., *et al.* (1991). Emery–Dreifuss muscular dystrophy (EDMD) with atrial tachycardia and apparent autosomal dominant transmission. Proceedings of the VIIIth International Congress on Human Genetics. *American Journal of Human Genetics* **49** (Suppl.), 151 (Abstract).

Michal, V. (1972). Psychika ditete s progresivni svalovou dystrofi. *Ceskoslovenska Psychiatrie* **68**, 226–30.

Michelson, A. M., Russell, E. S., and Harman, P. J. (1955). Dystrophia muscularis: a hereditary primary myopathy in the house mouse. *Proceedings of the National Academy of Sciences, USA* **41**, 1079–84.

Miciak, A., Keen, A., Jadayel, D., *et al.* (1992). Multiple mutation in an extended Duchenne muscular dystrophy family. *Journal of Medical Genetics* **29**, 123–6.

Milhorat, A. T. and Wolff, H. G. (1943). Studies in diseases of muscle. *Archives of Neurology and Psychiatry* **49**, 641–54.

Miller, A. D. (1992). Human gene therapy comes of age. *Nature* **357**, 455–60.

Miller, E. D., Sanders, D. B., Rowlingson, J. C., Berry, F. A., Sussman, M. D., and Epstein, R. M. (1978). Anaesthesia-induced rhabdomyolysis in a patient with Duchenne's muscular dystrophy. *Anesthesiology* **48**, 146–8.

Miller, G. and Dunn, N. (1982). An outline of the management and prognosis of Duchenne muscular dystrophy in Western Australia. *Australian Paediatric Journal* **18**, 277–82.

——, Tunnecliffe, M., and Douglas, P. S. (1985). IQ, prognosis and Duchenne muscular dystrophy. *Brain and Development* **7**, 7–9.

Miller, J. R. (1990). *X-linked traits: a catalog of loci in nonhuman mammals.* Cambridge University Press.

Miller, R. G., Layzer, R. B., Mellenthin, M. A., Golabi, M., Francoz, R. A., and Mall, J. C. (1985). Emery–Dreifuss muscular dystrophy with autosomal dominant transmission. *Neurology* **35**, 1230–3.

Milne, B. and Rosales, J. K. (1982). Anaesthetic considerations in patients with muscular dystrophy undergoing spinal fusion and Harrington rod insertion. *Canadian Anaesthetists Society Journal* **29**, 250–3.

Minetti, C., Beltrame, F., Marcenaro, G., and Bonilla, E. (1992). Dystrophin at the plasma membrane of human muscle fibers shows a costameric localization. *Neuromuscular Disorders* **2**, 99–109.

Miranda, A. F. and Mongini, T. (1984). Duchenne muscle culture: current status and future trends. In *Neuromuscular diseases*, (ed. G. Serratrice *et al.*), pp. 365–71. Raven Press, New York.

——, Bonilla, E., Martucci, G., *et al.* (1988). Immunocytochemical study of dystrophin in muscle cultures from patients with Duchenne muscular dystrophy and unaffected control patients. *American Journal of Pathology* **132**, 410–16.

Miyatake, M., Miike, T., Zhao, J., *et al.* (1989). Possible systemic smooth muscle layer dysfunction due to a deficiency of dystrophin in Duchenne muscular dystrophy. *Journal of the Neurological Sciences* **93**, 11–17.

Miyoshi, K. (1991). Echocardiographic evaluation of fibrous replacement in the myocardium of patients with Duchenne muscular dystrophy. *British Heart Journal* **66**, 452-5.

Mohr, C. H. and Hill, N. S. (1990). Long-term follow-up of nocturnal ventilatory assistance in patients with respiratory failure due to Duchenne-type muscular dystrophy. *Chest* **97**, 91-6.

Mokri, B. and Engel, A. G. (1975). Duchenne dystrophy: electron microscopic findings pointing to a basic defect or early abnormality in the plasma membrane of the muscle fiber. *Neurology* **25**, 1111-20.

Mokuno, K., Riku, S., Matsuoka, Y., Sobue, I., and Kato, K. (1984). Serum muscle-specific enolase in progressive muscular dystrophy and other neuromuscular diseases. *Journal of the Neurological Sciences* **63**, 345-52.

Monaco, A. P., Bertelson, C. J., Middlesworth, W., *et al.* (1985). Detection of deletions spanning the Duchenne muscular dystrophy locus using a tightly linked DNA segment. *Nature* **316**, 842-5.

——, Neve, R. L., Colletti-Feener, C., Bertelson, C. J., Kurnit, D. M., and Kunkel, L. M. (1986). Isolation of candidate cDNAs for portions of the Duchenne muscular dystrophy gene. *Nature* **323**, 646-50.

——, Bertelson, C. J., Liechti-Gallati, S., Moser, H., and Kunkel, L. M. (1988). An explanation for the phenotypic differences between patients bearing partial deletions of the DMD locus. *Genomics* **2**, 90-5.

——, Walker, A. P., Millwood, I., Larin, Z., and Lehrach, H. (1992). A yeast artificial chromosome contig containing the complete Duchenne muscular dystrophy gene. *Genomics* **12**, 465-73.

Monckton, G., Hoskin, V., and Warren, S. (1982). Prevalence and incidence of muscular dystrophy in Alberta, Canada. *Clinical Genetics* **21**, 19-24.

Mongini, T., Ghigo, D., and Doriguzzi, C. (1988). Free cytoplasmic Ca^{++} at rest and after cholinergic stimulus is increased in cultured muscle cells from Duchenne muscular dystrophy patients. *Neurology* **38**, 476-80.

Moosa, A., Brown, B. H., and Dubowitz, V. (1972). Quantitative electromyography —carrier detection in Duchenne type muscular dystrophy using a new automatic technique. *Journal of Neurology, Neurosurgery and Psychiatry* **35**, 841-4.

Morandi, L., Mora, M., Gussoni, E., *et al.* (1990). Dystrophin analysis in Duchenne and Becker muscular dystrophy carriers: correlation with intracellular calcium and albumin. *Annals of Neurology* **28**, 674-9.

Morgan, G. (1975). Effects of genetic counselling in Duchenne muscular dystrophy. In *Recent advances in myology*, (ed. W. G. Bradley, D. Gardner-Medwin, and J. N. Walton), pp. 477-8. Excerpta Medica, Amsterdam.

Morrell, R. M. (1959). Abnormal hepatic tests in muscular disease. *Archives of Internal Medicine* **104**, 83-90.

Morton, N. E. (1959). Genetic tests under incomplete ascertainment. *American Journal of Human Genetics* **11**, 1-16.

—— (1969). Segregation analysis. In *Computer applications in genetics*, (ed. N. E. Morton), pp. 129-39. University of Hawaii Press, Honolulu.

—— and Chung, C. S. (1959). Formal genetics of muscular dystrophy. *American Journal of Human Genetics* **11**, 360-79.

Moseley, C. F. (1984). Natural history and management of scoliosis in Duchenne muscular dystrophy. In *Neuromuscular diseases*, (ed. G. Serratrice *et al.*), pp. 545-9. Raven Press, New York.

Moser, H. (1971). Trisomie 21 bei einem Knaben mit progressiver Muskeldystrophie Duchenne. *Zeitschrift für Kinderheilkunde* **109**, 318–25.

—— (1977). Heterozygotenerfassung und genetische Beratung bei der progressiven Muskeldystrophie Duchenne. *Schweizerische Rundschau für Medizin Praxis* **66**, 814–22.

—— (1984). Duchenne muscular dystrophy: pathogenetic aspects and genetic prevention. *Human Genetics* **66**, 17–40.

—— and Emery, A. E. H. (1974). The manifesting carrier in Duchenne muscular dystrophy. *Clinical Genetics* **5**, 271–84.

—— and Vogt, J. (1974). Follow-up study of serum creatine kinase in carriers of Duchenne muscular dystrophy. *Lancet* **ii**, 661–2.

—— and Wiesmann, U. (1971). Serum-Creatin-Kinase und Sulfhydril-Konzentration nach ischämischer Arbeitsbelastung der Vorderarmmuskulatur bei Patienten und Konduktorinnen der progressiven Muskeldystrophie Duchenne. *Klinische Wochenschrift* **49**, 488–94.

——, Wiesmann, U., Richterich, R., and Rossi, E. (1964). Progressive Muskeldystrophie. VI. Häufigkeit, Klinik und Genetik der Duchenne-form. *Schweizerische Medizinische Wochenschrift* **94**, 1610–21.

——, Wiesmann, U., Richterich, R., and Rossi, E. (1966). Progressive Muskeldystrophie. VII. Häufigkeit, Klinik und Genetik der Typen I und II. *Schweizerische Medizinische Wochenschrift* **96**, 169–74, 205–11.

Moss, D. W., Whitaker, K. B., Parmar, C., *et al.* (1981). Activity of creatine kinase in sera from healthy women, carriers of Duchenne muscular dystrophy and cord blood, determined by the 'European' recommended method with NAC-EDTA activation. *Clinica Chimica Acta* **116**, 209–16.

Mossman, J., Blunt, S., Stephens, R., Jones, E. E., and Pembrey, M. (1983). Hunter's disease in a girl: association with X:5 chromosome translocation disrupting the Hunter gene. *Archives of Disease in Childhood* **58**, 911–15.

Mostacciuolo, M. L., Lombardi, A., Cambissa, V., Danieli, G. A., and Angelini C. (1987). Population data on benign and severe forms of X-linked muscular dystrophy. *Human Genetics* **75**, 217–20.

Moxley, R. T. (1984). Skeletal muscle blood flow and exercise. In *Neuromuscular diseases*, (ed. G. Serratrice *et al.*), pp. 51–6. Raven Press, New York.

MRC (1943). *Aids to the investigation of peripheral nerve injuries*. MRC War Memorandum No. 7, (2nd edn). HMSO, London.

Mueller, O. T., Hartsfield, Jr., J. K., Gallardo, L. A., *et al.* (1991). Lowe oculocerebrorenal syndrome in a female with a balanced X;20 translocation: mapping of the X chromsome breakpoint. *American Journal of Human Genetics* **49**, 804–10.

Müller, B., Dechant, C., Meng, G., *et al.* (1992). Estimation of the male and female mutation rates in Duchenne muscular dystrophy (DMD). *Human Genetics* **89**, 204–6.

Müller, E., Siciliano, B., Mostacciuolo, M. L., *et al.* (1991). Linkage analysis in one family with recurrence of Emery-Dreifuss muscular dystrophy. In *Muscular dystrophy research: from molecular diagnosis toward therapy*, (ed. C. Angelini, G. A. Danieli, and D. Fontanari), p. 239. Excerpta Medica, Amsterdam.

Mukoyama, M., Kondo, K., Hizawa, K., Nishitani, H., and the DMDR Group. (1987). Life spans of Duchenne muscular dystrophy patients in the hospital care program in Japan. *Journal of the Neurological Sciences* **81**, 155–8.

Murphy, E. A. (1973). Probabilities in genetic counselling. *Birth Defects Original Article Series* **9**, 19–33.

—— and Mutalik, G. S. (1969). The application of Bayesian methods in genetic counselling. *Human Heredity* **19**, 126–51.

Murphy, E. G. and Thompson, M. W. (1969). Manifestations of Duchenne muscular dystrophy in carriers. In *Progress in neurogenetics*, (ed. A. Barbeau and J. R. Brunette), pp. 162–8. Excerpta Medica, Amsterdam.

——, Thompson, M. W., Corey, P. N. J., and Conen, P. E. (1965). Varying manifestations of Duchenne muscular dystrophy in a family with affected females. In *Muscle*, (ed. W. M. Paul, E. E. Daniel, C. M. Kay, and G. Monckton), pp. 529–45. Pergamon Press, New York.

Murray, J. M., Davies, K. E., Harper, P. S., Meredith, L., Mueller, C. R., and Williamson, R. (1982). Linkage relationship of a cloned DNA sequence on the short arm of the X chromosome to Duchenne muscular dystrophy. *Nature* **300**, 69–71.

Musch, B. C., Papapetropoulos, T. A., McQueen, D. A., Hudgson, P., and Weightman, D. (1975). A comparison of the structure of small blood vessels in normal, denervated and dystrophic human muscle. *Journal of the Neurological Sciences* **26**, 221–34.

Mussini, E., Cornelio, F., Colombo, L., *et al.* (1984). Increased myofibrillar protein catabolism in Duchenne muscular dystrophy measured by 3-methylhistidine excretion in the urine. *Muscle and Nerve* **7**, 388–91.

Mutton, D. E., Chown, K., Thomson, L., Berry, A. C., Botcherby, P. K., and Bobrow, M. (1988). PRUFILE: a clinical and laboratory database for the genetics centre. *Clinical Genetics* **34**, 209–18.

Nadas, A. S. (1963). *Pediatric cardiology*, (2nd edn), p. 71. Saunders, Philadelphia.

Nakagawa, M., Nakahara, K., Yoshidome, H., *et al.* (1991). Epidemiology of progressive muscular dystrophy in Okinawa, Japan. *Neuroepidemiology* **10**, 185–91.

Nance, W. E. (1990). Invited editorial: do twin Lyons have larger spots? *American Journal of Human Genetics* **46**, 646–8.

Narazaki, O., Hanai, T., Ueki, Y., and Mitsudome, A. (1985). Duchenne muscular dystrophy in a female with an X-autosome translocation. (Japanese.) *Clinical Neurology* **25**, 432–6.

Nasse, C. F. (1820). Von einer erblichen Neigung zu tödlichen Blutungen. *Arch Med Erfahrung Geb Praktischen Med Staatsarzneikunde*, p. 385.

Nassi, P., Liguri, G., Landi, N., *et al.* (1985). Acylphosphatase from human skeletal muscle: purification, some properties and levels in normal and myopathic muscles. *Biochemical Medicine (New York)* **34**, 166–75.

Nayler, W. G. (1980). The pharmacological protection of the ischaemic heart: the use of calcium and beta-adrenoceptor antagonists. *European Heart Journal* **1** (Suppl. B), 5–13.

Neerunjun, J. S., Allsop, J., and Dubowitz, V. (1979). Hypoxanthine-guanine phosphoribosyltransferase activity of blood and muscle in Duchenne dystrophy. *Muscle and Nerve* **2**, 19–23.

Neligan, G. and Prudham, D. (1969). Norms for four standard developmental milestones by sex, social class and place in family. *Developmental Medicine and Child Neurology* **11**, 413–22.

Neville, H. E. and Harrold, S. (1985). Protein degradation in cultured skeletal muscle from Duchenne muscular dystrophy patients. *Muscle and Nerve* **8**, 253–7.

Nevin, N. C., Hughes, A. E., Calwell, M., and Lim, J. H. K. (1986). Duchenne muscular dystrophy in a female with a translocation involving Xp21. *Journal of Medical Genetics* **23**, 171–3.

Newberry, P. E. (1893). Beni Hasan, Part II. In *Archaeological survey of Egypt*, (ed. F. L. Griffith). Kegan Paul, Trench, Trübner and Co., London.

Newman, R. J., Bore, P. J., Chan, L., *et al.* (1982). Nuclear magnetic resonance studies of forearm muscle in Duchenne dystrophy. *British Medical Journal* **284**, 1072–4.

Newsom-Davis, J. (1980). The respiratory system in muscular dystrophy. *British Medical Bulletin* **36**, 135–8.

Newton, C. R., Graham, A., Heptinstall, L. E., *et al.* (1989). Analysis of any point mutation in DNA. The amplification refractory mutation system (ARMS). *Nucleic Acids Research* **17**, 2503–16.

Nguyen thi Man, Ellis, J. M., Love, D. R., *et al.* (1991). Localization of the DMDL gene-encoded dystrophin-related protein using a panel of nineteen monoclonal antibodies: presence at neuromuscular junctions, in the sarcolemma of dystrophic skeletal muscle, in vascular and other smooth muscles, and in proliferating brain cell lines. *Journal of Cell Biology* **115**, 1695–1700.

Nicholson, G. A. and Sugars, J. (1982). An evaluation of lymphocyte capping in Duchenne muscular dystrophy. *Journal of the Neurological Sciences* **53**, 511–18.

——, Gardner-Medwin, D., Pennington, R. J. T., and Walton, J. N. (1979). Carrier detection in Duchenne muscular dystrophy: assessment of the effect of age on detection-rate with serum-creatine-kinase-activity. *Lancet* **i**, 692–4.

——, Lane, R. J. M., Gardner-Medwin, D., and Walton, J. N. (1981). Carrier testing in families of isolated cases of Duchenne muscular dystrophy. *Journal of the Neurological Sciences* **51**, 29–42.

Nicholson, L. V. B. (1981). Serum myoglobin in muscular dystrophy and carrier detection. *Journal of the Neurological Sciences* **51**, 411–26.

——, Davison, K., Falkous, G., *et al.* (1989a). Dystrophin in skeletal muscle. I. Western blot analysis using a monoclonal antibody. *Journal of the Neurological Sciences* **94**, 125–36.

——, Davison, K., Johnson, M. A., *et al.* (1989b). Dystrophin in skeletal muscle. II. Immunoreactivity in patients with Xp21 muscular dystrophy. *Journal of the Neurological Sciences* **94**, 137–46.

——, Johnson, M. A., Gardner-Medwin, D., Bhattacharya, S., and Harris, J. B. (1990). Heterogeneity of dystrophin expression in patients with Duchenne and Becker muscular dystrophy. *Acta Neuropathologica* **80**, 239–50.

——, Bushby, K. M. D., Johnson, M. A., den Dunnen, J. T. Ginjaar, I. B., and van Ommen, G. J. B. (1992a). Predicted and observed sizes of dystrophin in some patients with gene deletions that disrupt the open reading frame. *Journal of Medical Genetics* (In press.)

——, Johnson, M. A., Davison, K., *et al.* (1992b). Dystrophin or a 'related protein' in Duchenne muscular dystrophy? *Acta Neurologica Scandinavica* (In press.)

——, Johnson, M. A., Bushby, K. M. D., and Gardner-Medwin, D. (1992c). The functional significance of dystrophin-positive fibres in Duchenne muscular dystrophy. *European Journal of Pediatrics* (In press.)

Niebrój-Dobosz, I. (1984). Surface membrane enzymes in human dystrophic muscle. in *Neuromuscular diseases*, (ed. G. Serratrice *et al.*), pp. 115–18. Raven Press, New York.

Nigris, P. (1984). Personal communication to G. A. Danieli (1984).

Nigro, G. (1986). Conte or Duchenne? *Cardiomyology* 5, 3-6.

——, Comi, L. I., Limongelli, F. M., *et al.* (1983). Prospective study of X-linked progressive muscular dystrophy in Campania. *Muscle and Nerve* 6, 253-62.

——, Comi, L. I., Politano, L., *et al.* (1984). Electrocardiographic evaluation of the P-type stage of dystrophic cardiomyopathy. *Cardiomyology* 3, 45-58.

——, Comi, L. I., Politano, L., and Bain, R. J. I. (1990a). The incidence and evolution of cardiomyopathy in Duchenne muscular dystrophy. *International Journal of Cardiology* 26, 271-7.

——, Comi, L. I., Politano, L., *et al.* (1990b). Treatment of cardiac involvement in late stage of Duchenne muscular dystrophy. *Acta Cardiomiologica* II(l), 13-24.

Nigro, V., Politano, L., Nigro, G., *et al.* (1992). Detection of a nonsense mutation in the dystrophin gene by multiple SSCP. *Human Molecular Genetics* 1, 517-20.

Nishio, H., Wada, H., Matsuo, T., *et al.* (1990). Glucose, free fatty acid and ketone body metabolism in Duchenne muscular dystrophy. *Brain and Development* 12, 390-402.

Nordenskjöld, M., Nicholson, L. V. B., Edström, L., *et al.* (1990). A normal male with an inherited deletion of one exon within the DMD gene. *Human Genetics* 84, 207-9.

Norman, A. and Harper, P. (1989). A survey of manifesting carriers of Duchenne and Becker muscular dystrophy in Wales. *Clinical Genetics* 36, 31-7.

——, Thomas, N., Coakley, J., and Harper, P. (1989a). Distinction of Becker from limb-girdle muscular dystrophy by means of dystrophin cDNA probes. *Lancet* i, 466-8.

Norman, A. M., Hughes, H. E., Gardner-Medwin, D., and Nicholson, L. V. B. (1989b). Dystrophin analysis in the diagnosis of muscular dystrophy. *Archives of Disease in Childhood* 64, 1501-3.

Northrup, H., Wheless, J. W., Lewis, R. A., *et al.* (1990). Monozygotic twins discordant for tuberous sclerosis. *American Journal of Human Genetics* 47, A69 (Abstract).

Nowak, T. V., Ionasescu, V., and Anuras, S. (1982). Gastrointestinal manifestations of the muscular dystrophies. *Gastroenterology* 82, 800-10.

Nudel, U., Zuk, D., Einat, P., *et al.* (1989). Duchenne muscular dystrophy gene product is not identical in muscle and brain. *Nature* 337, 76-8.

——, Zuk, D., Barnea, E., *et al.* (1992). Tissue and cell type distribution of transcripts of the Duchenne muscular dystrophy gene. In *Neuromuscular development and disease* (ed. A. M. Kelly and H. M. Blau), pp. 341-9. Raven Press, New York.

Nutting, D. F., MacPike, A. D., and Meier, H. (1980). The calcium content of various tissues from myodystrophic and dystrophic mice. *Journal of Heredity* 71, 15-18.

O'Brien, T., Sibert, I. R., and Harper, P. S. (1983). Implications of diagnostic delay in Duchenne muscular dystrophy. *British Medical Journal* 287, 1106-7.

Ogasawara, A. (1989). Similarity of IQs of siblings with Duchenne progressive muscular dystrophy. *American Journal of Mental Retardation* 93, 548-50.

Ohlendieck, K., Ervasti, J. M., Snook, J. B., and Campbell, K. P. (1991). Dystrophin-glycoprotein complex is highly enriched in isolated skeletal muscle sarcolemma. *Journal of Cell Bilogy* 112, 135-48.

Oka, S., Igarashi, Y., Takagi, A., *et al.* (1982). Malignant hyperpyrexia and

Duchenne muscular dystrophy: a case report. *Canadian Anaesthetists Society Journal* 29, 627-9.

Olson, B. J. and Fenichel, G. M. (1982). Progressive muscle disease in a young woman with family history of Duchenne's muscular dystrophy. *Archives of Neurology* 39, 378-80.

Olsson, T., Henriksson, K. G., Klareskog, L., and Forsum, U. (1984). HLA-DR expression, T lymphocyte phenotypes, OKM 1 and OKT 9 reactive cells in inflammatory myopathy. *Acta Neurologica Scandinavica* 69 (Suppl. 98), 200-1.

Orita, M., Suzuki, Y., Sekiya, T., and Hayashi, K. (1989). Rapid and sensitive detection of point mutations and DNA polymorphisms using the polymerase chain reaction. *Genomics* 5, 874-9.

Ørstavik, K. H., Kloster, R., Lippestad, C., *et al.* (1990). Emery-Dreifuss syndrome in three generations of females, including identical twins. *Clinical Genetics* 38, 447-51.

Ortaggio, F., Guidetti, D., Motti, L., Marcello, N., Solime, F., and Lucci, B. (1984). Studio longitudinale della funzionalita respiratoria nella distrofia muscolare di Duchenne. *Cardiomyology* 3, 73-83.

Oswald, A., Goldblatt, J., Horak, A., and Beighton, P. (1987). Lethal cardiac conduction defects in Emery-Dreifuss muscular dystrophy. *South African Medical Journal* 72, 567-70.

——, Heilig, R., Hanauer, A., and Mandel, J. L. (1991). Nonradioactive assay for new microsatellite polymorphisms at the 5' end of the dystrophin gene, and estimation of intragenic recombination. *American Journal of Human Genetics* 49, 311-19.

Oudet, C., Hanauer, A., Clemens, P., Caskey, T., and Mandel, J-L. (1992). Two hot spots of recombination in the DMD gene correlate with the deletion prone regions. *Human Molecular Genetics* 1, 599-603.

Panayiotopoulos, C. P. (1975). The neural hypothesis. In *Recent advances in myology*, (ed. W. G. Bradley, D. Gardner-Medwin, and J. N. Walton), pp. 159-62. Excerpta Medica, Amsterdam.

Park, Y. C., Kameda, N., Kobayashi, T., and Tsukagoshi, H. (1991). Developmental study of the expression of dystrophin in cultured human muscle aneurally and innervated with fetal rat spinal cord. *Brain Research* 565, 280-9.

Parry, R. (1984). Basic counselling techniques. In *Psychological aspects of genetic counselling*, (ed. A. E. H. Emery and I. M. Pullen), pp. 11-21. Academic Press, London.

Partridge, T. A., Morgan, J. E., Coulton, G. R., Hoffman, E. P., and Kunkel, L. M. (1989). Conversion of mdx myofibres from dystrophin-negative to -positive by injection of normal myoblasts. *Nature* 337, 176-9.

Passos, M. R., Gonzalez, C. H., and Zatz, M. (1985). Creatine-kinase and pyruvate-kinase activities in normal children: implications in Duchenne muscular dystrophy carrier detection. *American Journal of Medical Genetics* 22, 255-62.

Passos-Bueno, M. R., Rabbi-Bortolini, E., Azevêdo E., and Zatz, M. (1989*a*). Racial effect on serum creatine-kinase: implications for estimation of heterozygosity risks for females at-risk for Duchenne dystrophy. *Clinica Chimica Acta* 179, 163-8.

——, Otto, P. A., and Zatz, M. (1989*b*). Estimates of conditional heterozygosity risks for young females in Duchenne muscular dystrophy. *Human Heredity* 39, 202-11.

——, Rapaport, D., Love, D., *et al.* (1990*a*). Screening of deletions in the dystrophin gene with the cDNA probes Cf23a, Cf56a, and Cf115. *Journal of Medical Genetics* **27**, 145–50.

——, Lima, M. A., and Zatz, M. (1990*b*). Estimate of germinal mosaicism in Duchenne muscular dystrophy. *Journal of Medical Genetics* **27**, 727–8.

——, Vainzof, M., Pavanello, R. de C. M., *et al.* (1991). Limb-girdle syndrome: a genetic study of 22 large Brazilian families: comparison with X-linked Duchenne and Becker dystrophies. *Journal of the Neurological Sciences* **103**, 65–75.

——, Bakker, E., Kneppers, A. L. J., *et al.* (1992). Different mosaicism frequencies for proximal and distal Duchenne muscular dystrophy (DMD) mutations indicate difference in etiology and recurrence risk. *American Journal of Human Genetics* **51** (In press.)

Patel, K., Voit, T., Dunn, M. J., Strong, P. N., and Dubowitz, V. (1988). Dystrophin and nebulin in the muscular dystrophies. *Journal of the Neurological Sciences* **87**, 315–26.

Patterson, M., Ong, H., and Drake, A. (1964). Intestine absorption in muscular dystrophy patients. *Archives of Internal Medicine* **114**, 67–70.

Patterson, V., Morrison, O., and Hicks, E. (1991). Mode of death in Duchenne muscular dystrophy. *Lancet* **337**, 801–2.

Paulson, O. B., Engel, A. G., and Gomez, M. R. (1974). Muscle blood flow in Duchenne type muscular dystrophy, limb-girdle dystrophy, polymyositis and in normal controls. *Journal of Neurology, Neurosurgery and Psychiatry* **37**, 685–90.

Pearce, J. and Harriman, D. G. F. (1966). Chronic spinal muscular atrophy. *Journal of Neurology, Neurosurgery and Psychiatry* **29**, 509–20.

Pearn, J. H. (1990). Spinal muscular atrophies. In *Principles and practice of medical genetics*, (2nd edn), (ed. A. E. H. Emery and D. L. Rimoin), Vol. 1, pp. 565–78. Churchill Livingstone, Edinburgh.

—— and Hudgson, P. (1979). Anterior-horn cell degeneration and gross calf hypertrophy with adolescent onset. *Lancet* **i**, 1059–61.

Pearson, C. M. (1962). Histopathological features of muscle in the preclinical stages of muscular dystrophy. *Brain* **85**, 109–20.

——, Fowler, W. M., and Wright, S. W. (1963). X-chromosome mosaicism in females with muscular dystrophy. *Proceedings of the National Academy of Sciences, USA* **50**, 24–31.

Pellié, C., Feingold, J., and Démos, J. (1973). Age parental et mutation. A propos d'une enquête sur la myopathie de Duchenne de Boulogne. *Journal de Génétique Humaine* **21**, 33–41.

Pembrey, M. E., Davies, K. E., Winter, R. M., *et al.* (1984). Clinical use of DNA markers linked to the gene for Duchenne muscular dystrophy. *Archives of Disease in Childhood* **59**, 208–16.

Pena, S. D. J., Karpati, G., Carpenter, S., and Fraser, F. C. (1982). The clinical consequences of X-chromosomal inactivation: Duchenne muscular dystrophy in one of monozygotic twins. *Neurology* **32**, A83 (Abstract).

——, Karpati, G., Carpenter, S., and Fraser, F. C. (1987). The clinical consequences of X-chromosome inactivation: Duchenne muscular dystrophy in one of monozygotic twins. *Journal of the Neurological Sciences* **79**, 337–44.

Penn, A. S., Lisak, R. P., and Rowland, L. P. (1970). Muscular dystrophy in young girls. *Neurology* **20**, 147–59.

Pennington, R. J. T. (1962). Some enzyme studies in muscular dystrophy.

Proceedings of the Association of Clinical Biochemists **2**, 17–18.

—— (1977*a*). Serum enzymes. In *Pathogenesis of human muscular dystrophies*, (ed. L. P. Rowland), pp. 341–9. Excerpta Medica, Amsterdam.

—— (1977*b*). Proteinases of muscle. In *Proteinases in mammalian cells and tissues*, (ed. A. J. Barrett), pp. 515–43. Elsevier/North-Holland, Amsterdam.

—— (1980). Clinical biochemistry of muscular dystrophy. *British Medical Bulletin* **36**, 123–6.

—— (1988). Biochemical aspects of muscle disease with particular reference to the muscular dystrophies. In *Disorders of voluntary muscle*, (5th edn), (ed. J. N. Walton), pp. 455–86. Churchill Livingstone, Edinburgh.

Pennington, R. J. and Robinson, J. E. (1968). Cathepsin activity in normal and dystrophic human muscle. *Enzymologia Biologica et Clinica* **9**, 175–82.

Penrose, L. S. (1951). Measurement of pleiotropic effects in phenylketonuria. *Annals of Eugenics (London)* **16**, 134–41.

—— (1955). Parental age and mutation. *Lancet* **ii**, 312–13.

Percy, M. E., Andrews, D. F., and Thompson, M. W. (1982). Serum creatine kinase in the detection of Duchenne muscular dystrophy carriers: effects of season and multiple testing. *Muscle and Nerve* **5**, 58–64.

——, Pichora, G. A., Chang, L. S., Manchester, K. E., and Andrews, D. F. (1984). Serum myoglobin in Duchenne muscular dystrophy carrier detection: a comparison with creatine kinase and hemopexin using logistic discrimination. *American Journal of Medical Genetics* **18**, 279–87.

Perez Vidal, M. T., Grau, E. S., Viñas, J. P., Bayona, T. V., and Rustein, P. (1983). Distrofia muscular tipo Duchenne en una hembra con una translocación equilibrada X/6. *Revista de Neurologia (Barcelona)* **XI** (51), 155–8.

Perloff, J. K., De Leon, A. C., and O'Doherty, D. (1966). The cardiomyopathy of progressive muscular dystrophy. *Circulation* **33**, 625–48.

——, Roberts, W. C., De Leon, A. C., and O'Doherty, D. (1967). The distinctive electrocardiogram of Duchenne's progressive muscular dystrophy. *American Journal of Medicine* **42**, 179–88.

——, Henze, E., and Schelbert, H. R. (1984). Alterations in regional myocardial metabolism, perfusion, and wall motion in Duchenne muscular dystrophy studied by radionuclide imaging. *Circulation* **69**, 33–42.

Pescia, G. and The, N. G. (eds) (1986). *Chorionic villi sampling (CVS)*. Contributions to gynecology and obstetrics, Vol. 15. Karger, Basel.

Peter, J. B., Worsfold, M., and Pearson, C. M. (1969). Erythrocyte ghost adenosine triphosphatase (ATPase) in Duchenne dystrophy. *Journal of Laboratory and Clinical Medicine* **74**, 103–8.

Peterson, R., Masurovsky, E. B., Spiro, A. J., and Crain, S. M. (1986). Duchenne dystrophic muscle develops lesions in long-term coculture with mouse spinal cord. *Muscle and Nerve* **9**, 787–808.

Petty, R. K. H., Thomas, P. K., and Landon, D. N. (1986). Emery–Dreifuss syndrome. *Journal of Neurology* **233**, 108–14.

Phelan, M. C., Morton, C. C., Swenson, B. A., *et al.* (1980). Evidence for Lyonization of G-6-PD in a monozygotic twin pair. *American Journal of Human Genetics* **32**, 123A (Abstract).

Philip, J., Vogelius Andersen, C. H., Dreyer, V., *et al.* (1969). Colour vision deficiency in one of two presumably monozygotic twins with secondary amenorrhoea. *Annals of Human Genetics* **33**, 185–95.

Pickard, N. A., Gruemer, H. D., Verrill, H. L., *et al.* (1978). Systemic membrane defect in the proximal muscular dystrophies. *New England Journal of Medicine* **299**, 841-6.

Pillers, D. M., Weleber, R. G., Powell, B. R., Hanna, C. E., Magenis, R. E., and Buist, N. R. M. (1990*a*). Åland Island eye disease (Forsius-Eriksson ocular albinism) and an Xp21 deletion in a patient with Duchenne muscular dystrophy, glycerol kinase deficiency, and congenital adrenal hypoplasia. *American Journal of Medical Genetics* **36**, 23-8.

——, Towbin, J. A., Chamberlain, J. S., *et al.* (1990*b*). Deletion mapping of Åland Island eye disease to Xp21 between DXS67 (B24) and Duchenne muscular dystrophy. *American Journal of Human Genetics* **47**, 795-801.

——, Weleber, R. G., Musarella, M. A., *et al.* (1992). Abnormal eye findings documented by electroretinography in Duchenne/Becker muscular dystrophy. *Science* (In press.)

Pöch, H. and Becker, P. E. (1955). Eine Muskeldystrophie auf einem altägyptischen Relief. *Nervenarzt* **26**, 528-30.

Pöche, H. and Schulze, H. (1985). Ribosomal protein synthesis in altered skin fibroblast cells obtained from patients with Duchenne muscular dystrophy. *Journal of the Neurological Sciences* **70**, 295-304.

Poore, G. V. (1883). *Selections from the clinical works of Dr. Duchenne de Boulogne.* The New Sydenham Society, London.

Prelle, A., Chianese, L., Moggio, M., *et al.* (1991). Appearance and localization of dystrophin in normal human fetal muscle. *International Journal of Developmental Neuroscience* **9**, 607-12.

Prior, T. W. (1991). Genetic analysis of the Duchenne muscular dystrophy gene. *Archives of Pathology and Laboratory Medicine* **115**, 984-90.

——, Highsmith, W. E., Friedman, K. J., Perry, T. R., Scheuerbrandt, G., and Silverman, L. M. (1990). A model for molecular screening of newborns: simultaneous detection of Duchenne/Becker muscular dystrophies and cystic fibrosis. *Clinical Chemistry* **36**, 1756-9.

——, Papp, A. C., Snyder, P. J., and Mendell, J. R. (1992). Case of the month: Germline mosaicism in carriers of Duchenne muscular dystrophy. *Muscle and Nerve* **15**, 960-3.

Prosser, E. J., Murphy, E. G., and Thompson, M. W. (1969). Intelligence and the gene for Duchenne muscular dystrophy. *Archives of Disease in Childhood* **44**, 221-30.

Prot, J. (1971). Genetic-epidemiological studies in progressive muscular dystrophy. *Journal of Medical Genetics* **8**, 90-6.

Pullen, I. M. (1984). Physical handicap. In *Psychological aspects of genetic counselling*, (ed. A. E. H. Emery and I. M. Pullen), pp. 107-24. Academic Press, London.

Radhakrishnan, K., El-Mangoush, M. A., and Gerryo, S. E. (1987). Descriptive epidemiology of selected neuromuscular disorders in Benghazi, Libya. *Acta Neurologics Scandinavica* **75**, 95-100.

Radu, H. and Sarközi, A. (1978). Personal communication to P. Becker (1980).

——, Migea, S., Török, Z., Bordeianu, L., and Radu, A. (1968). Carrier detection in X-linked Duchenne type muscular dystrophy. A pluridimensional investigation. *Journal of the Neurological Sciences* **6**, 289-300.

Rapaport, D., Colletto, G. M. D. D., Vainzof, M., Duaik, M. C., and Zatz, M.

(1991*a*). Short stature in Duchenne muscular dystrophy. *Growth Regulation* **1**, 11–15.

——, Passos-Bueno, M. R., Brandão, L., *et al.* (1991*b*). Apparent association of mental retardation and specific patterns of deletions screened with probes Cf56a and Cf23a in Duchenne muscular dystrophy. *American Journal of Medical Genetics* **39**, 437–41.

——, Passos-Bueno, M. R., Takata, R. I., *et al.* (1992). A deletion including the brain promoter of the Duchenne muscular dystrophy gene is not associated with mental retardation. *Neuromuscular Disorders* **2**, 117–20.

Ray, P. N., Belfall, B., Duff, C., *et al.* (1985). Cloning of the breakpoint of an X;21 translocation associated with Duchenne muscular dystrophy. *Nature* **318**, 672–5.

Read, A. P., Storrar, L. K., Mountford, R. C., Elles, R. G., and Harris, R. (1986). A register based system for gene tracking in Duchenne muscular dystrophy. *Journal of Medical Genetics* **23**, 581–6.

Récan, D., Chafey, P., Leturcq, F., *et al.* (1992). Are cysteine-rich and COOH-terminal domains of dystrophin critical for sarcolemmal localization? *Journal of Clinical Investigation* **89**, 712–16.

Reddy, B. K., Anandavalli, T. E., and Reddi, O. S. (1984). X-linked Duchenne muscular dystrophy in an unusual family with manifesting carriers. *Human Genetics* **67**, 460–2.

Renier, W. O., Nabben, F. A. E., Hustinx, T. W. J., *et al.* (1983). Congenital adrenal hypoplasia, progressive muscular dystrophy, and severe mental retardation, in association with glycerol kinase deficiency, in-male sibs. *Clinical Genetics* **24**, 243–51.

Rennie, M. J., Edwards, R. H. T., Millward, D. L., Wolman, S. L., Halliday, D. H., and Matthews, D. E. (1982). Effects of Duchenne muscular dystrophy on muscle protein synthesis. *Nature* **296**, 165–7.

Révész, T., Schuler, D., Goldschmidt, B., and Elödi, S. (1972). Christmas disease in one of a pair of monozygotic twin girls, possibly the effect of Lyonization. *Journal of Medical Genetics* **9**, 396–400.

Riad, N. (1955). *La médecine au temps des Pharaons*, p. 242. Librairie Maloine, Paris.

Ribeiro, M. C. M., Melaragno, M. I., Schmidt, B., Brunoni, D., Gabbai, A. A., and Hackel, C. (1986). Duchenne muscular dystrophy in a girl with an (X;15) translocation. *American Journal of Medical Genetics* **25**, 231–6.

Richards, C. S., Watkins, S. C., Hoffman, E. P., *et al.* (1990). Skewed X inactivation in a female MZ twin results in Duchenne muscular dystrophy. *American Journal of Human Genetics* **46**, 672–81.

Richards, R. I. and Friend, K. (1991). Determination of Duchenne muscular dystrophy carrier status by single strand conformation polymorphism analysis of deleted regions of the dystrophin locus. *Journal of Medical Genetics* **28**, 856–9.

——, Friend, K., and Haan, E. A. (1992). Informative microsatellite markers allow carrier detection in a Duchenne muscular dystrophy deletion pedigree in the absence of DNA from an affected boy. *American Journal of Human Genetics* **50**, 448–9.

Richards, W. C. (1972). Anaesthesia and serum creatine phosphokinase levels in patients with Duchenne's pseudohypertrophic muscular dystrophy. *Anaesthesia and Intensive Care* **1**, 150-3.

Rideau, Y. M. (1979). *Outlines of muscular dystrophy*, (edited, revised, and translated from the French). Serem, Poitiers.

Rideau, Y. (1986). Prophylactic surgery for scoliosis in Duchenne muscular dystrophy. *Developmental Medicine and Child Neurology* **28**, 398-9.

——, Glorion, B., and Duport, G. (1983*a*). Prolongation of ambulation in the muscular dystrophies. *Acta Neurologica* (New Series) **5**, 390-7.

——, Gatin, G., Bach, J., and Ginies, G. (1983*b*). Prolongation of life in Duchenne's muscular dystrophy. *Acta Neurologica* (New Series) **5**, 118-24.

——, Glorion, B., DeLaubier, A., Tarle, O., and Bach, J. (1984). The treatment of scoliosis in Duchenne muscular dystrophy. *Muscle and Nerve* **7**, 281-6.

Ried, T., Mahler, V., Vogt, P., Blonden, L., van Ommen, G. J. B., Cremer, T., and Cremer, M. (1990). Direct carrier detection by in situ suppression hybridization with cosmid clones of the Duchenne/Becker muscular dystrophy locus. *Human Genetics* **85**, 581-6.

Riggs, J. E., Romano, J. T., Schochet, S. S., and Gutmann, L. (1988). Humeropelviperoneal muscular dystrophy with contractures: a genetically heterogeneous phenotype. *Archives of Neurology* **45**, 374-5.

Ringel, S. P., Carroll, J. E., and Schold, S. C. (1977). The spectrum of mild X-linked recessive muscular dystrophy. *Archives of Neurology* **34**, 408-16.

Robert, J. M. and Vignon, E. (1972). Les formes tardives des dystrophies musculaires liées a l'X. *Sciences Medicales* **3**, 397-402.

Roberts, R. G., Bentley, D. R., Barby, T. F. M., Manners, E., and Bobrow, M. (1990). Direct diagnosis of carriers of Duchenne and Becker muscular dystrophy by amplification of lymphocyte RNA. *Lancet* **336**, 1523-6.

——, Barby, T. F. M., Manners, E., Bobrow, M., and Bentley, D. R. (1991). Direct detection of dystrophin gene rearrangements by analysis of dystrophin mRNA in peripheral blood lymphocytes. *American Journal of Human Genetics* **49**, 298-310.

——, Bobrow, M., and Bentley, D. R. (1992). Point mutations in the dystrophin gene. *Proceedings of the National Academy of Sciences, USA* **89**, 2331-5.

Robin, G. C. (1976). Scoliosis in Duchenne muscular dystrophy. In *Muscular dystrophy 1976*, (ed. G. C. Robin and G. Falewski de Leon), pp. 119-22. Karger, Basel.

—— and Falewski, G. de L. (1963). Acute gastric dilatation in progressive muscular dystrophy. *Lancet* **ii**, 171-2.

Rodeck, C. H. and Morsman, J. M. (1983). First-trimester chorion biopsy. *British Medical Bulletin* **39**, 338-42.

Roddie, A. and Bundey, S. (1992). Racial distribution of Duchenne muscular dystrophy in the West Midlands region of Britain. *Journal of Medical Genetics* **29**, 555-7.

Rojas, C. V. and Hoffman, E. P. (1991). Recent advances in dystrophin research. *Current Opinion in Neurobiology* **1**, 420-9.

Ronan, J. A., Perloff, J. K., Bowen, P. J., and Mann, O. (1972). The vectorcardiogram in Duchenne's progressive muscular dystrophy. *American Heart Journal* **84**, 588-96.

Ronzoni, E., Berg, L., and Landau, W. (1960). Enzyme studies in progressive muscular dystrophy. *Research Publications — Association for Research in Nervous and Mental Disease* **38**, 721–9.

Ropers, H-H., Wienker, T. F., Grimm, T., Schroetter, K., and Bender, K. (1977). Evidence for preferential X-chromosome inactivation in a family with Fabry disease. *American Journal of Human Genetics* **29**, 361–70.

——, Zuffardi, O., Bianchi, E., and Tiepolo, L. (1982). Agenesis of corpus callosum, ocular and skeletal anomalies (X-linked dominant Aicardi's syndrome) in a girl with balanced X/3 translocation. *Human Genetics* **61**, 364–8.

Rosalki, S. B. (1967). An improved procedure for serum creatine phosphokinase determination. *Journal of Laboratory and Clinical Medicine* **69**, 696–705.

Roses, A. D. and Appel, S. H. (1976). Erythrocyte spectrin peak II phosphorylation in Duchenne muscular dystrophy. *Journal of the Neurological Sciences* **29**, 185–93.

——, Herbstreith, M. H., and Appel, S. H. (1975). Membrane protein kinase alteration in Duchenne muscular dystrophy. *Nature* **254**, 350–1.

——, Herbstreith, M., Metcalf, B., and Appel, S. H. (1976a). Increased phosphorylated components of erythrocyte membrane spectrin band II with reference to Duchenne dystrophy. *Journal of the Neurological Sciences* **30**, 167–78.

——, Roses, M. J., Miller, S. F., Hull, K. L., and Appel, S. H. (1976b). Carrier detection in Duchenne muscular dystrophy. *New England Journal of Medicine* **294**, 193–8.

——, Roses, M. J., Metcalf, B. S., *et al.* (1977). Pedigree testing in Duchenne muscular dystrophy. *Annals of Neurology* **2**, 271–8.

Rosman, N. P. (1970). The cerebral defect and myopathy in Duchenne muscular dystrophy. A comparative clinicopathological study. *Neurology* **20**, 329–35.

—— and Kakulas, B. A. (1966). Mental deficiency associated with muscular dystrophy. A neuropathological study. *Brain* **89**, 769–88.

Rossiter, B. J. F., Stirpe, N. S., and Caskey, C. T. (1992). Report of the MDA Gene Therapy Conference, Tucson, Arizona, September 27–28, 1991. *Neurology* (In press).

Rott, H-D., and Rödl, W. (1985). Imaging techniques in muscular dystrophies. *Clinical Genetics* **28**, 179–80.

Rotthauwe, H. W. and Kowalewski, S. (1966). Gutartige recessiv X-chromosomal vererbte Muskeldystrophie. I. Untersuchungen bei Merkmalsträgern. *Humangenetik* **3**, 17–29.

——, Mortier, W., and Beyer, H. (1972). Neuer Typ einer recessiv X-chromosomal vererbten Muskeldystrophie: scapulo-humero-distale Muskeldystrophie mit frühzeitigen Kontrakturen und Herzrhythmusstörungen. *Humangenetik* **16**, 181–200.

Rowe, D., Isenberg, D. A., and Beverley, P. C. L. (1983). Monoclonal antibodies to hunan leucocyte antigens in polymyositis and muscular dystrophy. *Clinical and Experimental Immunology* **54**, 327–36.

Rowland, L. P. (1976). Pathogenesis of muscular dystrophies. *Archives of Neurology* **33**, 315–21.

—— (1980). Biochemistry of muscle membranes in Duchenne muscular dystrophy. *Muscle and Nerve* **3**, 3–20.

—— (1984). Myoglobinuria, 1984. *Canadian Journal of Neurological Sciences* **11**, 1–13.

—— (1988). Clinical concepts of Duchenne muscular dystrophy: the impact of molecular genetics. *Brain* **111**, 479–95.

——, Fetell, M., Olarte, M., Hays, A., Singh, N., and Wanat, F. E. (1979). Emery-

Dreifuss muscular dystrophy. *Annals of Neurology* 5, 111–7.

Ruitenbeek, W. (1979). Membrane-bound enzymes of erythrocytes in human muscular dystrophy. ($Na^+ + K^+$)-ATPase, CA^{2+}-ATPase, K^+ and Ca^{2+}-P-Nitrophenylphosphatase. *Journal of the Neurological Sciences* 41, 71–80.

Russman, B. S. (1984). Comprehensive management of children with muscular disorders. *Pediatric Annals* 13, 103–12.

——, Melchreit, R., and Drennan, J. C. (1983). Spinal muscular atrophy: the natural course of disease. *Muscle and Nerve* 6, 179–81.

Saito, F., Tonomura, A., Kimura, S., Misugi, N., and Sugita, H. (1985). High resolution banding study of an X/4 translocation in a female with Duchenne muscular dystrophy. *Human Genetics* 71, 370–2.

——, Goto, J., Kakinuma, H., *et al.* (1986). Inherited Xp21 deletion in a boy with complex glycerol kinase deficiency syndrome. *Clinical Genetics* 29, 92–3.

Salih, M. A. M., Omer, M. I. A., Bayoumi, R. A., Karrar, O., and Johnson, M. (1983). Severe autosomal recessive muscular dystrophy in an extended Sudanese kindred. *Developmental Medicine and Child Neurology* 25, 43–52.

Samaha, F. J. and Congedo, C. Z. (1977). Two biochemical types of Duchenne dystrophy: sarcoplasmic reticulum membrane proteins. *Annals of Neurology* 1, 125–30.

——, Davis, B., and Nagy, B. (1981). Duchenne muscular dystrophy: adenosine triphosphate and creatine phosphate content in muscle. *Neurology* 31, 916–19.

Sanyal, S. K. and Johnson, W. W. (1982). Cardiac conduction abnormalities in children with Duchenne's progressive muscular dystrophy: electrocardiographic features and morphologic correlates. *Circulation* 66, 853–63.

——, Johnson, W. W., Dische, M. R., Pitner, S. E., and Beard, C. (1980). Dystrophic degeneration of papillary muscle and ventricular myocardium. A basis for mitral valve prolapse in Duchenne's muscular dystrophy. *Circulation* 62, 430–8.

Sarfarazi, M. and Williams, H. (1986). A computer programme for estimation of genetic risk in X linked disorders, combining pedigree and DNA probe data with other conditional information. *Journal of Medical Genetics* 23, 40–5.

Saviranta, P., Lindlöf, M., Lehesjoki, A-E., *et al.* (1988). Linkage studies in a new X-linked myopathy, suggesting exclusion of DMD locus and tentative assignment to distal Xq. *American Journal of Human Genetics* 42, 84–8.

Schanne, F. A. X., Kane, A. B., Young, E. E., and Farber, J. L. (1979). Calcium dependence of toxic cell death: a final common pathway. *Science* 206, 700–2.

Schapira, F., Dreyfuss J. C., Schapira, G., and Démos, J. (1960). Étude de l'aldolase et de la créatine kinase du sérum chez les mères de myopathes. *Revue Française Études Cliniques et Biologiques* 5, 990–4.

Schapira, G. and Dreyfuss J. C. (1963). Biochemistry of progressive muscular dystrophy. In *Muscular dystrophy in man and animals*, (ed. G. H. Bourne and M. N. Golarz), pp. 48–87. Hafner, New York.

Scheuerbrandt, G., Hammerschmidt, M., and Mortier, W. (1984). Voluntary CK screening programme for the early detection of Duchenne muscular dystrophy in infants. In *Research into the origin and treatment of muscular dystrophy*, (ed. L. P. ten Kate, P. L. Pearson, and A. M. Stadhouders), pp. 73–7. Excerpta Medica, Amsterdam.

——, Lundin, A., Lövgren, T., and Mortier, W. (1986). Screening for Duchenne muscular dystrophy: an improved screening test for creatine kinase and its application in an infant screening program. *Muscle and Nerve* 9, 11–23.

Schiaffino, S., Gorza, L., Dones, I., Cornelio, F., and Sartore, S. (1986). Fetal myosin immunoreactivity in human dystrophic muscle. *Muscle and Nerve* **9**, 51–8.

Schiffer, D., Bertolotto, A., De Marchi, M., *et al*. (1981). Epidemiology of Duchenne muscular dystrophy in the province of Turin. *Italian Journal of Neurological Sciences* **2**, 81–4.

——, Doriguzzi, C., Mongini, T., and Palmucci, L. (1984). Quantitative analysis of muscle biopsy. Results in 30 female controls and in 51 Duchenne carriers. *Italian Journal of Neurological Sciences* **5** (Suppl. 1), 175–6.

Schliephake, E. (1929). Der Kardio-intestinale Symptomenkomplex bei der progressiven Muskeldystrophie. II. Graphische Untersuchungen. *Zeitschrift für Kinderheilkunde* **47**, 85–93.

Schmalbruch, H. (1982). The muscular dystrophies. In *Skeletal muscle pathology*, (ed. F. L. Mastaglia and J. N. Walton), pp. 235–65. Churchill Livingstone, Edinburgh.

Schmidt, C. C. (1838). Krankhafte Hypertrophie des Muskelsystems. Mittheilung von den DDr. Coste und Gioja! In *Schmidt's Jahrbücher der in- und ausländischen gesamten Medizin* **24**, 176.

Scholte, H. R. and Busch, H. F. M. (1980). Decreased phosphorylase activity in leucocytes of Duchenne carriers. *Clinica Chimica Acta* **105**, 137–9.

Schorer, C. E. (1964). Muscular dystrophy and the mind. *Psychosomatic Medicine* **26**, 5–13.

Schröder, J. M. (1982). *Pathologie der Muskulatur*. Springer, Berlin.

Schrödinger, E. (1944). *What is life*? Cambridge University Press.

Schwartz, L. S., Tarleton, J., Popovich, B., Seltzer, W., and Hoffman, E. P. (1992). Fluorescent multiplex linkage analysis and carrier detection for Duchenne muscular dystrophy. *American Journal of Human Genetics* **51**, 721–9.

Scott, M. O., Sylvester, J. E., Heiman-Patterson, T., *et al*. (1988). Duchenne muscular dystrophy gene expression in normal and diseased human muscle. *Science* **239**, 1418–20.

Scott, O. M., Hyde, S. A., Goddard, C., Jones, R., and Dubowitz, V. (1981). Effect of exercise in Duchenne muscular dystrophy. *Physiotherapy* **67**, 174–6.

——, Hyde, S. A., Goddard, C., and Dubowitz, V. (1982). Quantitation of muscle function in children: a prospective study in Duchenne muscular dystrophy. *Muscle and Nerve* **5**, 291–301.

——, Hyde, S. A., Vrbová G., and Dubowitz, V. (1990). Therapeutic possibilities of chronic low frequency electrical stimulation in children with Duchenne muscular dystrophy. *Journal of the Neurological Sciences* **95**, 171–82.

Seay, A. R., Ziter, F. A., and Thompson, J. A. (1978). Cardiac arrest during induction of anesthesia in Duchenne muscular dystrophy. *Journal of Pediatrics* **93**, 88–90.

Seeger, B. R., Sutherland, A. D. A., and Clark, M. S. (1984). Orthotic management of scoliosis in Duchenne muscular dystrophy. *Archives of Physical and Medical Rehabilitation* **65**, 83–6.

Seltzer, W. K., Angeline, C., Dhariwal, G., Ringel, S. P., and McCabe, E. R. B. (1989). Muscle glycerol kinase in Duchenne dystrophy and glycerol kinase deficiency. *Muscle and Nerve* **12**, 307–13.

Serratrice, G. and Pouget, J. (1986). Maladie d'Emery–Dreifuss ou syndrome d'amyotrophie avec rétractions précoces et troubles secondaires de la conduction cardiaque d'heredité variable. *Revue Neurologique (Paris)* **142**, 766–70.

——, Pouget, J., Pellissier, J. F., Gastaut, J. L., and Cros, D. (1982). Les atteintes musculaires à transmission récessive liées à l'X avec rétractions musculaires précoces et troubles de la conduction cardiaque. *Revue Neurologique (Paris)* **138**, 713-24. (*See also* Serratrice, G. and Pouget, J. (1986).)

——, Pellissier, J. F., Pouget, J., and Desnuelle, C. (1984). Des formes précoces aux formes tardives des amyotrophies spinales chroniques. À propos de quatre-vingt-quatorze observations. *Semaine des Hôpitaux de Paris* **60**, 2867-74.

——, Guastalla, B., and Pellisier, J. F. (1988). À propos de la maladie d'Emery-Dreifuss. Discussion de deux nouvelles observations. *Revue de Médecine Interne* **9**, 365-8.

Sethna, N. F., Rockoff, M. A., Worthen, H. M., and Rosnow, J. M. (1988). Anesthesia-related complications in children with Duchenne muscular dystrophy. *Anesthesiology* **68**, 462-5.

Shalev, O., Leida, M. N., Hebbel, R. P., Jacob, H. S., and Eaton, J. W. (1981). Abnormal erythrocyte calcium homeostasis in oxidant-induced hemolytic disease. *Blood* **58**, 1232-5.

Shapiro, F. and Bresnan, M. J. (1982). Orthopaedic management of childhood neuromuscular disease. Part III. Diseases of muscle. *Journal of Bone and Joint Surgery* **64A**, 1102-7.

——, Sethna, N., Colan, S., Wohl, M. E., and Specht, L. (1992). Spinal fusion in Duchenne muscular dystrophy: a multidisciplinary approach. *Muscle and Nerve* **15**, 604-14.

Shaw, R. F. and Dreifuss, F. E. (1969). Mild and severe forms of X-linked muscular dystrophy. *Archives of Neurology* **20**, 451-60.

Sherwin, A. C. and McCully, R. S. (1961). Reactions observed in boys of various ages (10-14) to a crippling progressive and fatal illness (muscular dystrophy). *Journal of Chronic Diseases* **13**, 59-68.

Shoji, S. (1981). Calcium flux of erythrocytes in Duchenne muscular dystrophy. *Journal of the Neurological Sciences* **51**, 427-35.

Shokeir, M. H. K. and Kobrinsky, N. L. (1976). Autosomal recessive muscular dystrophy in Manitoba Hutterites. *Clinical Genetics* **9**, 197-202.

—— and Rozdilsky, B. (1985). Muscular dystrophy in Saskatchewan Hutterites. *American Journal of Medical Genetics* **22**, 487-93.

Shomrat, R., Driks, N., Legum, C., and Shiloh, Y. (1992). Use of dystrophin genomic and cDNA probes for solving difficulties in carrier detection and prenatal diagnosis of Duchenne muscular dystrophy. *American Journal of Medical Genetics* **42**, 281-7.

Shumate, J. B., Carroll, J. E., Brooke, M. H., and Choksi, R. M. (1982). Palmitate oxidation in human muscle: comparison to CPT and carnitine. *Muscle and Nerve* **5**, 226-31.

Sibert, J. R., Harper, P. S., Thompson, R. J., and Newcombe, R. G. (1979). Carrier detection in Duchenne muscular dystrophy. *Archives of Disease in Childhood* **54**, 534-7.

Sibley, J. A. and Lehninger, A. L. (1949). Aldolase in the serum and tissues of tumour-bearing animals. *Journal of the National Cancer Institute* **9**, 303-9.

Sidler, A. (1944). Beitrag zur Vererbung der progressiven Muskeldystrophie. *Archiv Julius Klaus Stiftung* **19**, 213-23.

Siegel, I. M. (1977a). *The clinical management of muscular disease*. Heinemann, London.

—— (1977*b*). Fractures of long bones in Duchenne muscular dystrophy. *Journal of Trauma* **17**, 219–22.

—— (1978). The management of muscular dystrophy: a clinical review. *Muscle and Nerve* **1**, 453–60.

—— (1980). Maintenance of ambulation in Duchenne muscular dystrophy. *Clinical Pediatrics* **19**, 383–8.

—— and Kornfeld, M. S. (1980). Kinetic family drawing test for evaluating families having children with muscular dystrophy. *The Journal of the American Physical Therapy Association* **60**, 293–8.

——, Miller, J. E., and Ray, R. D. (1968). Subcutaneous lower limb tenotomy in the treatment of pseudohypertrophic muscular dystrophy. *Journal of Bone and Joint Surgery* **50A**, 1437–43.

——, Miller, J. E., and Ray, R. D. (1974). Failure of corticosteroid in the treatment of Duchenne (pseudohypertrophic) muscular dystrophy. Report of a clinically matched three year double blind study. *Illinois Medical Journal* **145**, 32–6.

Silverman, L. M., Mendell, J. R., Sahenk, Z., and Fontana, M. B. (1976). Significance of creatine phosphokinase isoenzymes in Duchenne dystrophy. *Neurology* **26**, 561–4.

Simpson, A. C., Holmes, D., and Pennington, R. J. T. (1979). Dilution effect on serum creatine kinase in carriers of Duchenne muscular dystrophy. *Annals of Clinical Biochemistry* **16**, 54–5.

Skinner, R., Emery, A. E. H., Scheuerbrandt, G., and Syme, J. (1982). Feasibility of neonatal screening for Duchenne muscular dystrophy. *Journal of Medical Genetics* **19**, 1–3.

Sklar, R. M. and Brown, R. H. (1991). Methylprednisolone increases dystrophin levels by inhibiting myotube death during myogenesis of normal human muscle in vitro. *Journal of the Neurological Sciences* **101**, 73–81.

——, Beggs, A. H., Lev, A. A., *et al.* (1990). Defective dystrophin in Duchenne and Becker dystrophy myotubes in cell culture. *Neurology* **40**, 1854–8.

Skolnick, M., Carmelli, D., and Tyler, F. (1977). A two-locus selection hypothesis for Duchenne muscular dystrophy. *Theoretical Population Biology* **12**, 230–45.

Skyring, A. and McKusick V. A. (1961). Clinical, genetic and electrocardiographic studies in childhood muscular dystrophy. *American Journal of Medical Sciences* **242**, 534–47.

Slater, C. R. and Nicholson, L. V. B. (1991). Is dystrophin labelling always discontinuous in Becker muscular dystrophy? *Journal of the Neurological Sciences* **101**, 187–92.

Slucka, C. (1968). The electrocardiogram in Duchenne progressive muscular dystrophy. *Circulation* **38**, 933–40.

Smith, C. A. B. and Kilpatrick, S. J. (1958). Estimates of the sex ratio of mutation rates in sex-linked conditions by the method of maximum likelihood. *Annals of Human Genetics* **22**, 244–9.

Smith, C. L. and Bush, G. H. (1985). Anaesthesia and progressive muscular dystrophy. *British Journal of Anaesthesia* **57**, 1113–18.

Smith, I., Elton, R. A., and Thomson, W. H. S. (1979). Carrier detection in X-linked recessive (Duchenne) muscular dystrophy: serum creatine phosphokinase values in premenarchal, menstruating and postmenopausal and pregnant normal women. *Clinics Chimica Acta* **98**, 207–16.

Smith, P. E. M., Carty, A., Owen, R., and Edwards, R. H. T. (1986). Quantitative computerized tomography scanning of psoas and erector spinae in muscular dystrophy. *Muscle and Nerve* **9** (Suppl.), 243 (Abstract).

——, Calverley, P. M. A., Edwards, R. H. T., Evans, G. A., and Campbell, E. J. M. (1987). Practical problems in the respiratory care of patients with muscular dystrophy. *New England Journal of Medicine* **316**, 1197–1205.

——, Edwards, R. H. T., and Calverley, P. M. A. (1989*a*). Oxygen treatment of sleep hypoxaemia in Duchenne muscular dystrophy. *Thorax* **44**, 997–1001.

——, Edwards, R. H. T., and Calverley, P. M. A. (1989*b*). Protriptyline treatment of sleep hypoxaemia in Duchenne muscular dystrophy. *Thorax* **44**, 1002–5.

——, Edwards, R. H. T., and Calverley, P. M. A. (1991). Mechanisms of sleep-disordered breathing in chronic neuromuscular disease: implications for management. *Quarterly Journal of Medicine* (New Series 81) **296**, 961–73.

Smith, R. A., Rogers, M., Bradley, D. M., Sibert, J. R., and Harper, P. S. (1989). Screening for Duchenne muscular dystrophy. *Archives of Disease in Childhood* **64**, 1017–21.

——, Sibert, J. R., and Harper, P. S. (1990*a*). Early development of boys with Duchenne muscular dystrophy. *Developmental Medicine and Child Neurology* **32**, 519–27.

——, Williams, D. K., Sibert, J. R., and Harper, P. S. (1990*b*). Attitudes of mothers to neonatal screening for Duchenne muscular dystrophy. *British Medical Journal* **300**, 1112.

Sollee, N. D., Latham, E. E., Kindlon, D. J., and Bresnan, M. J. (1985). Neuropsychological impairment in Duchenne muscular dystrophy. *Journal of Clinical and Experimental Neuropsychology* **7**, 486–96.

Solti, F., Zádory, E., and Bekény, G. (1963). Electrocardiographic and circulatory changes in progressive muscular dystrophy. *Acta Medica Academiae Scientiarum Hungaricae* **19**, 1–10.

Somer, H. (1980). Enzyme release from isolated erythrocytes and lymphocytes in Duchenne muscular dystrophy. *Journal of the Neurological Sciences* **48**, 445–52.

——, Donner, M., Murros, J., and Konttinen, A. (1973). A serum isozyme study in muscular dystrophy. Particular reference to creatine kinase, aspartate aminotransferase and lactic dehydrogenase isozymes. *Archives of Neurology* **29**, 343–5.

——, Willner, J., DeCresce, R. P., Willner, J., and Somer, M. (1980). Duchenne carriers: lactate dehydrogenase isoenzyme 5 in serun and muscle. *Neurology* **30**, 206–9.

——, Voutilainen, A., Knuutila, S., Kaitila, I., Rapola, J., and Leinonen, H. (1985). Duchenne-like muscular dystrophy in two sisters with normal karyotypes: evidence for autosomal recessive inheritance. *Clinical Genetics* **28**, 151–6.

——, Laulumaa, V., Paljärvi, L., *et al.* (1991). Benign muscular dystrophy with autosomal dominant inheritance. *Neuromuscular Disorders* **1**, 267–73.

Sood, S. C. and Goyal, B. G. (1969). An unusual form of progressive muscular dystrophy. *Indian Journal of Pediatrics* **36**, 219–23.

Spector, E. B., Baumbach, L. L., Seltzer, W. K., Hoffman, E. P., Crandall, B. F., and Smith, A. C. M. (1990). X-linked muscular dystrophy affecting both females and males in a large caucasian family. *American Journal of Human Genetics* **47**, A236 (Abstract).

Speer, M. C., Yamaoka, L. H., Gilchrist, J. H., *et al.* (1992). Confirmation of genetic heterogeneity in limb girdle muscular dystrophy: linkage of an autosomal dominant form to chromosome 5q. *American Journal of Human Genetics* **50**, 1211–17.

Spencer, G. E. and Vignos, P. J. (1962). Bracing for ambulation in childhood progressive muscular dystrophy. *Journal of Bone and Joint Surgery* **44A**, 234–42.

Spiegler, A. W. J. and Herrmann F. H. (1983). Erfassung und humangenetische Betreuung von Risikofamilien mit progressiver Muskeldystrophie der Typen Duchenne (DMD) und Becker–Kiener (BMD) im Bezirk Erfurt. *Deutsche Gesundheitswesen* **38**, 994–9.

——, Hausmanowa-Petrusewicz, I., Borkowska, J., and Herrmann, F. H. (1987). Atypical form of X-linked proximal pseudohypertrophic muscular dystrophy. *Journal of Neurology* **234**, 163–71.

Spillane, J. D. (1981). *The doctrine of the nerves – chapters in the history of neurology*. Oxford University Press.

Spowart, G., Buckton, K. E., Skinner, R., and Emery, A. E. H. (1982). X-chromosome in Duchenne muscular dystrophy. *Lancet* i, 1251.

Staples, D. (1977). Intellect and psychological problems. In *Severe childhood neuromuscular disease – the management of Duchenne muscular dystrophy and spinal muscular atrophy*, (ed. D. H. Bossingham, E. Williams, and P. J. R. Nichols), pp. 30–7. Muscular Dystrophy Group of Great Britain and Northern Ireland, London.

Stark, P., Maves, C., and Wertz, R. A. (1988). Acute gastric dilatation as a manifestation of Duchenne's muscular dystrophy. *ROFO Fortschritte auf dem Gebiete der Röntgenstrahlen und der Nuklearmedizin* **149**, 554–5.

Starr, J., Lamont, M., Iselius, L., *et al.* (1990). A linkage study of a large pedigree with X linked centronuclear myopathy. *Journal of Medical Genetics* **27**, 281–3.

Statham, H. E. and Dubowitz, V. (1979). Duchenne muscular dystrophy: ^{45}Ca exchange in cultured skin fibroblasts and the effect of calcium ionophore A23187. *Clinica Chimica Acta* **96**, 225–31.

Stedman, H. H., Sweeney, H. L., Shrager, J. B., *et al.* (1991). The *mdx* mouse diaphragm reproduces the degenerative changes of Duchenne muscular dystrophy. *Nature* **352**, 536–9.

Stephens, F. E. and Tyler, F. H. (1951). Studies in disorders of muscle. V. The inheritance of childhood progressive muscular dystrophy in 33 kindreds. *American Journal of Human Genetics* **3**, 111–25.

Stern, L. M., Caudrey, D. J., Clark, M. S., Perrett, L. V., and Boldt, D. W. (1985). Carrier detection in Duchenne muscular dystrophy using computed tomography. *Clinical Genetics* **27**, 392–7.

Stern, L. Z. (1984). Criteria for therapeutic trials in Duchenne muscular dystrophy. In *Neuromuscular diseases*, (ed. G. Serratrice *et al.*), pp. 525–8. Raven Press, New York.

Stern, R. and Eldridge, R. (1975). Attitudes of patients and their relatives to Huntington's disease. *Journal of Medical Genetics* **12**, 217–23.

——, Godbold, J. H., Chess, Q., and Kagen, L. J. (1984). ECG abnormalities in polymyositis. *Archives of Internal Medicine* **144**, 2185–9.

Stevenson, A. C. (1953). Muscular dystrophy in Northern Ireland. *Annals of Eugenics (London)* **18**, 50–91.

—— (1958). Muscular dystrophy in Northern Ireland. IV. Some additional data. *Annals of Human Genetics* **22**, 231–4.

Sugita, H. and Tyler, F. H. (1963). Pathogenesis of muscular dystrophy. *Trans-*

actions of the Association of American Physicians **76**, 231–43.

——, Ishiura, S., and Kohama, K. (1984). Lysosomal and nonlysosomal enzymes and amino acid fluxes in catabolic states. In *Neuromuscular diseases*, (ed. G. Serratrice *et al.*), pp. 143–7. Raven Press, New York.

——, Arahata, K. Ishiguro, T., *et al.* (1988). Negative immunostaining of Duchenne muscular dystrophy (DMD) and mdx muscle surface membrane with antibody against synthetic peptide fragment predicted from DMD cDNA. *Proceedings of the Japan Academy* **64**, 37–9.

Sussman, M. D. (1984). Advantage of early spinal stabilization and fusion in patients with Duchenne muscular dystrophy. *Journal of Pediatric Orthopedics* **4**, 532–7.

—— (1985). Treatment of scoliosis in Duchenne muscular dystrophy. *Developmental Medicine and Child Neurology* **27**, 522–4.

Sutherland, D. H., Olshen, R., Cooper, L., *et al.* (1981). The pathomechanics of gait in Duchenne muscular dystrophy. *Developmental Medicine and Child Neurology* **23**, 3–22.

Suthers, G. K., Manson, J. I., Stern, L. M., *et al.* (1989). Becker muscular dystrophy (BMD) and Klinefelter's syndrome: a possible cause of variable expression of BMD within a pedigree. *Journal of Medical Genetics* **26**, 251–4.

Swash, M. and Schwartz, M. S. (1988). *Neuromuscular diseases—a practical approach to diagnosis and management*, (2nd edn). Springer, Berlin.

——, Schwartz, M. S., Carter, N. D., Heath, R., Leak, M., and Rogers, K. L. (1983). Benign X-linked myopathy with acanthocytes (McLeod syndrome). Its relationship to X-linked muscular dystrophy. *Brain* **106**, 717–33.

Swinyard, C. A., Deaver, G. G., and Greenspan, L. (1957). Gradients of functional ability of importance in rehabilitation of patients with progressive muscular and neuromuscular diseases. *Archives of Physical and Medical Rehabilitation* **38**, 574–9.

Szibor, R. and Steinbicker, V. (1983). Untersuchungen zu genetischen und diagnostischen Problemen bei Patienten mit Duchenne'scher Muskeldystrophie und bei Konduktorinnen. Unpublished dissertation, Magdeburg.

——, Till, U., Lösche, W., and Steinbicker, V. (1981). Red cell response to A23187 and valinomycine in Duchenne muscular dystrophy. *Acta Biologica et Medica Germanica* **40**, 1187–90.

Tachi, N., Tachi, M., Sasaki, K., *et al.* (1990). Dystrophin analysis in the differential diagnosis of autosomal recessive muscular dystrophy of childhood and Duchenne muscular dystrophy. *Pediatric Neurology* **6**, 265–8.

Taft, L. T. (1973). The care and management of the child with muscular dystrophy. *Developmental Medicine and Child Neurology* **15**, 510–18.

Takagi, A. (1984). Sarcoplasmic reticulum of Duchenne muscular dystrophy: a study on skinned muscle fiber. In *Neuromuscular diseases*, (ed. G. Serratrice *et al.*), pp. 123–5. Raven Press, New York.

—— and Nonaka, I. (1981). Duchenne muscular dystrophy: unusual activation of single fibers *in vitro*. *Muscle and Nerve* **4**, 10–15.

——, Shimada, Y., and Mozai, T. (1970). Studies on plasma free fatty acid and ketone bodies in young patients with muscular atrophy. *Neurology* **20**, 904–8.

Takamoto, K., Hirose, K., Uono, M., and Nonaka, I. (1984). A genetic variant of Emery-Dreifuss disease: muscular dystrophy with humeropelvic distribution, early joint contracture, and permanent atrial paralysis. *Archives of Neurology* **41**, 1292–3.

Takeshita, K., Yoshino, K., Kitahara, T., Nakashima, T., and Kato, N. (1977). Survey of Duchenne type and congenital type of muscular dystrophy in Shimane, Japan. *Japanese Journal of Human Genetics* **22**, 43–7.

——, Kasagi, S., Mito, T., *et al.* (1987). Decreased incidence of Duchenne muscular dystrophy in Western Japan 1956–80. *Neuroepidemiology* **6**, 130–8.

Tanaka, K., Yoshimura, T., Muratani, H., *et al.* (1989). Familial myopathy with scapulohumeral distribution, rigid spine, cardiopathy and mitochondrial abnormality. *Journal of Neurology* **236**, 52–4.

Tangsrud, S-E. and Halvorsen, S. (1988). Child neuromuscular disease in Southern Norway. Prevalence, age and distribution of diagnosis with special reference to 'non-Duchenne muscular dystrophy'. *Clinical Genetics* **34**, 145–52.

Tanzer, M. L. and Gilvarg, C. (1959). Creatine and creatine kinase measurement. *Journal of Biological Chemistry* **234**, 3201–4.

Tay, J. S. H., Low, P. S., Lee, W. S., *et al.* (1990). Dystrophin function: calcium related rather than mechanical. *Lancet* **335**, 983.

Templeton, A. R. and Yokoyama, S. (1980). Effect of reproductive compensation and the desire to have male offspring on the incidence of a sex-linked lethal disease. *American Journal of Human Genetics* **32**, 575–81.

Thomas, A., Bax, M., Coombes, K., Goldson, E., Smyth, D., and Whitmore, K. (1985). The health and social needs of physically handicapped young adults: Are they being met by the statutory services? *Developmental Medicine and Child Neurology* **27** (Suppl. 50[4]).

Thomas, N. S. T., Williams, H., Elsas, L. J., Hopkins, L. C., Sarfarazi, M., and Harper, P. S. (1986). Localization of the gene for Emery–Dreifuss muscular dystrophy to the distal long arm of the X-chromosome. *Journal of Medical Genetics* **23**, 596–8.

——, Williams, H., Cole, G., *et al.* (1990). X linked neonatal centronuclear/ myotubular myopathy: evidence for linkage to Xq28 DNA marker loci. *Journal of Medical Genetics* **27**, 284–7.

Thomas, P. K., Calne, D. B., and Elliott, C. F. (1972). X-linked scapuloperoneal syndrome. *Journal of Neurology, Neurosurgery and Psychiatry* **35**, 208–15.

——, Schott, G. D., and Morgan-Hughes, J. A. (1975). Adult onset scapuloperoneal myopathy. *Journal of Neurology, Neurosurgery and Psychiatry* **38**, 1008–15.

Thompson, C. E. (1978). Reproduction in Duchenne dystrophy. *Neurology* **28**, 1045–7.

Thompson, M. W. (1984). Genetic management of pregnancies of carriers and possible carriers of Duchenne muscular dystrophy. In *Neuromuscular diseases*, (ed. G. Serratrice *et al.*), pp. 21–3. Raven Press, New York.

——, Ludvigsen, B., and Monckton, G. (1962). Some problems in genetics of muscular dystrophy. *Revue Canadienne de Biologie* **21**, 543–50.

Thompson, W. H. S. (1968). Determination and statistical analyses of the normal ranges for five serum enzymes. *Clinica Chimica Acta* **21**, 469–78.

—— (1971). Serum enzyme studies in acquired disease of skeletal muscle. *Clinica Chimica Acta* **35**, 193–9.

——, Sweetin, J. C., and Elton, R. A. (1974). The neurogenic and myogenic hypotheses in human (Duchenne) muscular dystrophy. *Nature* **249**, 151–2.

Tippett, P. A., Dennis, N. R., Machin, D., Price, C. P., and Clayton, B. E. (1982). Creatine kinase activity in the detection of carriers of Duchenne muscular dystrophy: comparison of two methods. *Clinica Chimica Acta* **121**, 345–59.

Tomelleri, G., Orrico, D., De Grandis, D., and Fiaschi, A. (1980). Emery–Dreifuss muscular dystrophy in two brothers. In *Muscular dystrophy research: advances and new trends*, (ed. C. Angelini, G. A. Danieli, and D. Fontanari), pp. 307-8. Excerpta Medica, Amsterdam.

Toop, J. (1975). The histochemical development of human skeletal muscle and its motor innervation. In *Recent advances in myology*, (ed. W. G. Bradley, D. Gardner-Medwin, and J. N. Walton), pp. 322-9. Excerpta Medica, Amsterdam.

—— and Emery, A. E. H. (1974). Muscle histology in fetuses at risk for Duchenne muscular dystrophy. *Clinical Genetics* **5**, 230-3.

Topaloğlu, H., Yalaz, K., Renda, Y., *et al.* (1989). Congenital muscular dystrophy (non-Fukuyama type) in Turkey: a clinical and pathological evaluation. *Brain and Development* **11**, 341-4.

Torres, L. F. B., and Duchen, L. W. (1987). The mutant *mdx*: inherited myopathy in the mouse. *Brain* **110**, 269-99.

Totsuka, T., Watanabe, K., and Uramoto, I. (1983). A bone–muscle imbalance hypothesis for the pathogenesis of murine muscular dystrophy. In *Muscular dystrophy: biomedical aspects*, (ed. S. Ebashi and E. Ozawa), pp. 29-38. Springer, Berlin.

Turner, P. R., Fong, P., Denetclaw, W. F., and Steinhardt, R. A. (1991). Increased calcium influx in dystrophic muscle. *Journal of Cell Biology* **115**, 1701-12.

Turpin, J. C., Berriche, S., Intrator, S., and Lucotte, G. (1989). La maladie d'Emery-Dreifuss. A propos d'un cas de dystrophie musculaire scapulo-huméro-péronière. *Semaine des Hôpitaux de Paris* **65**, 894-7.

Tyler, F. H. (1950). Studies in disorders of muscle. III. 'Pseudohypertrophy' of muscle in progressive muscular dystrophy and other neuromuscular diseases. *Archives of Neurology and Psychiatry* **63**, 425-32.

—— and Wintrobe, M. M. (1950). Studies in disorders of muscle. I. The problems of progressive muscular dystrophy. *Annals of Internal Medicine* **32**, 72-9.

Tzvetanova, E. (1971). Aldolase isoenzymes in serum and muscle from patients with progressive muscular dystrophy and from human foetus. *Journal of the Neurological Sciences* **14**, 483-9.

Upadhyaya, M., Smith, R. A., Thomas, N. S. T., Norman, A. M., and Harper, P. S. (1990). Intragenic deletions in 164 boys with Duchenne muscular dystrophy (DMD) studied with dystrophin cDNA. *Clinical Genetics* **37**, 456-62.

Usuki, F., Nakazato, O., Osame, M., and Igata, A. (1985). Hyperestrogenemia in Duchenne muscular dystrophy (DMD). *Clinical Neurology* **25**, 711-5.

Vainzof, M., Zatz, M., and Otto, P. A. (1985). Serum CK-MB activity in progressive muscular dystrophy: Is it of nosologic value? *American Journal of Medical Genetics* **22**, 81-7.

——, Pavanello, R. C. M., Pavanello-Filho, I., *et al.* (1990). Dystrophin immunostaining in muscles from patients with different types of muscular dystrophy: a Brazilian study. *Journal of the Neurological Sciences* **98**, 221-33.

——, Pavanello, R. C. M., Pavanello-Filho, I., *et al.* (1991a). Screening of male patients with autosomal recessive Duchenne dystrophy through dystrophin and DNA studies. *American Journal of Medical Genetics* **39**, 38-41.

——, Pavanello, R. C. M., Pavanello, I., *et al.* (1991b). Dystrophin immunofluorescence pattern in manifesting and asymptomatic carriers of Duchenne's and Becker muscular dystrophies of different ages. *Neuromuscular Disorders* **1**, 177-83.

——, Passos-Bueno, M. R., Pavanello, R. C. M., Schreiber, R., and Zatz, M. (1992). A model to estimate the expression of the dystrophin gene in muscle from female Becker muscular dystrophy carriers. *Journal of Medical Genetics* **29**, 476-9.

Valentine, B. A., Cooper, B. J., Cummings, J. F. and deLahunta, A. (1986). Progressive muscular dystrophy in a golden retriever dog: light microscope and ultrastructural features at 4 and 8 months. *Acta Neuropathologica (Berlin)* **71**, 301-10.

——, Cooper, B. J., Cummings, J. F. and deLahunta, A. (1990). Canine X-linked muscular dystrophy: morphologic lesions. *Journal of the Neurological Sciences* **97**, 1-23.

——, Winand, N. J., Pradhan, D., *et al.* (1992). Canine X-linked muscular dystrophy as an animal model of Duchenne muscular dystrophy: a review. *American Journal of Medical Genetics* **42**, 352-6.

Van Voorhis, B. J., Williamson, R. A., Gerard, J. L., Hammitt, D. C., and Syrop, C. H. (1992). Use of oocytes from anonymous, matched, fertile donors for prevention of heritable genetic diseases. *Journal of Medical Genetics* **29**, 398-9.

Vasari, G. (1568). *Lives of the artists.* (Translated and reprinted in *Penguin*, London, 1981.)

van der Ven, P. F. M., Jap, P. H. K., Wetzels, R. H. W., *et al.* (1991). Postnatal centralization of muscle fibre nuclei in centronuclear myopathy. *Neuromuscular Disorders* **1**, 211-20.

Verellen, C., De Meyer, R., Freund, M., Laterre, C., Scholberg, B., and Frédéric, J. (1977). Progressive muscular dystrophy of the Duchenne type in a young girl associated with an aberration of chromosome X. In *Proceedings of the 5th International Congress on Birth Defects*, p. 42 (Abstract). Excerpta Medica, Amsterdam.

——, Markovic, V., De Meyer, R., Freund, M., Laterre, C., and Worton, R. (1978). Expression of an X-linked recessive disease in a female due to non-random inactivation of the X chromosome. *American Journal of Human Genetics* **30**, 97A (Abstract).

Verellen-Dumoulin, C., Freund, M., De Meyer, R., *et al.* (1984). Expression of an X-linked muscular dystrophy in a female due to a translocation involving Xp21 and non-random inactivation of the normal X chromosome. *Human Genetics* **67**, 115-91.

Verga, V., Hall, B. K., Wang, S., *et al.* (1991). Localization of the translocation breakpoint in a female with Menkes syndrome to Xq13.2-q13.3 proximal to PGK-1. *American Journal of Human Genetics* **48**, 1133-8.

Vignos, P. J. (1977a). Intellectual function and educational achievement in Duchenne muscular dystrophy. In *Muscular dystrophy*, 1976, (ed. G. C. Robin and G. Falewski de Leon), pp. 131-8. Karger, Basel.

—— (1977b). Respiratory function and pulmonary infection in Duchenne muscular dystrophy. In *Muscular dystrophy, 1976*, (ed. G. C. Robin and G. Falewski de Leon), pp. 123-30. Karger, Basel.

—— (1979). Rehabilitation in the myopathies. In *Handbook of clinical neurology*, (Vol. 41), (ed. P. J. Vinken and G. W. Bruyn), pp. 457-500. Elsevier/North-Holland, Amsterdam.

—— and Lefkowitz, M. (1959). A biochemical study of certain skeletal muscle constituents in human progressive muscular dystrophy. *Journal of Clinical Investigation* **38**, 873-81.

—— and Watkins, M. P. (1966). The effect of exercise in muscular dystrophy. *Journal of the American Medical Association* **197**, 121–6.

——, Spencer, G. E., and Archibald, K. C. (1963). Management of progressive muscular dystrophy of childhood. *Journal of the American Medical Association* **184**, 89–96.

de Visser, M. and Verbeeten, B. (1985*a*). Computed tomography of the skeletal musculature in Becker-type muscular dystrophy and benign infantile spinal muscular atrophy. *Muscle and Nerve* **8**, 435–44.

—— and Verbeeten, B. (1985*b*). Computed tomographic findings in manifesting carriers of Duchenne muscular dystrophy. *Clinical Genetics* **27**, 269–75.

Vitiello, L., Mostacciuolo, M. L., Oliviero, S., Schiavon, F., Nicoletti, L., Angelini, C., and Danieli, G. A. (1992). Screening for mutations in the muscle promoter region and for exonic deletions in a series of 115 DMD and BMD patients. *Journal of Medical Genetics* **29**, 127–30.

Vlietinck, R. F. and van den Berghe, H. (1976). The Belgian national register. In *Registers for the detection and prevention of genetic disease*, (ed. A. E. H. Emery and J. R. Miller), pp. 65–71. Stratton Intercontinental, New York.

Vogel, F. (1990). Mutation in man. In *Principles and practice of medical genetics*, (2nd edn), (ed. A. E. H. Emery and D. L. Rimoin), Vol. 1, pp. 53–76. Churchill Livingstone, Edinburgh.

Voit, T., Krogmann, O., Lennard, H. G., *et al.* (1988). Emery–Dreifuss muscular dystrophy: disease spectrum and differential diagnosis. *Neuropediatrics* **19**, 62–71.

——, Haas, K., Léger, J. O. C., *et al.* (1991*a*). Xp2l dystrophin and 6q dystrophin-related protein: comparative immunolocalization using multiple antibodies. *American Journal of Pathology* **139**, 969–76.

——, Stuettgen, P., Cremer, M., and Goebel, H. H. (1991*b*). Dystrophin as a diagnostic marker in Duchenne and Becker muscular dystrophy. Correlation of immunofluorescence and Western blot. *Neuropediatrics* **22**, 152–62.

Wadia, R. S., Wadgaonkar, S. U., Amin, R. B., and Sardesai, H. V. (1976). An unusual family of benign 'X' linked muscular dystrophy with cardiac involvement. *Journal of Medical Genetics* **13**, 352–6.

Walton, J. N. (1955). On the inheritance of muscular dystrophy. *Annals of Human Genetics* **20**, 1–38.

—— (1956). Amyotonia congenita, a follow-up study. *Lancet* **i**, 1023–7.

—— (1957). The inheritance of muscular dystrophy. *Acta Genetica* (*Basel*) **7**, 318–20.

—— (1969). Muscular dystrophies and their management. *British Medical Journal* **3**, 639–42.

—— (ed.) (1988). *Disorders of voluntary muscle*, (5th edn). Churchill Livingstone, Edinburgh.

—— (1990). *Method in medicine*. The Harveian oration. Royal College of Physicians, London.

—— and Gardner-Medwin, D. (1988). The muscular dystrophies. In *Disorders of voluntary muscle*, (5th edn), (ed. J. N. Walton), pp. 519–68. Churchill Livingstone, Edinburgh.

—— and Nattrass, F. J. (1954). On the classification, natural history and treatment of the myopathies. *Brain* **77**, 169–231.

—— and Warrick, C. J. (1954). Osseous changes in myopathy. *British Journal of*

Radiology **27**, 1-15.

Waters, D. D., Nutter, D. O., Hopkins. L. C., and Dorney, E. R. (1975). Cardiac features of an unusual X-linked humeroperoneal neuromuscular disease. *New England Journal of Medicine* **293**, 1017-22.

Watters, G., Karpati, G., and Kaplan, B. (1977). Post-anaesthetic augmentation of muscle damage as a presenting sign in three patients with Duchenne muscular dystrophy. *Canadian Journal of Neurological Sciences* **4**, 228 (Abstract).

Wehnert, M., Machill, G., Grimm, T., *et al.* (1991). Evidence supporting tight linkage of X-linked Emery–Dreifuss muscular dystrophy to the factor VIII:C gene. In *Muscular dystrophy research: from molecular diagnosis toward therapy*, (ed. C. Angelini, G. A. Danieli, and D. Fontanari), pp. 260-1. Excerpta Medica, Amsterdam.

Weiller, C. (1985). Muskeldystrophie Duchenne. Ein Fallbericht. *Pathologe* **6**, 32-7.

Weller, B., Karpati, G., Lehnert, S., Carpenter, S., Ajdukovic, B., and Holland, P. (1991). Inhibition of myosatellite cell proliferation by gamma irradiation does not prevent the age-related increase of the number of dystrophin-positive fibers in soleus muscles of mdx female heterozygote mice. *American Journal of Pathology* **138**, 1497-1502.

Wells, D. J., Wells, K. E., Walsh, F. S., *et al.* (1992). Human dystrophin expression corrects the myopathic phenotype in transgenic *mdx* mice. *Human Molecular Genetics* **1**, 35-40.

Werner, W. and Spiegler, A. W. J. (1988). Inherited deletion of subband Xp21.13 in a male with Duchenne muscular dystrophy. *Journal of Medical Genetics* **25**, 377-82.

Wessels, A., Ginjaar, I. B., Moorman, A. F. M., and van Ommen, G. J. B. (1991). Different localization of dystrophin in developing and adult human skeletal muscle. *Muscle and Nerve* **14**, 1-7.

Whelan, T. B. (1987). Neuropsychological performance of children with Duchenne muscular dystrophy and spinal muscle atrophy. *Developmental Medicine and Child Neurology* **29**, 212-20.

Wiegand, V., Rahlf, G., Meinck, M., and Kreuzer, H. (1984). Kardiomyopathie bei Trägerinnen des Duchenne-Gens. *Zeitschrift für Kardiologie* **73**, 188-91.

Wieme, R. J. and Herpol, J. E. (1962). Origin of the lactate dehydrogenase iso-enzyme pattern found in the serum of patients having primary muscular dystrophy. *Nature* **194**, 287-8.

Wilcox, D. E., Affara, N. A., Yates, J. R. W., Ferguson-Smith, M. A., and Pearson, P. L. (1985). Multipoint linkage analysis of the short arm of the human X chromosome in families with X-linked muscular dystrophy. *Human Genetics* **70**, 365-75.

——, Cooke, A., Colgan, J., *et al.* (1986). Duchenne muscular dystrophy due to a familial Xp21 deletion detectable by DNA analysis and flow cytometry. *Human Genetics* **73**, 175-80.

Williams, E. A., Read, L., Ellis, A., Galasko, C. S. B., and Morris, P. (1984). The management of equinus deformity in Duchenne muscular dystrophy. *Journal of Bone and Joint Surgery* **66B**, 546-50.

Williams, W. R., Thompson, M. W., and Morton, N. E. (1983). Complex segregation analysis and computer-assisted genetic risk assessment for Duchenne muscular dystrophy. *American Journal of Medical Genetics* **14**, 315-33.

Willner, J., Nakagawa, M., and Wood, D. (1984). Drug-induced fiber necrosis in

Duchenne dystrophy. *Italian Journal of Neurological Sciences* Suppl. 3 (Muscular Dystrophy Facts and Perspectives), 117–21.

Winchester, B., Young, E., Geddes, S., *et al.* (1990). Mucopolysaccharidosis II (Hunter disease) in a female twin. *Journal of Medical Genetics* 27, 645 (Abstract).

Winter, R. M. (1980). Estimation of male to female ratio of mutation rates from carrier-detection tests in X-linked disorders. *American Journal of Human Genetics* 32, 582–8.

Witkowski, J. A. and Dubowitz, V. (1985). Duchenne muscular dystrophy: studies of cell motility *in vitro. Journal of Cell Science* 76, 225–34.

Witt, T. N., Garner, C. G., Pongratz, D., and Baur, X. (1988). Autosomal dominant Emery–Dreifuss syndrome: evidence of a neurogenic variant of the disease. *European Archives of Psychiatry and Neurological Sciences* 237, 230–6.

Wohlfart, G., Fex, J., and Eliasson, S. (1955). Hereditary proximal spinal muscular atrophy—a clinical entity simulating progressive muscular dystrophy. *Acta Psychiatrica et Neurologica (Copenhagen)* 30, 395–406.

Wolff, J. A., Malone, R. W., Williams, P., *et al.* (1990). Direct gene transfer into mouse muscle in vivo. *Science* 247, 1465–8.

Wood, D. S. (1984). Excitation-contraction coupling in Duchenne muscular dystrophy. In *Neuromuscular diseases*, (ed. G. Serratrice *et al.*), pp. 185–90. Raven Press, New York.

Wood, S. and McGillivray, B. C. (1988). Germinal mosaicism in Duchenne muscular dystrophy. *Human Genetics* 78, 282–4.

Worden, D. K. and Vignos, P. J. (1962). Intellectual function in childhood progressive muscular dystrophy. *Pediatrics* 29, 968–77.

Worton, R. G. and Thompson, M. W. (1988). Genetics of Duchenne muscular dystrophy. *Annual Review of Genetics* 22, 601–29.

——, Duff, C., Sylvester, J. E., Schmickel, R. D., and Willard, H. F. (1984). Duchenne muscular dystrophy involving translocation of the *dmd* gene next to ribosomal RNA genes. *Science* 224, 1447–9.

Wrogemann, K. and Pena, S. D. J. (1976). Mitochondrial calcium overload: a general mechanism for cell-necrosis in muscle diseases. *Lancet* i, 672–4.

Wulfsberg, E. A. and Skoglund, R. R. (1986). Duchenne muscular dystrophy in a 46 XY female. *Clinical Pediatrics* 25, 276–8.

Wyse, D. G., Nath, F. C., and Brownell, A. K. W. (1987). Benign X-linked (Emery–Dreifuss) muscular dystrophy is not benign. *PACE* 10, 533–7.

Yasin, R., Van Beers, G., Nurse, K. C. E., *et al.* (1977). A quantitative technique for growing human adult skeletal muscle in culture starting from mononucleated cells. *Journal of the Neurological Sciences* 32, 347–60.

Yasuda, N. and Kondo, K. (1980). No sex difference in mutation rates of Duchenne muscular dystrophy. *Journal of Medical Genetics* 17, 106–11.

—— and Kondo, K. (1982). The effect of parental age on rate of mutation for Duchenne muscular dystrophy. *American Journal of Medical Genetics* 13, 91–9.

Yates, J. R. W. and Emery, A. E. H. (1985). A population study of adult onset limb-girdle muscular dystrophy. *Journal of Medical Genetics* 22, 250–7.

——, Affara, N. A., Jamieson, D. M., *et al.* (1986). Emery–Dreifuss muscular dystrophy: localisation to Xq27.3 → qter confirmed by linkage to the factor VIII gene. *Journal of Medical Genetics* 23, 587–90.

Yoshioka, M., Okuno, T., Honda, Y., and Nakano, Y. (1980). Central nervous system involvement in progressive muscular dystrophy. *Archives of Disease in Childhood* **55**, 589–94.

——, Itagaki, Y., Saida, K., and Nishitani, Y. (1986). Clinical and genetic studies of muscular dystrophy in young girls. *Clinical Genetics* **29**, 137–42.

——, Saida, K., Itagaki, Y., and Kamiya, T. (1989). Follow up study of cardiac involvement in Emery-Dreifuss muscular dystrophy. *Archives of Disease in Childhood* **64**, 713–15.

Yotsukura, M., Miyagawa, M., Tsuya, T., Ishihara, T., and Ishikawa, K. (1988). Pulmonary hypertension in progressive muscular dystrophy of the Duchenne type. *Japanese Circulation Journal* **52**, 321–6.

Young, A., Johnson, D., O'Gorman, E., Macmillan, T., and Chase, A. P. (1984). A new spinal brace for use in Duchenne muscular dystrophy. *Developmental Medicine and Child Neurology* **26**, 808–13.

Young, I. D. (1991). *Introduction to risk calculation in genetic counselling.* Oxford University Press.

Yu, Y. L. and Murray, N. M. F. (1984). A comparison of concentric needle electromyography, quantitative EMG and single fibre EMG in the diagnosis of neuromuscular diseases. *Electroencephalography and Clinical Neurophysiology* **58**, 220–5.

Zalman, F., Perloff, J. K., Durant, N. N., and Campion, D. S. (1983). Acute respiratory failure following intravenous verapamil in Duchenne's muscular dystrophy. *American Heart Journal* **105**, 510–11.

Zatz, M. (1983). Effects of genetic counseling on Duchenne muscular dystrophy families in Brazil. *American Journal of Medical Genetics* **15**, 483–90.

——, Frota-Pessoa, O., Levy, J. A., and Peres, C. A. (1976). Creatine phosphokinase (CPK) activity in relatives of patients with X-linked muscular dystrophies. A Brazilian study. *Journal de Génétique Humaine* **24**, 153–68.

——, Shapiro, L. J., Campion, D. S., Oda, E., and Kaback, M. M. (1978). Serum pyruvate kinase (PK) and creatine phosphokinase (CPK) in progressive muscular dystrophies. *Journal of the Neurological Sciences* **36**, 349–62.

——, Vianna-Morgante, A. M., Campos, P., and Diament, A. J. (1981*a*). Translocation (X;6) in a female with Duchenne muscular dystrophy: implications for the localisation of the DMD locus. *Journal of Medical Genetics* **18**, 442–7.

——, Betti, R. T. B., and Levy, J. A. (1981*b*). Benign Duchenne muscular dystrophy in a patient with growth hormone deficiency. *American Journal of Medical Genetics* **10**, 301–4 (and also *American Journal of Medical Genetics* **24**, 567–72 (1986)).

——, Rapaport, D., Vainzof, M., *et al.* (1988). Relation between height and clinical course in Duchenne muscular dystrophy. *American Journal of Medical Genetics* **29**, 405–10.

——, Passos-Bueno, M. R., and Rapaport, D. (1989). Estimate of the proportion of Duchenne muscular dystrophy with autosomal recessive inheritance. *American Journal of Medical Genetics* **32**, 407–10.

——, Rapaport, D., Vainzof, M., *et al.* (1991*a*). Serum creatine-kinase (CK) and pyruvate-kinase (PK) activities in Duchenne (DMD) as compared with Becker (BMD) muscular dystrophy. *Journal of the Neurological Sciences* **102**, 190–6.

——, Passos-Bueno, M. R., Rapaport, D., *et al.* (1991*b*). Familial occurrence of Duchenne dystrophy through paternal lines in four families. *American Journal of Medical Genetics* **38**, 80–4.

Zellweger, H. (1975). Family counselling in Duchenne muscular dystrophy. In *Recent advances in myology*, (ed. W. G. Bradley, D. Gardner-Medwin, and J. N. Walton), pp. 469–71. Excerpta Medica, Amsterdam.

—— and Antonik, A. (1975). Newborn screening for Duchenne muscular dystrophy. *Pediatrics* **55**, 30–4.

—— and Hanson, J. W. (1967*a*). Slowly progressive X-linked recessive muscular dystrophy (Type IIIB). *Archives of Internal Medicine* **120**, 525–35.

—— and Hanson, J. W. (1967*b*). Psychometric studies in muscular dystrophy type IIIa (Duchenne). *Developmental Medicine and Child Neurology* **9**, 576–81.

—— and Niedermeyer, E. (1965). Central nervous system manifestations in childhood muscular dystrophy. I. Psychometric and electroencephalographic findings. *Annals of Paediatrics* **205**, 25–42.

——, Hanson, J. W., and Markowitz, E. (1970). Age- and sex-dependent differences of serum enzymes in normal controls. In *Muscle diseases*, (International Congress Series, No. 199), (ed. J. N. Walton, N. Canal, and G. Scarlato), pp. 445–9. Excerpta Medica, Amsterdam.

——, Ionasescu, V., Simpson, J., Waziri, M., and Antonik, A. (1975). Screening of the newborn for Duchenne muscular dystrophy. *British Medical Journal* **3**, 767.

Zerres, K. (1989). *Klassifikation und Genetik Spinaler Muskelatrophien*. Thieme, Stuttgart.

——, Rudnik-Schöneborn, S., and Rietschel, M. (1990). Heterogeneity in proximal spinal muscular atrophy. *Lancet* **336**, 749–50.

Zhao, J., Yoshioka, K., Miike, T., Kageshita, T., and Arao, T. (1991). Nerve growth factor receptor immunoreactivity on the intramuscular blood vessels in childhood muscular dystrophies. *Neuromuscular Disorders* **1**, 135–41.

Zietkiewicz, E., Simard, L. R., Melançon, S. B., Vanasse, M., and Labuda, D. (1992). Carrier status diagnosis in Duchenne muscular dystrophy with 'conformational' DNA polymorphism. *Lancet* **339**, 134.

Ziter, F. A., Allsop, K. G., and Tyler, F. H. (1977). Assessment of muscle strength in Duchenne muscular dystrophy. *Neurology* **27**, 981–4.

Zneimer, S. M., Schneider, N. R., and Richards, C. S. (1990). *In situ* hybridization shows direct evidence of skewed X inactiviation in monozygotic twin females discordant for Duchenne muscular dystrophy. *American Journal of Human Genetics* **47** (Suppl.), A45 (Abstract).

Zubrzycka-Gaarn, E. E., Bulman, D. E., Karpati, G., *et al.* (1988). The Duchenne muscular dystrophy gene product is localized in sarcolemma of human skeletal muscle. *Nature* **333**, 466–9.

Zupan, A. (1992). Long-term electrical stimulation of muscles in children with Duchenne and Becker muscular dystrophy. *Muscle and Nerve* **15**, 362–7.

Index

Aarskog syndrome 172 (*table*)
A bands 2 (*fig.*), 5 (*fig.*)
abortion, therapeutic 252
acetylcholine 203
Achilles tenotomy 264, 267
achondroplasia, mutation rate 160 (*table*)
aconitase 131 (*table*)
actin 127
  erythrocyte 192 (*fig.*), 193
  myosin binding with 202
action potentials 51
  muscular dystrophy 52, 53–4
acyl phosphatase 131 (*table*), 132
adenosine diphosphate 45
adenosine monophosphate (AMP)
    deaminase 49, 131, 132, 132 (*table*)
adenosine triphosphate (ATP) 45–6, 128–9
adenosine triphosphate:creatine
    phosphotransferase, *see* creatine kinase
adenylate kinase 49, 132, 132 (*table*), 136
adenylosuccinate 131 (*table*)
adolescents, serum creatine kinase 46
adrenal hypoplasia 185
  X-linked 173
adrenal insufficiency 109
adults, serum creatine kinase 46
age at death 30 (*table*), 34–5, 35 (*table*), 39
    (*table*), 42 (*table*), 43–4
  social class of parents 39–40
age of onset 41–3
  percentiles 28
age of onset/confined wheelchair
    correlation 34–5, 163–4, 166 (*table*)
aids for the disabled 270
Åland Island eye disease, Duchenne
    muscular dystrophy, association 173,
    173 (*fig.*)
alanine aminotransferase (glutamic–pyruvic
    transaminase) 49, 199
albinism, mutation rate 160 (*table*)
albumin 130, 205–6, 205 (*table*)
aldolase 46, 48, 132 (*table*), 136
  molecular weight 49
alkaline phosphatase 131 (*table*)
alleles 23, 178
allopurinol 282 (*table*)
ambulation, prolongation 267–9
amino acids
  therapeutic trial 282 (*table*)

urinary excretion 143 (*table*)
aminotransferases 131 (*table*), 132
amniocentesis, transabdominal 244 (*fig.*)
amyotonia congenita (myotonia congenita,
    Oppenheim disease) 26–7
amyotrophic lateral sclerosis 102
anabolic steroids 282 (*table*)
anaesthetic risks 273–5
anhidrotic ectodermal dysplasia 170 (*table*)
animal models 143–6
ankyrin 191, 192 (*fig.*)
antibody response to membranes 142
antigens
  HLA class I 206
  MHC class I 206
arthrogryposis multiplex congenita 103
    (*table*)
aspartate aminotransferase (glutamic–
    oxaloacetic transaminase) 49, 199
aspirin 282 (*table*)
assisted ventilation 41, 276–7
atrial natriuretic peptide 110
autoimmune response 206–8
autophagy, X-linked myopathy with 90
autosomal dominant muscular
    dystrophies 22 (*table*)
  Emery–Dreifuss type dystrophy
    compared 94–5 (*table*)
autosomal recessive limb girdle muscular
    dystrophy
  of adult onset 85
  of childhood 91–7, 101, 107
autosomal recessive muscular
    dystrophies 22 (*table*)
  dystrophin studies 97
  Emery–Dreifuss type dystrophy
    compared 94–5 (*table*)
  Réunion type 97
azathioprine 290

'back mutation' 74–5, 87–8
back supports 265 (*fig.*), 267
Bacon, Francis (1561–1626), quoted 21
ballistocardiography 111
barbiturates 275
basal lamina (muscle fibre) 1
basic fibroblast growth factor (bFGF) 205,
    207 (*fig.*)

Becker, Peter E. 22, 23 (*fig.*)
Becker type muscular dystrophy 22 (*table*),
    23, 82–6, 106–7
  blood flow in tibialis anterior
      muscle 114–15
  cardiac abnormalities 114
  Duchenne muscular dystrophy
      compared 84–5, 86 (*table*)
  dystrophin studies 74, 77
  Klinefelter's syndrome, association 82
  linkage to DXS7, DXS9, other DNA
      markers 178
  muscle pathology 59, 63
  in same family as Duchenne 87
  serum creatine kinase 47, 84
  verbal IQ 118
behaviour 118
Bell, Charles (1774–1842) 9, 10 (*fig.*)
benign congenital hypotonia 27
biochemistry 125–47
  molecular basis 126
  selection of material, patients,
      controls 125–6
  see also muscle, biochemistry
biopsy, *see specific tissues*
blastocyst biopsy 249
blood, DNA studies 69–70
blood vessels, *see* vascular system
body jackets 266 (*fig.*), 267
bone 120–1
'bone dystrophy' 120–1
brain 115–20
branching, nerve fibres 68
breathing exercises 276
British Clinical Genetics Society 213
brothers, affected 28–9, 97

C-terminal, *see* dystrophin, C-terminal
Ca^{2+}-ATPase 196, 202, 207 (*fig.*)
calcium
  abnormalities 199–203
  binding to troponin C 202
  efflux 196
  exchange in cultured skin fibroblasts
      196
  increase in muscle fibres 59, 130–1, 139,
      199–202
  influx and cell death 205 (*fig.*)
  intracellular 199–202
  leak channels 203, 207 (*fig.*)
  release from sarcoplasmic reticulum 4
calcium-activated protease(s) 133, 204
calcium blockers 261, 282 (*table*)
calcium-positive fibres 59, 130–1, 139,
      199–202
calf sizes, female controls/carriers of

  Duchenne and Becker muscular
      dystrophies 219 (*table*)
capillaries
  diffusion capacity 114
  nail bed 114
  number per unit of muscle fibre 114
  size 114
carbon dioxide tension 38
carbonic anhydrase III 48
carboxy-terminal, *see* dystrophin,
    C-terminal
cardiac glycosides 277, 278, 282 (*table*)
cardiac *see* heart
cardiomyopathy
  in carriers 220–1
  X-linked 185
carnitine 130
carnitine palmityltransferase 133 (*table*)
  deficiency 34, 81 (*table*)
carriers
  abnormalities 217–22
    cardiac 220–1
  biological considerations 215
  childhood 223, 225
  definition of carrier status 215
  detection 215–18
  familial 219
  heterozygous advantage 150
  manifesting 97–101, 218–21
    woman with limb girdle muscular
        dystrophy compared 99–100
  methodological considerations 216–17
  serum creatine kinase, *see* creatine kinase
      (and serum levels, SCK), carriers
  tests 217–18
cat, muscular dsytrophy in 146
cataract
  congenital 253
  infantile 80
catecholamines 282 (*table*)
cathepsins 133
cell death 205 (*fig.*), 206
cell membrane, *see* membrane
central core disease 81 (*table*)
central nervous system 115–20
centronuclear (myotubular) myopathy 81
    (*table*), 82
cerebral atrophy 120
chest deformity 38
chest infections 276
cholesterol 134
choline plasmalogen 134
chorion biopsy 244 (*fig.*), 245
'CIDD' grade scale for upper limbs 35, 303
circulation time, peripheral 114
circumcision, exemption (Talmud) 19
classification

clinical/genetical, of muscular dystrophies
22 (*table*)
spinal muscular atrophies 103 (*table*)
clinical features 26–44
atrophy 37
early signs 32–4
inability to rise with arms folded 32
later stages 37–41
onset 26–30, 42 (*table*)
delayed 30
progression 34–41
stiffness 33
club foot, Egyptian wall painting 7
coenzyme Q 282 (*table*)
collateral reinnervation 55, 88, 103
colour blindness
Duchenne muscular dystrophy and 149
Emery-Dreifuss muscular dystrophy
linked 178
complement 130, 205–6, 205 (*table*)
complex segregation analysis 150
computed tomography (CT scanning) 77
mental defect 120
computer programs, calculating risk of
carrier status 236
congenital cataract 253
congenital deafness 253
congenital fibre type disproportion 81
(*table*)
congenital heart disease 41, 80
congenital muscular dystrophies 22 (*table*),
26, 80–1
congenital myopathies 81–2
electromyography 53
congestive heart failure 278
consanguinity 156
Conte, Gaetano (b. 1798) 9–10
content-orientated genetic counselling 253
contiguous gene syndromes 173–4, 173
(*fig.*)
contraception 252
contraceptives, serum creatine kinase in
carriers 223
contraction, muscle 4
contractures 37–8
physiotherapy 263
coping process, genetic counselling 254–5
Cornelio scoring system 35
counselling, *see* genetic counselling
coupled reactions, serum creatine kinase
estimation 45
cramp 33
creatine, urinary excretion 129–30, 142
creatine kinase (and serum levels, SCK) 24
(*table*), 44–7, 132 (*table*), 144
assay 44–5
bioluminescence 210

fluorimetric/electrophoretic 210
carriers 24 (*table*), 222–8
genetic factors 226
pregnancy/post-partum 224
congenital muscular dystrophy 80–1
efflux from skeletal muscle 199
genetic factors 224
inhibitor? 142
isoenzymes 48
BB 137
linked DNA markers 231
male relative 149–50
molecular weight 49
neonatal screening 156
normal serum levels 46
storage of specimens 223
creatine phosphate 45, 128
creatinine excretion 129–30, 142
cryostat section 56
C-terminal, *see* dystrophin, C-terminal
CT scanning 77
cuirass, with associated ventilation 277
cystic fibrosis 295
cytochrome oxidase 131 (*table*)
cytoskeletal proteins 191–2

dantrolene 282 (*table*)
Davies, Kay 25 (*fig.*)
deafness, congenital 253
death 39–41, 110
age at confinement to wheelchair related
35 (*table*), 43–4
causes 39
mode of 41
see also age at death
'dedifferentiation' 134–7, 207 (*fig.*)
definition of muscular dystrophy 21
dehydrogenases, NADP-linked 132–3, 133
(*table*)
deletion region, high frequency, central and
proximal 183
denervation 65, 65 (*fig.*)
depolarization of surface membrane,
myofibre 4
dermatomyositis, muscle pathology 64
diabetes mellitus 41
diagnosis
confirmation 45–79
DNA 69–73
dystrophin 74–7
flanking markers 71
gene specific (cDNA) probe 71
of Morgagni 15
serum creatine kinase 69
diaphragmatic function 39–40
diarrhoea, recurrent 122

diet 260
diethylstilboestrol 141
digitalis 282 (*table*)
digitoxin 277
dimethylarginines 142
direct carrier detection 238–41
Disability Information Trust 282
distribution, muscle involvement 31–2,
    66–8, 67 (*table*)
diuretics 278
DNA 69–73
  fetal 244–5
  haplotypes, study of mutation rates 165
  isolation of sequence 176–7
  markers 173
    linked 175–9, 228, 237–8
  sequencing 24 (*table*), 169
    automated 240
dog, muscular dystrophy model 146
drug therapy 282–90
drug trials
  design 284–9
  evaluation 283–4
  statistical considerations 285–9
Dubowitz, V., quoted 32
Duchenne, Guillaume Benjamin Armand
    (1806–75) 12–15
  obituary (*Lancet*, 1875) 297–8
  on *Transfiguration* (Raphael) 7
dynamometry 285, 286 (*fig.*)
dystrophia muscularis progressiva 19
dystrophin 24, 187–8
  'back mutation' 74–5
  Becker muscular dystrophy 87–8
  calcium and 199
  C-terminal 87–8, 88 (*fig.*)
    fetus 246
  deletions 71, 72 (*fig.*), 180–2
  duplications 71–2, 72 (*fig.*), 180–1
  dystrophin–glycoprotein complex 88,
    202–3, 207 (*fig.*)
  dystrophin-like protein (utrophin) 75–6,
    191
  fetal muscle 245–6
  'illegitimate transcription' 140
  immunohistochemistry 71–2, 72 (*fig.*),
    241–3
  isoforms 188
  mild phenotypes 184–5
  minigene 293
  monoclonal antibodies 74, 75 (*fig.*)
  muscle biopsy 74–7
  muscle culture 139–40
  mutations 88, 88 (*fig.*)
  myoblast transfer 290–2
  phenotype 123
  prognostic value 76–7

  studies 24 (*table*), 74–7
  utrophin 75–6, 191
dystrophin–glycoprotein complex 189

echinocytes 194, 194 (*fig.*), 195 (*fig.*)
echocardiography 111, 113
educational needs 280–1
Egyptian wall paintings, possible muscular
    dystrophy in 6–7
electrical stimulation, chronic low
    frequency 264
electrocardiography (ECG) 53, 54 (*fig.*), 77,
    111–13
  Duchenne muscular dystrophy *vs* Becker
    muscular dystrophy 85
electroencephalography (EEG) 120
electromyography 50–5
  muscular dystrophy 52–3, 55 (*table*)
  normal 51–2
electronmicroscopy 68–9, 70 (*fig.*)
Emery–Dreifuss muscular dystrophy 22
    (*table*), 88–90, 92–5 (*table*)
  colour blindness linked 178
  DNA markers linked 178
emotional disturbance 118
endomysium 1
enolase 48, 132 (*table*), 136
  β-enolase 48
enzymes
  in dystrophic muscle 131–3
  efflux 49, 198, 207 (*fig.*)
  membrane 133–4, 191–3
  serum 45–50, 141–2
eosinophilic fibres 56–7, 79, 199, 200 (*fig.*)
epilepsy 118
Erb, Wilhelm H. (1840–1921) 19, 20 (*fig.*)
  scapulohumeral dystrophy 22 (*table*)
ergometry 35, 285, 286 (*fig.*)
erythrocytes
  actin 193
  calcium concentrations 204, 205 (*table*)
  calcium pumped out 196
  echinocytes 194 (*fig.*), 195 (*fig.*)
  ghost protein 193
  intramembranous particles 194, 196 (*fig.*)
  membrane-associated abnormalities 193
    (*table*)
  membrane proteins 192 (*fig.*)
  membrane rigidity 194
European Alliance of Muscular Dystrophy
    Associations 213
  Respiratory insufficiency in
    neuromuscular disorders 277
  Surgical treatment of spinal
    deformities 273
exercise 261–4

effect on serum creatine kinase in carriers 223, 224–5

Fabry's disease 219
facioscapulohumeral (Landouzy–Dejerine) dystrophy 22 (*table*), 103 (*table*), 108
  serum creatine kinase (SCK) 47
  verbal IQ 118
failure to thrive 27
'familial clustering', serum creatine kinase in carriers 226
family, psychological effects within 279–80
Family Care Officers 294
family drawing test 279
fatty acids
  long chain derivatives 130
  oxidation 131, 140
  plasma free 129
fetus
  dystrophin, C-terminal region 246
  loss 150
  male at risk 201 (*table*)
fibrillation potentials 53
fibroblasts
  cultures 140
    calcium exchange 196
    calcium levels 204
  membrane-associated abnormalities 193 (*table*)
fibrosis, myocardial 111
field inversion electrophoresis, direct carrier detection 239
flanking markers 178, 234
flexion contractures, *see* contractures
floppy babies 26
fractures 275
frame-shift hypothesis 182
frozen section 56
fructose 131
fructose 1,6-diphosphatase 131 (*table*)
Fukuyama congenital muscular dystrophy 80, 81
fumarase 132 (*table*)
functional ability, assessment 35

gait 29–30, 31
gastrointestinal system 121–2
Gaussian curves, overlap 84–5
gene (gene cluster) (Duchenne)
  deletions 24 (*table*), 71–3, 180–6
  duplications 71, 72 (*fig.*), 180–1
  isolation 179–82
  localization 169–75
  micro-inversions 181
  penetrance 149–50

pleiotropic effects 116, 122 (*fig.*), 123
  reading frame (RF) 87–8, 183–4, 184 (*fig.*), 185 (*fig.*)
  restored by mutation 74–5, 87–8
  transfer, direct 24 (*table*)
genes, isolation/cloning 126
gene specific probes 71
gene therapy 293–4
  reporter genes 293
  viral vector 293
genetic counselling 251–9
  effects 256–8
  timing 254–5
  to whom offered 255–6
genetic heterogeneity 165–7
genetic registers 212–13
genetics 148–67
  calculation of risks 229–38
  incidence, *see* incidence
  mode of inheritance 85, 148–50
  see also pedigrees
'giant' action potentials 53
Gioja, L. (Neapolitan physician) 9
girls with muscular dystrophy 91–6, 169–72, 219
α_2-globulin 141
glucose-6-phosphate dehydrogenase 132, 133 (*table*)
glucose tolerance curve 129
glutamic-oxaloacetic transaminase (aspartate aminotransferase) 49, 199
glutamic-pyruvic transaminase (alanine aminotransferase) 49, 199
γ-glutamyltransferase 141
glutathione reductase 133 (*table*)
gluteus muscles, weakness 32
glyceraldehyde-3-phosphate dehydrogenase 191
glycerol kinase deficiency 109, 173 (*fig.*), 185
glycine 282 (*table*)
glycogenoses 81 (*table*)
glycogen phosphorylase 132 (*table*)
glycogen synthetase 132 (*table*)
glycolysis 131
  defective 140
glycolytic enzymes 131
glycoprotein, in autosomal recessive limb girdle muscular dystrophy of childhood 97
glycosides 277, 278, 282 (*table*)
glyoxalase II 131 (*table*)
Gowers, William R. (1845–1915) 5, 9, 15–19
  manoeuvre (sign) 17, 32
grading systems, motor ability 35–7
grandparents, ages 161, 162 (*table*)

granulomatous disease, chronic 109, 172,
    173 (*fig.*)
group atrophy 63
growth factor
    basic fibroblast (bFGF) 205, 207 (*fig.*)
    nerve 191
growth hormone 283 (*table*), 290
    deficiency 290
growth hormone inhibitor 283 (*table*)

haemolytic anaemia, non-spherocytic 132
haemopexin 141, 228
haemophilia 19, 108
    A and B, mutation rates 160 (*table*)
Hammersmith motor ability score 35, 302
Harrington rods 270
Harvey, William (1578-1657) 9
hearing acuity 118
heart
    abnormalities in carriers 220-1
    arrhythmias 110
    catheterization 111
    congential heart disease 41, 80
    disease, sudden death from 110
    failure 278
    murmurs 110
    muscle 39, 41, 109-14
        creatine kinase isoenzyme 48
        Emery-Dreifuss muscular dystrophy 90
        troponin-T 134
    see also cardiomyopathy
hepatic tests 122
hepatocytes, rat 204, 204 (*table*)
hereditary myopathy
    females (Henson) 22 (*table*)
    males (De Coster) 22 (*table*)
heterogeneity 165-7
heterozygous advantage/fetal loss 150
hexokinase 131 (*table*)
high frequency deletion region, central and
    proximal 183
history of muscular dystrophy 6-24
HLA class I antigens 206
Hoffman, Eric 25 (*fig.*)
hospital treatment, effect on age at death
    40-1
Hunter's syndrome 172 (*table*)
Huntington's chorea, mutation rate 160
    (*table*)
hydrogen electrode technique, blood
    flow 114
hydronephrosis 41
α-hydroxybutyrate dehydrogenase 49
hyperhidrosis 80
hyperkalaemia, postoperative 275
hyperlordosis 265

hyperoestrogenaemia 122
hypertrophy 30
hypocalcaemia 47
hypogonadism 80
hypothyroidism 47
hypoxanthine-guanine
    phosphoribosyltransferase 136-7
hypoxia 278
    nocturnal 227

I bands 2 (*fig.*), 5 (*fig.*)
IgG 130
'illegitimate transcription' 140
immunocytochemistry 74, 76
immunological mapping 246
impairment of intellect, *see* mental defect
    (handicap)
inbreeding 156
incidence 150-8
    changes in recent years 156-8, 158 (*table*)
    neonatal screening of serum creatine
        kinase 156
incontinentia pigmenti 172 (*table*)
infantile spinal muscular atrophy
    (Werdnig-Hoffmann disease) 26,
    65-6, 103-5, 103 (*table*), 253
inflammatory infiltration, polymyositis 64
influenza, vaccination 275-6
inheritance, mode of 148-50
insertion activity (EMG) 50, 51
in situ hybridization, direct carrier
    detection 239-40
intelligence quotient (IQ) 115-18
    partition 117-18
    see also mental defect
intercostal muscles, weakness 38
interference pattern, EMG 51-2
International Units, serum creatine
    kinase 46
intravital staining 68
ischaemic muscle necrosis, acute, serum
    creatine kinase 47
isocitrate dehydrogenase 133, 133 (*table*),
    136
isolated cases, incidence 158

junction fragments, direct carrier detection
    238-9
juvenile progressive bulbar palsy 103 (*table*)

Kearn-Sayre syndrome 81 (*table*)
Kennedy syndrome 103 (*table*), 106
ketoacids 283 (*table*)
kidney, *see* renal

Kiener, Franz 23
Klinefelter's syndrome, Becker type
  muscular dystrophy, association 82
Kunkel, Lou 25 (*fig.*)
kyphoscoliosis, *see* scoliosis

lactate dehydrogenase 48, 132 (*table*), 199
  isoenzymes 134-6, 136 (*fig.*)
Laevadosin 283 (*table*)
lag period, Becker muscular dystrophy 83
Landouzy-Dejerine's dystrophy, *see*
  facioscapulohumeral
  (Landouzy-Dejerine) dystrophy
learning difficulties, *see* mental defect
  (handicap)
lecithin 134
left ventricular abnormalities 113
leucine 283 (*table*)
leucocytes, peripheral blood 140
Leyden-Möbius' pelvifemoral muscular
  dystrophy 21
limb blood flow 114
limb girdle muscular dystrophy 22 (*table*)
  females 99, 100 (*table*), 191 (*table*)
  manifesting carrier of Duchenne
    dystrophy compared 99-100
  serum creatine kinase 47
  verbal IQ 118
lipid peroxidation 133 (*table*)
lithium carbonate 141
Little, W. J. 11
liver
  cells, rat 204, 204 (*table*)
  enzyme release from 141
  tests 122
Lowe's syndrome 172 (*table*)
lumbar lordosis 33
Luque operation 270-3
lymphocytes
  calcium level 204
  capping 163, 193 (*table*), 194, 197 (*fig.*),
    198
  cytotoxic 206
  RNA, direct carrier detection 240
lysolecithin phospholipase 131 (*table*)
lysosomal acid hydrolases 133

Mabry type muscular dystrophy 22 (*table*),
  88
McArdle's syndrome, *see* carnitine
  palmityltransferase, deficiency
McLeod syndrome 172, 173 (*fig.*)
macroglossia 30
macrophages 206
Magendie, François 9
magnetic resonance imaging (MRI) 120

magnetic resonance spectroscopy, *see*
  nuclear magnetic resonance
malabsorption 122
malate dehydrogenase 49, 133, 133 (*table*),
  136
male infant deaths 151
malignant hyperpyrexia 47, 274
management 260-96
  aids for the disabled 270
  comprehensive 294-5
  prolongation of ambulation 267-9
manifesting carriers, *see* carriers,
  manifesting
marital problems, parents 279
maximum inspiratory/expiratory pressures
  276
Medical Research Council (MRC) grading
  of muscle strength 35, 299
membrane 191-8
  binding sites 191-3
  enzymes 133-4, 191-3
  reduced fluidity 194
memory 115
Menkes syndrome 172 (*table*)
menstrual cycle, serum creatine kinase in
  carriers 223
mental defect (handicap) 34, 115-20
  Becker type muscular dystrophy 83
  dystrophin gene 123
  genetic deletions 184
  heterotopias in cerebral cortex 120
  severe 167
  see also intelligence quotient
Meryon, Edward (1809-80) 11-12, 15 (*fig.*)
methylene blue 68
3-methylhistidine 130
methylthioadenosine nucleosidase 131
  (*table*)
MHC class I antigens 206
mice, *see* mouse
micro-inversions 181
milestones, delayed 27-8
MIND, *see* National Association for Mental
  Health
minicore (multicore) disease 81 (*table*)
minipolymyoclonus 90, 106
misclassification, percentage 84-5
mitochondrial calcium overload 204
mitochondrial myopathy 81
mitral valve prolapse 110, 113
  in carrier 220
molecular pathology 168-89
  Duchenne gene
    isolation 179-82
    localization 166-72
  linked DNA markers 175-9
monoamine oxidase 131 (*table*)

monoclonal antibodies
  dystrophin studies 74
  to T-lymphocytes 206
mononuclear cells 206
mosaicism
  germ-line 246-8
  somatic (in carriers) 100
motor ability, assessment 35-7
motor development delayed 27
motor end-plate 68
motor neurone disease 102
  serum creatine kinase 47
motor unit 50 (*fig.*)
mouse
  genotypic dwarf-dystrophic 290
  mdx 145-6
  mutants 144-6
multi-centre trials 289
multicore (minicore) disease 81 (*table*)
multiplex method, detection of
    deletions 71-2
muscle
  amount in human body 1
  biochemistry 126-40
  biopsy 56, 57 (*fig.*), 78, 125
    by G. B. A. Duchenne 15
    open 64
  blood flow 114
  cardiac 109-14
  culture 137-40
  development, by weeks of gestation 134
    (*fig.*)
  fast/slow 191
  fetal, tissue culture 137-40
  fibre, see muscle fibres
  glycogenoses 81 (*table*)
  histochemistry 64-8, 205-6, 205 (*table*)
  innervation 68
  involvement distribution 31-2, 66-8, 67
    (*table*)
  membrane-associated abnormalities 193
    (*table*)
  microcirculation 190
  pathology, see muscle pathology
  proteins 127-8, 130-1
  pseudohypertrophy 30
  ribosomal protein synthesis 130
  smooth 109
  strength assessment 35
  wasting, biochemistry 127-31
muscle fibres (myofibres) 1-4
  abnormalities in carriers 221-2
  calcium-positive 59, 130-1, 139, 199-202
  classification 64-5, 66
  depolarization of surface membrane 4
  development 221
  eosinophilic 199, 200 (*fig.*)

glycogen granules 3
histochemical reactions in Duchenne
    muscular dystrophy 64-8, 145
    (*table*), 205-6
lipid bodies 3
mitochondria 3
ribosomes 3
'skinned' 133-4
muscle pathology 55-64
  later stages 61-4
  preclinical stage 56-61
muscular dystrophy associations/groups 4,
    304-7
  MDA of America
    colloquium 289
    monthly abstracts 4
  MDG of Great Britain and Northern
    Ireland 281, 294
Muscular dystrophy handbook 281
mutation(s)
  different in same family 149
  new, proportion ('x') 161-5, 166 (*table*)
  point mutations 73, 181
  restoring reading frame 74-5, 87-8
mutation rate 159-65
  direct estimation 159-60
  grandparental ages 161, 162 (*table*)
  indirect estimation 159
  parental age 160-1
  sex difference 161-5
myasthenia gravis 293-4
myoblasts
  cultured 137-40
  stem cells 1
  transfer 24 (*table*), 290-2
myocardial fibrosis 111
myocardial infarction 47
myocardium, see heart,
    muscle
myofibres, see muscle fibres
myofibrils 1-3
myofilaments 3
myogenic factors 139 (*fig.*)
myoglobin 49, 127, 141, 228
myoglobinaemia 273
myoglobinuria (rhabdomyolysis)
  postoperative 273, 274 (*table*)
  succinylcholine-induced 273
myometry 285, 286 (*fig.*)
myopathy + glycerol kinase
    deficiency + adrenal
    insufficiency 173
myosin 127
  binding with actin 202
  fetal 134, 137
myositis, absence 33
myotonia 21